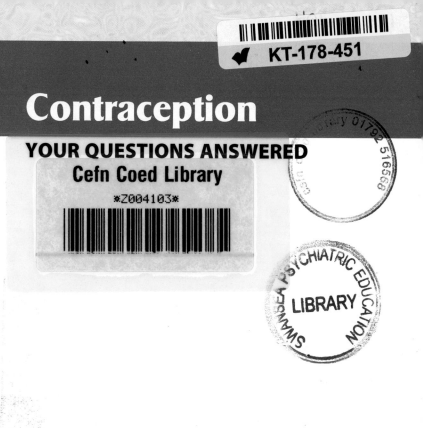

✔ KT-178-451

Contraception

YOUR QUESTIONS ANSWERED

Commissioning Editor: Pauline Graham
Development Editor: Lulu Stader
Project Manager: Emma Riley
Designer: George Ajayi

Contraception

YOUR QUESTIONS ANSWERED

FIFTH EDITION

John Guillebaud MA FRCSEd FRCOG Hon FFSRH Hon FCOG (SA)

Emeritus Professor of Family Planning and Reproductive Health, University College London, UK

Trustee of the Margaret Pyke Memorial Trust

Formerly Medical Director of the Margaret Pyke Family Planning Centre, London, UK

Surgeon, Elliot-Smith Vasectomy Clinic, Oxford, UK

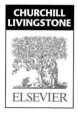

Edinburgh London New York Oxford Philadelphia St Louis Sydney Toronto 2009

ELSEVIER
CHURCHILL
LIVINGSTONE

An imprint of Elsevier Limited
© Pearson Professional Ltd 1996
© 1999, 2004, Elsevier Ltd.
© 2009, 1993, 1985 Professor John Guillebaud.
Published by Elsevier Ltd. All rights reserved.

First edition 1985 (Pitman Publishing Ltd)
  Reprinted 1986, 1987 (twice), 1988
  Revised and reprinted 1989
  Reprinted 1991, 1992
Second edition 1993
  Revised and reprinted 1994
  Reprinted 1995 (twice), 1997
Third edition 1999
  Reprinted 2000, 2001
Fourth Edition 2004
  Revised and reprinted 2005
Fifth edition 2009

ISBN-13: 978 0 443 06908 6

British Library Cataloguing in Publication Data
A catalogue record for this book is available from
the British Library

**Library of Congress Cataloging in Publication
Data**
A catalog record for this book is available from
the Library of Congress

Note
Knowledge and best practice in this field are
constantly changing. As new research and
experience broaden our knowledge, changes in
practice, treatment and drug therapy may become
necessary or appropriate. Readers are advised to
check the most current information provided (i)
on procedures featured or (ii) by the
manufacturer of each product to be administered,
to verify the recommended dose or formula, the
method and duration of administration, and
contraindications. It is the responsibility of the
practitioner, relying on their own experience and
knowledge of the patient, to make diagnoses, to
determine dosages and the best treatment for each
individual patient, and to take all appropriate
safety precautions. To the fullest extent of the law,
neither the Publisher nor the Author assumes any
liability for any injury and/or damage to persons
or property arising out or related to any use of the
material contained in this book.

The Publisher

Working together to grow
libraries in developing countries

www.elsevier.com | www.bookaid.org | www.sabre.org

ELSEVIER **BOOK AID** International **Sabre Foundation**

ELSEVIER your source for books,
journals and multimedia
in the health sciences

www.elsevierhealth.com

Printed in China

Contents

Preface

We have not inherited the earth from our grandparents – we have borrowed it from our grandchildren

(Kashmiri proverb)

The world has enough for everyone's need (1) But not enough for everyone's greed! (2)

(Mahatma Gandhi, 1869–1948)

Frighteningly, we now have over 6 800 000 000 humans on the planet and all of them seeking (very reasonably) either to escape from poverty or, in the affluent 'North', to remain out of poverty. There is only one way to do either, namely to consume energy and other resources. Hence on a finite planet, Gandhi's statement (2) is so true! But his first statement (1) may, very soon, no longer be true: through the arrival of 'too many everyones' for our fragile earth to be able to resource all of them so they can live a decent life, not in poverty. Population is certainly not the only world problem. But it is the most neglected one, the *taboo* one: and *the great multiplier* of most other world problems. Human numbers are relevant to climate change, 'peak oil' and most other threats that face our grandchildren in this century.

And what is so tragic as well as so avoidable is that, among the rich as well as the poor . . . 'most humans are still caused by accidents' (*see Q 1.20*). Consider poverty: children who are never born unintendedly (through voluntary family planning) do not die miserably in infancy. Maternal mortality (one per minute worldwide): you cannot die of a pregnancy you don't have. Environment: an *absent human* has no environmental footprint, will not require the equivalent in carbon dioxide production of one million miles of driving to get them out of poverty, or, in the UK, 3 million miles' worth to keep them in the manner to which UK people have become accustomed (*Q 1.3*). Mass migrations, violence between young men (especially) between and within countries, habitat destruction, species extinctions, all these and more can be linked to human numbers. Moreover, all can be ameliorated by that amazing but undervalued technology (available and accessible contraception (*Q 1.2*)) which gives us an opportunity to avoid the fate of all other species: namely, Nature's inevitable cull when the carrying capacity of environments is exceeded. Maybe, if the world were run by biologists rather than economists, humankind would have heard this wake-up call sooner.

There are hopeful signs. Couples in most countries are now choosing family sizes which will lead (with a lag-time of up to 60 years) to replacement fertility or below. Moreover, in comparison with the not-very-distant past, contraceptive technology is approaching closer to a 'contraceptive utopia'. If only every couple in the world could have access to the full range – not true (for many astoundingly bad reasons) for hundreds of millions – it ought in theory to be possible to offer a method to suit everyone. Yet even in the UK, where the choice is wider than in most countries (with recent brilliant additions, notably the LNG-IUS, Implanon, Cerazette, Evra, and, shortly, NuvaRing), almost 200 000 pregnancies are terminated annually – and from a large survey (Farrow et al 2002, *see* Q 5.62 in this book) it seems that almost one-third of children still owe their arrival more to carelessness and chance than to caring choice.

Is not the prime purpose of contraception 'orgasms but without babies'? Pretty basic, but we forget that too often. Sexuality and communication influence crucially both strong and weak motivation for effective contraception. There are other crucial interfaces: e.g. the parallel need to avoid sexually transmitted infections ('Double Dutch', Q 1.15). Why in primary care do we so often neglect to take a simple sexual history (Qs 1.13, 1.14)? Or fail to detect psychosexual unhappiness through the hidden clues, verbal and by body language: particularly at the 'moment of truth' before, during and after a genital examination? Moreover, as the NHS gets ever more stressful, we need to remind ourselves to discuss the full range of choices, especially the long-acting reversible contraceptives (LARCs) even when the woman asks for the pill – as she usually will, since that is everyone's expectation. However, note that I have taken as my remit the technology of *reversible* birth control, with little discussion of male and female sterilization or (safe) induced abortion – indeed, with respect to the latter, part of my motivation in this business is to work towards a world where induced abortion will not be needed and instead will be seen as a transient historical aberration of the 20th and 21st centuries. Other essential subjects – such as counselling, social factors affecting contraceptive use, medico-legal aspects, sexual problems and health screening – are rather briefly mentioned, mainly in the final chapter, but they are amplified by other texts and on websites that are referenced here.

The prime readership of this book has proved to be General Practitioners and Practice Nurses, so I proudly record that I am an ex-GP and I think profited by the experience: during my training years I worked as a locum in places as diverse as Barnsley, Cambridge, Luton and Eltham (SE London).

For help with the first edition back in 1985, I am most grateful to the following: Toni Belfield, Walli Bounds, Ken Fotherby, Susan Hatwell, Sam

Hutt, Howard Jacobs, Pram Senanayake and Ali Kubba. Ray Phillips, Stuart Nightingale and Angela Scott helped with the illustrations. My select team of typists in those (pre-PC) days were Margaret Bailón, Diane Berry, Sue Nickells and Georgina Tregoning. I acknowledge some of the same people (especially Toni Belfield, see Chapter 11) for help with all later editions; with thanks additionally to Susan Brechin and staff of the Clinical Effectiveness Unit of the Faculty of Sexual and Reproductive Healthcare (FSRH), Elphis Christopher, Ron Kleinman, Hilary Luscombe, Anne MacGregor, Diana Mansour, Catherine Nelson-Piercy, Sam Rowlands, Anne Szarewski with other colleagues at the Margaret Pyke Centre and Joan Walsh; also my secretary Helen Prime and my son Jonathan Guillebaud. Through the 25 years of gestation of this latest edition the people I have worked with at my publishers, notably Howard Bailey, Miranda Bromage, Alyson Colley, Fiona Conn, Eleanor Flood, Ellen Green, Lucy Gardner, Emma Riley, Rachel Robson, Lulu Stader and Katherine Watts, have been as friendly as they were helpful. Above all, thanks to my wife Gwyneth for being so enormously supportive and usefully critical throughout.

But I remain happy to stand corrected by any reader, please! There is much truth in my former deputy Ali Kubba's spoof subtitle: 'Contraception – Your Answers Questioned'!

John Guillebaud

Glossary

adrenaline – epinephrine (adrenaline is previous name, still UK preference)
AIDS – acquired immune deficiency syndrome
ALO – *Actinomyces*-like organisms
AMI – acute myocardial infarction
AUC – area under the curve – in pharmacokinetic studies
BBD – benign breast disease
BBT – basal body temperature
bd – twice daily
BICH – benign intracranial hypertension
BME – bimanual examination
BMI – body mass index (weight in kg ÷ height in m^2)
BNF – *British National Formulary*
BP – blood pressure
BTB – breakthrough bleeding
BV – bacterial vaginosis
CDC – Centers for Disease Control
CGHFBC – Collaborative Group on Hormonal Factors in Breast Cancer
CHC – combined hormonal contraceptive
CIC – combined injectable contraceptive
CIN – cervical intraepithelial neoplasia
COC – combined oral contraceptive
CPA – cyproterone acetate
CSF – cerebrospinal fluid
CSM – Committee on Safety of Medicines
CVS – cardiovascular system
D&C – dilatation and curettage (superseded by hysteroscopy)
DES – diethylstilbestrol
DM – diabetes mellitus
DMPA – depot medroxyprogesterone acetate
DoH – Department of Health (DH)
DSG – desogestrel
DVT – deep venous thrombosis
E-3-G – estrone-3-glucuronide
EC – emergency contraception
ED – everyday (a COC variant)
EE – ethinylestradiol

epinephrine – adrenaline (old name, still preferred!)
EVA – ethylene vinyl acetate
FAQs – frequently asked questions
FDA – Food and Drug Administration (in the US)
FH – family history
FNH – focal nodular hyperplasia
FOC – functional ovarian cyst
FPA/fpa – Family Planning Association
FSH – follicle-stimulating hormone
FSRH/Faculty of SRH – Faculty of Sexual and Reproductive Healthcare
(a faculty of the RCOG since 1995). Formerly called the Faculty of Family
Planning and Reproductive Health Care (FFPRHC). (Name changed in 2007)
GSD – gestodene
GUM – genitourinary medicine
h – hour
hCG – human chorionic gonadotrophin
HDL-C – high-density lipoprotein–cholesterol
HELLP – hypertension, elevated liver enzymes, low platelets
HIV – human immunodeficiency virus
HPV – human papillomavirus (certain types can act as cervical
carcinogens)
HRT – hormone replacement therapy
IUD – intrauterine device
I.U.D. – intrauterine death
IMB – intermenstrual bleeding
INR – international normalized ratio (blood test for adequate
anticoagulation with warfarin)
IPPF – International Planned Parenthood Federation
IU – international unit
IUD – intrauterine device
IUS – intrauterine system (shortening of LNG-IUS below)
L – litre
LA – local anaesthesia
LAM – lactational amenorrhoea method
LARCs – long-acting reversible contraceptives (injections, implants,
intrauterine methods)
LDL-C – low-density lipoprotein–cholesterol
LH – luteinizing hormone
lidocaine – lignocaine
LMP – last menstrual period
LNG – levonorgestrel
LNG-IUS – levonorgestrel-releasing intrauterine system
LSCS – lower segment caesarean section

MHRA – Medicines and Healthcare products Regulatory Agency. New body which has taken over roles of the MDA and MCA (and CSM)

min – minute

MPA – medroxyprogesterone acetate

MRI – magnetic resonance imaging

N-9 – nonoxinol-9

NET – norethisterone (norethindrone in the US)

NET-EN – norethisterone enantate

NFP – natural family planning

NICE – National Institute of Clinical Excellence

OC – oral contraceptive

PCOS – polycystic ovary syndrome

PFI – pill-free interval

PG – prostaglandin

PGD – patient group directions (equates to protocols for nurse practitioners)

PGSI – prostaglandin synthetase inhibitor

PID – pelvic inflammatory disease

PIL – patient information leaflet (as produced by a manufacturer and officially approved)

PMS – premenstrual syndrome

POEC – progestogen-only emergency contraception

POP – progestogen-only pill

RCGP – Royal College of General Practitioners

RCOG – Royal College of Obstetricians and Gynaecologists

RCT – randomized controlled trial

SAH – subarachnoid haemorrhage

SEM – scanning electron microscope

SHBG – sex hormone-binding globulin

SLE – systemic lupus erythematosus

SPC – summary of product characteristics (as produced by a manufacturer, equates to Datasheet)

SRE – sex and relationships education

SRH – sexual and reproductive health

STI – sexually transmitted infection

SVT – superficial venous thrombosis

TIA – transient ischaemic attack

TSS – toxic shock syndrome

UC – ulcerative colitis

UKMEC – United Kingdom Medical Eligibility Criteria (Document of Faculty of SRH, see *Appendix B*)

UKSPR – United Kingdom Selected Practice Recommendations (Document of Faculty of SRH)

UN – United Nations
UPSI – unprotected sexual intercourse
US – United States (of America)
US scan – ultrasound scan
VTE – venous thromboembolism
VVs – varicose veins
WHO – World Health Organization
WHO 1, WHO 2, WHO 3, WHO 4 – WHO categories for contraindications, explained at *Q 5.121*
WHOMEC – WHO Medical Eligibility Criteria for contraceptive use (Document modified for UK as UKMEC))
WHOSPR – WHO Selected Practice Recommendations for contraceptive use (Document modified for UK as UKSPR)
WTB – withdrawal bleeding

List of figures

List of tables

How to use this book

The *Your Questions Answered* series aims to meet the information needs of GPs and other primary care professionals who care for women and men with long-term medical needs. It is designed to help them work with patients and their families, providing effective, evidence-based care and management.

The books are in an accessible question-and-answer format, with detailed contents lists at the beginning of every chapter and a complete index to help find specific information.

ICONS

Icons are used in the book to identify particular types of information:

 highlights important information

 highlights unwanted side-effect information

PATIENT QUESTIONS

At the end of relevant chapters there are sections of frequently asked patient questions, with easy-to-understand answers aimed at the non-medical reader.

NOTE

This book represents the personal opinions of John Guillebaud, based wherever possible on published and sometimes unpublished evidence. When (as is not infrequent) no epidemiological or other direct evidence is available, clinical advice herein is always as practical and realistic as possible and based, pending more data, on the author's judgment of other sources. These may include the opinions of Expert Committees and any existing Guidelines. In some instances the advice appearing in this book may even so differ appreciably from the latter, for reasons usually given in the text, and (since medical knowledge and practice are continually evolving) relates to the date of publication. Healthcare professionals must understand that they take ultimate responsibility for their patient and ensure that any clinical advice they use from this book is applicable to the specific circumstances that they encounter.

STATEMENT OF COMPETING INTERESTS

The author has received payments for research projects, lectures, ad hoc consultancy work and related expenses from the manufacturers of contraceptive products.

PROPRIETARY PRODUCTS

In this book, the relevant drug or device is signified by an initial capital letter.

Introduction: the population explosion, sexual and contraceptive history-taking and counselling – the importance of fertility control

1.1 What is the population explosion?

According to the Population Reference Bureau (www.prb.org), in mid-2008 the world's population was 6 705 000 000 (*Fig. 1.1*), rising by c 82 million per year. Every 10 seconds there are 44 births and 18 deaths, a net gain of 26. Every week an extra 1.5 million people need food and somewhere to live. This amounts to a huge new city each week, somewhere, which destroys wildlife habitats and augments world fossil fuel consumption. Every person born adds to greenhouse gas emissions, and escaping poverty is impossible without these increasing. Resourcing contraception therefore helps to combat climate change, though this is no let-out for the high emitters who must also greatly reduce their per capita emissions.

Because of demographic momentum, most of tomorrow's parents are children who have already been born (*see Q 1.6*) and so we must expect the

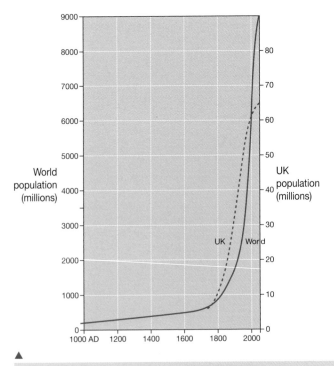

▲

Fig. 1.1 Estimated rate of population growth, AD 1750–2050. *Q 1.1*. Note that the UK differs from the rest of the world mainly by having had its 'population explosion' slightly earlier. The UK, too, was once covered by forest.

arrival of at least half as many again before the earliest date of stabilization. Yet even now, many of the existing millions are grossly deficient in the bare necessities of life: food, clean water, clothing, housing, healthcare, education and recreation. Is it quality of life we are after, or quantity of flesh?

We will never meet human needs on this finite planet until we stabilize human numbers.

1.2 So how is the world doing at present?

According to WHO figures (November 2006), out of over 180 million conceptions each year, at least 80 million are unwanted. This results in about 45 million abortions, of which 19 million are performed in unsafe circumstances. Around 540 000 women die each year from these pregnancies (equalling a jumbo jet of pregnant women crashing with no survivors every 6 h, or one woman dying this way every minute of the day) – either through complications of abortion or for lack of the basic requirements for safe delivery. At least 200 000 would not die if adequate services and supplies for contraception were available. They are killed by pregnancies they would have preferred not to have in the first place.

What infamous statistics! Such dreadful carnage! When you add the preventable deaths among children – as well as mothers – when births are too frequent, how is it that birth planning is so often stigmatized as anti-life? On the contrary:

Family planning could provide more benefits to more people at less cost than any other single 'technology' now available to the human race (James Grant, UNICEF Annual Report, 1992)

1.3 But isn't this primarily a problem of the 'developing' world?

That is where 99% of the population growth is occurring, yes, but on a finite planet everywhere is affected. The environmental crisis is the consequence of multiplying per-person consumption by ever more persons. The global consequences include climate change and the relentless destruction of the habitats of other animals and plants. For billions in the developing world there is no way out of poverty except by using energy – unavoidably worsening climate change, despite much less per person than in the 'developed' world. There, it has been calculated that every new birth is likely to lead, in the lifetime of that individual (depending on their 'environmental footprint', the consequence of affluence and the 'greenness' of available technology) to producing 200 times more carbon dioxide than an inhabitant of Chad. According to the Living Planet Report of the World Wide Fund for Nature (WWF – see URL www.panda.org/news_facts/publications/living_planet_report/index.cfm), humankind will by 2050 be trying to use 100% more resources than the whole biological capacity of the planet. Not possible: there is no suitable second planet available.

With respect to wildlife, according to the WWF, total extinction threatens one-quarter of all mammals, one bird species out of eight and almost one-third of terrestrial plants, and that's before considering some of the most dramatic losses occurring in the world's oceans. In 2002 it was calculated that already 97% of all the vertebrate biomass on land is human flesh plus our domestic and farm animals – leaving only 3% for all wild species, including all elephants and birds. A devastating statistic!

The rich 'north' ought to give far more and far more appropriate aid to the 'south', out of simple humanity. But even without that motivation, their own calculated self-interest should surely force voters, and therefore politicians, worldwide, massively to increase the aid they give to the poor countries – and, despite the numerous taboos, increase also the proportion of it given to reproductive health and the methods of voluntary birth control.

If we are not part of the solution, we *are* part of the problem (see www. ecotimecapsule.com, www.populationandsustainability.org, www. optimumpopulation.org and www.peopleandplanet.net for more details). One thought: in the UK, having one fewer children than one might have had would be the climate change equivalent of not driving 3 million miles by car – an economical hybrid car at that.

1.4 What changes birth rates?

As shown in *Fig. 1.2*, a great deal more is necessary than simply the provision of family planning. Although all are important, some need to be highlighted:

■ Better health and fewer child deaths: it has been calculated that in rural areas of India a couple need to have five children to have a 95% chance of one son reaching maturity. But there is a vicious circle here, because child mortality is itself greater in the absence of effective family spacing, and this is now being exacerbated by the worldwide decline in breastfeeding without enough alternative contraception.

■ A better deal for women: in too many societies worldwide, women remain second-class citizens and have little choice in their destiny or that of their family. They are forced by their male-dominated society in general, and their husbands in particular, as well as by their biology (*see Qs 2.1–2.10*), to have far more children than they desire. This was clearly shown by the World Fertility Survey and the Reproductive Health Surveys, which, in 60 countries in the developing world, found that even in the 1980s almost 50% of married women wanted no more

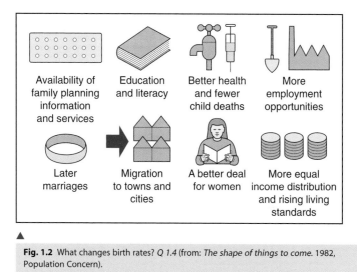

Fig. 1.2 What changes birth rates? *Q 1.4* (from: *The shape of things to come.* 1982, Population Concern).

children. So, for them at least, family planning had become a perceived unmet need – we should, and could (but did not), push at this open door. . . .

■ Implicit in the whole of *Fig. 1.2* are two slogans or sayings. The first is an ancient proverb referring to the inhabitants of rural areas:

Every mouth has got two hands.

In rural poverty, the hands are far more noticeable than the mouth, in that the labour and support that a child can give to its parents, especially in their old age or during disease, are far more important to them than the extra cost that might be incurred by having an extra child. It is hard for individuals to see how the macroproblems – burgeoning numbers in large tracts of the developing world leading to excessive tree-cutting, erosion and floods, desertification, salinization, habitat destruction and ultimately disaster – are in any way their business through decisions about childbearing.

Apart from the regrettable 'Big Brother' Chinese solution – enforcing one-child families – what can be done? Even the Chinese agree that this was a draconian measure forced on them mainly because they did not bring in a much less restrictive two-child policy when they had half as many people only 50 years ago. The best answer is summarized in the second slogan:

Take care of the people and the population will take care of itself.

■ Rising living standards: poverty should be eliminated. This should be done as a matter of social justice (*Fig. 1.2*) but, when coupled with the previous bulleted point, there is a vicious circle. Even if the gross domestic product (GDP) of a country like Burundi (the land of my birth) or of Rwanda, where I was brought up, does increase, the per capita GDP goes down if it is shared by more and more people. Ever more hardship results, and violence can be the outcome. When I was a child, there were only 2 million Rwandans; by the time of the appalling genocide in 1994 (in which several of my playmates and friends of the 1940s were slaughtered) the population was 8 million – four people sharing the available resources where before there had been one. This has to be relevant, though clearly not the whole story. 'The stork is the bird of war.'

1.5 Does this mean that development is the best contraceptive, so family planning doesn't matter?

Far from it; many people have misinterpreted the slogan in this way, claiming, for example, that improved child survival is always a prerequisite for family planning acceptance (although experience in Bangladesh and elsewhere has disproved this). The result is that in large areas of the world, in the slums and rural areas where people actually live, the basic tools for family planning are simply not being made available at a price that they can afford. 'Population will take care of itself' only when 'taking care of the people' includes every item in *Fig. 1.2* as part of an integrated solution. Family planning services must be provided locally, comprehensively and appropriately, as a human right, on an equal basis at least with all the other items illustrated. Instead of 'counting people' the emphasis must be 'people count', as highlighted at the UN world population conference in Cairo in 1994. The emphasis must be on choices in reproduction, education and the removal of a whole raft of barriers to women (including simple non-availability of a reasonable range of contraceptives and widespread misinformation about their risks).

At present, the proportion of aid for the developing world that is spent on the provision of voluntary birth control is around 1%. Family planning is no panacea and is not the whole answer, but it will surely provide much more than 1% of the answer!

1.6 If everything that could and should be done *was* done, what is the most likely future total world population at stabilization?

Realistically, at least 50% larger than now. Short of a cataclysm causing a massive increase in deaths, this is a demographic certainty. Why? Because, like a supertanker, world population has so much in-built momentum. Currently, 2000 million of the world's inhabitants are under 15, and that means very nearly all of tomorrow's parents are already born. They will have the offspring that will lead to a massive increase in total numbers even if they have an average of only two children each.

The world's population was 3000 million in 1960, when I first became aware of this problem (and, incidentally, it was this realization as a second-year medical student that drove me to specialize in contraception for men as well as women). We now have more than two worlds of that size. And everything we must do (and are not doing nearly well enough yet) in the provision of reproductive healthcare to the world is about stopping world number 4 from coming along: world number 3 is all but inevitable! Scientists can see some chance of a passable, if perilous, future for around 9000 million humans. More than that really does risk collapse of life-support mechanisms in the ecosystem and deaths and misery on an unheard-of scale.

1.7   Is the population crisis really that bad?

It is said that a frog dropped into boiling water jumps straight out, unscathed. If this (unethical) experiment is repeated with the same water, same container, same frog and same source of heat but starting from cold, the outcome is a boiled frog. The trouble about the population, development, resources and pollution story is that it is based on numerous interconnected adverse trends rather than on catastrophic events. Very like that frog, we humans have a poor track record for reacting vigorously to serious dangers (take cigarette smoke, for instance) if they are gradual and insidious. But we must. The crisis is caused much less by wilfulness than by carelessness and ignorance. It happens through millions of people 'doing their own thing'. All of us, rich and poor, whether clearing forests (130 000 km^2 per year) or producing greenhouse gases by driving to the shops, are using technology to improve our families' material environment: oblivious to the fact that, with more and more people doing the same and continuing for long enough, the consequences for our grandchildren could be horrendous. We must stop treating the fragile planet as an inexhaustible milch cow for our wants and as a bottomless cesspit for our wastes.

In the Preface I quoted the saying reportedly from Kashmir:

We have not inherited the world from our grandparents – we have borrowed it from our grandchildren.

I believe that our own children's children will brand this generation – living around the turn of the twenty-first century – as the worst ever, in that it was the last to have some chance of preventing the environmental wasteland that they will have inherited, but too little was done and too late. We will be seen as having selfishly mortgaged their future for our present gain.

1.8 Should we be apologizing for damaging this 'loan from our grandchildren'?

Because I felt the need to do just that, I devised the Environment Time Capsule project. Time capsules containing objects that were environmentally relevant to the year 1994 (including 'bad' items, like a car's petrol cap, or 'good' items, like a bicycle pump and – most relevantly – some packets of contraceptive pills and condoms), along with letters and poems written by 1000 people, mainly children, and addressed to the year 2044, were buried at strategic sites across the globe: in Mexico, UK (Kew Gardens, and Ness Gardens on the Wirral, Merseyside), South Africa, the Seychelles and Australia. As well as apologizing, there was this pledge: that all those involved would work tirelessly to ensure that, hopefully, those who dug up each time capsule in 2044 would wonder what we were on about, i.e. apologies would not be necessary! A reunion is held at Ness Gardens every year on the nearest Sunday to World Environment Day, June 5th – come along, I will be there! (See www.ecotimecapsule.com or my 'Personal View' in the *British Medical Journal* 1994;308:1377–1378 for more details.)

1.9 In view of the urgency, and the in-built momentum of population growth, why is so little being done?

Politicians across the globe don't act because voters, faced with the challenge of less 'jam' today so that their children can inherit a tolerable world in the future, invariably vote to have at least as much jam as they currently have, and preferably more. Human perspectives are remarkably insular in terms of space, and brief in terms of time. The following sayings summarize things well: 'my car is my car, everyone else's car is traffic'; 'my visit to the seaside is my holiday, but oh, the crowds on the beach'; and 'my baby is my baby, everybody else's baby is overpopulation'. These attitudes are reinforced by ignorance, by apathy and often by a hint of racism: 'The death of one baby in London is a tragedy; the death of millions of babies in Africa – that's a statistic.'

1.10 Is it all doom and gloom?

No, there are actually sound grounds for some optimism. Total fertility rates (average family sizes) are falling in almost every country. And there *is* enough money to tackle the problem. After all, smallpox was eradicated from the face of this planet by the equivalent amount of money that, at the time, was spent by the world's armed forces every 8 min. It has been estimated that the extra money required to provide adequate food, water, education, housing and health for the whole planet, including the means for each woman to control her fertility as she would choose, could be provided for as little as one month's spending on the world's armed forces. . . .

1.11 Against all the odds, anything I did would surely be just a drop in the ocean?

True, but:

The ocean is made up of drops.

As healthcare professionals, we should not underestimate our influence on those around us – our patients and our peer groups – and, through them, on the politicians. More immediately, knowledge is power. Here we come to my prime reason for writing this book: let us ensure that we are so well informed about the whole subject of contraception that we can answer the questions of the women and the men who come to us for contraceptive advice and help. In so far as we are able to influence events, the aim is simple: 'every child a wanted child'.

1.12 Is it enough just to answer the questions?

No – 1 g of *empathy* is worth 1 kg of *knowledge*. Moreover:

- There are techniques to be learnt and maintained: counselling skills and practical skills in the fitting of IUDs and the fitting and the training for women who wish to use female barrier methods.
- In reproductive healthcare, the correct non-directive counselling attitude and approach are vital. Couples must decide for themselves what aspects of the list in *Q 1.15* are most important in their situation. It has been well said that, in the matter of birth planning, 'we are advisers, we are the suppliers – but we are not the deciders' (*see Q 11.14*).
- Time is always a huge constraint, so doctors should work closely with other professionals, especially (family planning-trained) nurses. Appropriate delegation and teamwork ensure user-friendly services.
- Confidentiality should feel real to all clients (*see Qs 11.5, 11.6*).
- Examinations of breast and pelvis should be rare (*see Qs 6.3, 6.4*), and if either is indicated, always offer a chaperone.

1.13 Given that 'pregnancy is a sexually transmitted condition', presumably good contraceptive counselling should always include an adequate sexual history?

Absolutely, yet many providers in a family planning context claim to be too rushed (or could they still be too embarrassed?) to do this.

If the request is for 'emergency contraception', this should be seen as a marker of risk of a sexually transmitted infection (STI) having been passed along with the sperm. Indeed, there is increasing evidence that the sperm themselves can be 'bio-vectors' of *Chlamydia* and gonococci (although no *Chlamydia* test would be positive from that act, it would need repeating about 7 days later). Remember also that 'breakthrough bleeding' in pill-takers is often a sign of *Chlamydia* infection.

1.14 What are the best questions to ask?

If asked in a matter-of-fact way and non-judgmentally during the course of a consultation about periods and gynaecological symptoms, the following pair of questions are far less threatening than some:

■ 'When did you last have sex?' Followed by:
■ 'When did you last have sex with anybody different?'

A lot can be learned from this, whether the response is '19 years ago' or '3 months ago'. If the latter, it follows quite naturally to then query whether this was a change of partner during 'serial monogamy' or a 'one-night stand' outside a basically long-term relationship.

Some further questions may become highly relevant, depending on the tenor and the body language of the response:

■ Did you always use condoms with a new or casual partner?
■ Have you ever been checked or treated for an STI? Or:
■ Have you ever *thought about* having a sexual health screen?
■ Do you ever *wonder* whether your partner perhaps might have other sexual partner(s) (of either sex)?

Exceptionally, supplementary questions become important, e.g. whether (each) partner was male or female, or about oral or anal sex, or any possible abuse within a relationship. The answers will often show how wrong our assumptions are. The orange-haired young woman with multiple body piercings and tattoos might be in a mutually monogamous relationship while the 'pillar of society' might be having unsafe sex with multiple partners.

1.15 What are the features of the ideal contraceptive?

The list below is modified from Table 13 in my book *The Pill* (see Further Reading). The ideal method would be:

■ *100% effective* (with the default state as contraception)
■ *100% convenient* (forgettable, non-coitally-related)
   Comment: this will usually mean it being initiated by a single simple procedure and, ideally, not thereafter relying on the user's memory.

Taking into account the story at the start of Chapter 2 (which stresses the disjunction between the human brain and the genitalia!), the ideal has to be to switch off one's fertility at a certain time and then, maybe years later, to switch it on again when good and ready to conceive. Thus the 'default state' becomes one of staying contracepted, not conceiving! Note how the two most common methods used by young people – the pill and the condom – have the opposite and completely wrong 'default state'.

- *100% reversible*: reversed very simply, ideally without having to ask permission or get help to stop the method
- *100% safe*: without unwanted effects, whether fatal, dangerous or simply annoying
- *100% maintenance-free*: meaning it needs absolutely no medical or provider intervention (with potential pain or discomfort), whether initially or ongoing, or (as already said) to achieve reversal
- *Acceptable*: to every culture, religion and political view
- *Used by or obviously visible to the woman* (whose stakes in effective contraception are obviously greatest): although an effective non-condom reversible male option would be welcome!
- *Cheap and easy to distribute*
- *100% protective against STIs*
- *Having OTHER, non-contraceptive benefits*, e.g. to the dis-'eases' of the menstrual cycle. Couples are almost always ignorant about such established non-contraceptive benefits: less ovarian cancer with the pill or less blood loss with the levonorgestrel-releasing intrauterine system (LNG-IUS). Because good news is not 'news', almost by definition, these advantages get little publicity.

The most relevant benefit in today's world would be the penultimate bullet, protection against STIs, including viruses. So far, this can only (outside of monogamy) be adequately provided by condoms (male or female) and many couples have to be advised to supplement their non-coitally-related pregnancy-preventing method with a condom: the so-called 'double Dutch' approach.

1.16 **How do the available reversible methods perform when tested against the list in *Q 1.15*?**

No available method meets all these criteria, though the LNG-IUS gets closest.

Maximum effectiveness and independence from intercourse tend to go together and also, unfortunately, to be inversely linked with freedom from health risk. So, in practice, when counselling most couples, one can explain

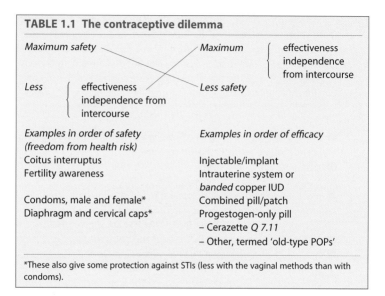

TABLE 1.1 The contraceptive dilemma

Maximum safety ⟍   ⟋ *Maximum*   { effectiveness
                                           independence
                                           from intercourse

Less   { effectiveness   ⟋ *Less safety*
        independence from
        intercourse

Examples in order of safety (freedom from health risk)	*Examples in order of efficacy*
Coitus interruptus	Injectable/implant
Fertility awareness	Intrauterine system or *banded* copper IUD
Condoms, male and female*	Combined pill/patch
Diaphragm and cervical caps*	Progestogen-only pill
	– Cerazette Q 7.11
	– Other, termed 'old-type POPs'

*These also give some protection against STIs (less with the vaginal methods than with condoms).

that there is always a dilemma, a bit of a 'Hobson's choice', as depicted in *Table 1.1*.

1.17 How is the effectiveness of any method commonly reported?

The data about efficacy, particularly of the non-medical methods, have shown extremely variable results. In clinical investigations an effort is usually made to make the (in practice very difficult) distinction between pregnancies that occurred despite the fact that the method was used correctly and consistently during every act of intercourse (perfect use) and those that resulted from incorrect use or non-use on one or more occasions (typical use). This process results in estimates of the consistent use or 'method-effectiveness' and of the more typical use-effectiveness:

- Method-effectiveness rates vary because of physiological differences between individuals, notably increasing age, which diminishes fertility.
- Typical use-effectiveness is a function of the motivation of the study population, the acceptability of another baby, the adequacy of counselling, the difficulty of using the method, the effect of experience through increasing duration of use, and other factors. Hence the findings are even more variable and it is very difficult to compare data from different studies among different populations.
- Extended use-effectiveness is a measure of all the pregnancies occurring in a large population based on their initial intention to use a particular

method. It includes individuals who abandon the method that they initially set out to use. Failure rates calculated on this basis tend to be very high indeed, even for a highly effective method such as the combined pill, because discontinuation due to side-effects or anxiety about side-effects or when a relationship ends can lead to it being abandoned, without any effective replacement, in a large proportion of the initial users.

1.18 How are the effectiveness rates measured and expressed?

They are usually expressed as failure rates/100 woman-years of exposure. The basis for many calculations is known as the Pearl pregnancy rate, calculated from the formula:

$$\text{Failure rate} = \frac{\text{Total accidental pregnancies} \times 1200}{\text{Total months of exposure}}$$

Every known conception must be included, whatever its outcome, when applying this formula. The figure 1200 is the number of months in 100 years. By convention, 10 months are deducted from the denominator for each full-term pregnancy and 4 months for any kind of abortion. If the relevant method is based on 28-day *cycles*, the appropriate multiplier is 1300.

Trussell (of Princeton, USA) points out that the usual convention of using the same denominator (total number of months) whether the numerator is the number of 'method failures' or 'user failures' is wrong because it fails to account for the fact that many contraceptive-users make errors and 'get away with it'. Any such method-failure rate is artificially lowered by the larger denominator. The true 'perfect use' (or 'consistent use') rate would use only the months of total compliance for the denominator. Very few studies, in which all users kept coital diaries, have included the option of computing this true rate. Moreover, because errors in compliance are so common and vary so widely, and the likelihood of 'getting away with it' also varies, this means that standard failure rates should ideally not be compared between populations. Yet in practice this is unavoidable (e.g. in preparing *Table 1.2*).

The risk of contraceptive failure tends to fall with the duration of use because of changes in the population under study, as women drop out for whatever reason. Long-term users obviously tend to be those who use the method efficiently and also include those of lower fertility (the more fertile ones are likely to leave the study by conceiving!) The life-table method of analysis is an attempt to overcome these problems. This takes into account all the reasons for contraceptive discontinuation, and permits the calculation of failure rates (or the rates for other events such as expulsion of an IUD) for specified intervals of use. The Pearl rate on the other hand pools the data and can give only one common measurement, not compensating for dropouts for varying reasons nor for different durations of use in different studies.

TABLE 1.2 Failure rates/100 women for different methods of contraception

	USA data used by WHO (Trussell): % of women having an unintended pregnancy within the first year of use		Oxford/FPA Study (Lancet report in 1982; all women married and aged above 25)		
	Typical use*	Perfect use†	Overall (any duration)	Age 25–34 (≤2 years use)	Age 35+ (≤2 years use)
Sterilization:					
Male (after azoospermia)	0.15	0.1	0.02	0.08	0.08
Female (Filshie clip)	0.5	0.5	0.13	0.45	0.08
Subcutaneous implant:					
Jadelle or Norplant	0.05	0.05	–	–	–
Implanon	<0.1‡	<0.1‡	–	–	–
Injectable (DMPA)	3	0.3	–	–	–
Combined pills:					
50 µg estrogen	8	0.3	0.16	0.25	0.17
<50 µg estrogen	8	0.3	0.27	0.38	0.23
Evra patch	8	0.3	–	–	–
Cerazette progestogen-only pill	–	0.17‡	–	–	–
Old-type POP	8	0.3	1.2	2.5	0.5
IUD (see Q 9.10):					
Levonorgestrel-releasing intrauterine system (LNG-IUS)	0.1	0.1	–	–	–
T-Safe Cu 380 A	0.8	0.6	–	–	–
Other >300-mm copper-wire IUDs (Nova-T 380, Multiload 375, Flexi-T 300)	≈1‡	≈1‡	–	–	–
Male condom	15	2	3.6	6.0	2.9
Female condom	21	5	–	–	–
Diaphragm (all caps believed similar, not all tested)	16	6	1.9	5.5	2.8

TABLE 1.2—cont'd

	USA data used by WHO (Trussell): % of women having an unintended pregnancy within the first year of use		Oxford/FPA Study (Lancet report in 1982; all women married and aged above 25)		
	Typical use*	Perfect use†	Overall (any duration)	Age 25–34 (≤2 years use)	Age 35+ (≤2 years use)
Coitus interruptus	27	4	6.7	–	–
Spermicides alone	29	18	11.9	–	–
Fertility awareness:					
Calendar	–	9	15.5	–	–
Ovulation (mucus) method	–	3	–	–	–
Sympto-thermal	–	2	–	–	–
Postovulation	–	1	–	–	–
Persona	6–?		–	–	–
No method, young women	80–90		–	–	–
No method at age 40	40–50		–	–	–
No method at age 45	10–20		–	–	–
No method at age 50 (if still having menses)	0–5		–	–	–

*<u>Typical use:</u> Among typical couples who initiate use of the method (not necessarily for the first time), the percentage who experience an accidental pregnancy during the first year if they do not stop use for any other reason.

†<u>Perfect use:</u> Among typical couples who initiate use of the method (not necessarily for the first time), and who then use it *perfectly* (both consistently and correctly), the percentage who experience an accidental pregnancy during the first year if they do not stop use for any other reason.

‡Data not available from Trussell, so best alternative data given (e.g. from manufacturer's studies).

Other Notes:

1. Note influence of age: all the rates in the fifth column being lower than those in the fourth column. Lower rates still may be expected above age 45.

2. Much better results also obtainable in other states of relative infertility, such as lactation.

3. Oxford/FPA users were established users at recruitment – greatly improving results for barrier methods (see Qs 1.19, 4.9).

4. The Implanon, Cerazette and Persona results come from pre-marketing studies by the manufacturer, giving an estimate of the Pearl 'method-failure' rate.

1.19 What effectiveness rates can be quoted for potential users?

Vested interests (especially by advertisers) and the distinct lack of comparative studies – let alone randomized controlled trials – readily lead to misuse of the data on the effectiveness of particular techniques. Failure rates need to be interpreted by the provider to each potential user, in the context of the woman's age and factors such as the steadiness of the relationship and the frequency of intercourse (*Table 1.2*).

Note how modern IUDs and the IUS have entirely comparable efficacy to female sterilization (*see Q 9.10*). Both vasectomy (after two negative sperm counts) and Implanon are more effective than female sterilization, and injectables beat the remainder (including the combined oral contraceptive [COC]) because of the user-failure problem. *Table 1.2* includes data from the Oxford/Family Planning Association (FPA) study, which are of interest as showing what motivated users can achieve with the included methods, and also the important (not unexpected) effect of increasing age. Note also how careful condom-users have been known to do better than poor pill-users. . . . But there are caveats (*see Q 4.9*) about the kind of women that the FPA study recruited, an untypically 'good' population.

In interpreting *Table 1.2* to couples at counselling, it is sometimes helpful to divide 100 by the figures given for the rates. This calculation gives the number of years of regular intercourse, using the method carefully, which would be expected to lead to one conception. For example, if per 100 woman-year rates of 10 and 1 were being compared, the couple could be told that regular use of the method would give an 'evens' chance of one pregnancy by the end of 10 years or 100 years of fertility, respectively. This clearly shows the difference, although for a full understanding it is very important to add that 'Of course, one pregnancy could occur in the very first year, with betting odds of 1 in 10 or 1 in 100, respectively.'

1.20 Given that, as you say, most accidents are caused by humans and most humans are still caused by accidents, what can I as a prescriber do about this?

It is no good just blaming the method-users. Prescribers can fail them in a number of ways, both by errors but more commonly by omissions, for example, simply not allowing enough time for basic instructions and for users to ask questions. 'You cannot make the horse drink' . . . but in the first place have we *properly* 'taken the horse to the water'? More on this follows in Chapter 11 (*see Qs 11.3–11.16*): we need first to be fully informed about the methods available (*Table 1.3*).

TABLE 1.3 Use of contraceptive methods by women aged 16–49 years living in Great Britain in 2005/2006

Method	Proportion*
Partner using the male condom	21%
Combined oral contraceptive (COC)	17%
Male partner sterilized	11%
Sterilized	10%
Copper IUD	5%
Progestogen-only pill (POP)	5%
Withdrawal	4%
Progestogen-only injectable	3%
Progestogen-only implant	1%
Cervical cap or diaphragm	1%
Emergency contraception	1%
Levonorgestrel-releasing intrauterine system (LNG-IUS)	1%
Natural family planning	1%
Female condom	<1%
Foams or gels	<1%
Using at least one method	74%

*Some women reported using more than one method; therefore the proportions sum to more than 74%.

Not using a method

Not currently in a heterosexual relationship	14%
Sterile after another operation, e.g. hysterectomy	3%
Wants to get pregnant	3%
Pregnant now	1%
Going without sex to avoid pregnancy	<1%
Unlikely to conceive because of menopause	2%
Possibly infertile	2%
Other reason	1%

*Some women reported more than one reason for no method; therefore the proportions sum to more than 26%.
Data from: National Statistics, 2006 http://www.statistics.gov.uk/STATBASE/Product. asp?vlnk=6988.
Note: Contraceptive method in use at that time (point prevalence) or reason for non-use was documented by a survey of nearly 5000 households in Great Britain (i.e. England, Scotland, and Wales), conducted in 2005 and 2006.

The Omnibus Survey of the Office for National Statistics will give readers access to all data they may desire regarding current contraception use in the UK (http://www.statistics.gov.uk/STATBASE/Product. asp?vlnk=6988).

Aspects of human fertility and fertility awareness: natural birth control

2

BACKGROUND CONSIDERATIONS

FERTILITY AWARENESS AND NATURAL FAMILY PLANNING: BACKGROUND AND MECHANISMS

Apparently, after God created the very first man, Adam, He said to him: 'I have some news for you: two bits of good news and one bit of bad news. Which would you like to hear first?' And Adam said, 'The good news first please, God.' So God said to Adam: 'The first good news is that I am going to create for you an Organ. This Organ is called the Brain. With this gift of mine you will be able to think, and to learn, and to feel – and to invent good names for all the beautiful animals and plants I am creating to be fruitful on land and in the seas.

'Thank you very much', said Adam. 'What's the other good news?'

'Well', said God, [*Note: you will not find a record of this particular conversation in available translations of either the Bible or Koran!*] I am going to create for you another Organ. This Organ is called the Penis. With it you will be able to give to your wife Eve much pleasure, and receive the same back from her – I want my creatures to enjoy themselves. But be aware it should only be with Eve, as my plan for you folks is monogamy. With my help as I am the Creator this second organ I am giving you will help you to have children and I'd like you to bring them up to steward and look after all this new creation of mine, of which I am very proud.'

'Thank you again', said Adam. 'I'll try. So, what's the bad news?'

<u>'You will never be able to use both at the same time', said God.</u>

This silly story is highly relevant to why contraceptives so often fail – especially whenever alcohol greatly potentiates the barrier between Organ 1 (with its sexual *knowledge* content) and Organ 2 (sexual *behaviour*). It also highlights the value of the LARCs, which are discussed later in Chapters 8 and 9. See www.nice.org.uk/guidance/CG30.

BACKGROUND CONSIDERATIONS

2.1 How fertile are human beings?

That story says it all: there is a complete disjunction, a great gulf fixed, between brain and genitalia – in both sexes, although undoubtedly men are the worse affected. . . . So it's not surprising that both the inventing and the practising of ideal contraception are difficult. We break no records in the animal kingdom but we are fertile enough to become – numerically – far and away the most successful vertebrate that this planet has ever known. Too successful for our own good (*see Chapter 1*).

The first half of this chapter deals with physiological factors that promote conception. We first consider aspects relating to intercourse, then the sperm, the ova, fertilization and implantation.

We can at least be grateful that the fertility of average couples is not as great as the human maximum, which must have been approached by the couple described in the *Guinness Book of Records*:

The greatest officially recorded number of children produced by a mother is 69 by the first of the two wives of Feodor Vasilyev (b. 1707), a peasant from Shuya, 241 km east of Moscow. In 27 confinements, she gave birth to 16 pairs of twins, 7 sets of triplets and 4 sets of quadruplets. . . . Almost all survived to their majority.

2.2 What features of human intercourse are particularly favourable to fertility?

■ The attraction between a man and a woman is frequently powerful and mutual, and the human female is exceptional in having no breeding season and in being potentially receptive on most days of the cycle.

■ Some indication of the power of the human sex instinct is provided by the calculation (never mind the assumptions) by WHO, in the early 1990s, that intercourse then took place about 42 000 million times per year. This worked out, somewhere in the world, to over 1300 ejaculations per second. With over 25% more sexually active adults now than then, I suppose that figure must now be 1600 per second . . . mind-boggling!

■ The drive towards copulation in both sexes is in 'real-time' – now – and feels irresistible. This frustrates forward planning and the successful use of intercourse-related methods of contraception. And men are the worst culprits – they omit to tell their partners important nuisance details (e.g. that the condom split!) and sometimes tell the most flagrant lies (whether about their undying love or their HIV status).

■ Some women report that maximum desire coincides with the most fertile phase, when there is an abundance of estrogenic mucus, which is very favourable to sperm survival; whereas minimum desire is unhelpfully often in the premenstrual 'safe' phase.

■ The outpouring of vaginal transudate described by Masters and Johnson raises the pH of the vagina so that it becomes favourable to sperm.

■ There is evidence that, at least in some women, there is a negative pressure in the uterus at orgasm. This might (though never proved) promote physical aspiration of sperm into the cervix and uterus. Sperm are certainly found in the cervix within 90 seconds of ejaculation.

2.3 How do the mechanics of intercourse interfere with the efficacy of vaginal methods of contraception?

■ The ballooning of the whole upper two-thirds of the vagina, also described by Masters and Johnson, leads to:
  – an increased risk of sperm passing over the rim of a diaphragm or other cervical cap
  – the risk of displacement of any cervical device into a fornix.

■ The penile thrusts themselves lead to:
  – the potential to dislodge all forms of female barrier, particularly in certain positions of intercourse
  – if a vaginal spermicide is used, it is probable that the spreading effect of intercourse means that there is ultimately too little spermicide around the external os of the cervix at ejaculation. This might in

part explain how spermicides have usually appeared far more effective in vitro than in vivo (*see Q 4.63*) – though they can be a good option for women who are less fertile through age or breastfeeding.

2.4 What are the relevant facts about cervical mucus?

Cervical mucus is only the most obvious component of the genital tract mucus and fluid, which extend right through the cavity of the uterus and both tubes. Under the influence of unopposed estrogen in the follicular phase it becomes increasingly fluid and receptive to sperm, with a marked Spinnbarkeit. It helps to capacitate sperm and provides an optimum environment for them to proceed to the upper tract. The ability to promote sperm survival for prolonged durations varies from woman to woman and from cycle to cycle, as does the length of time within the cycle that ovulatory mucus is present.

The characteristics of mucus change abruptly under the influence of progesterone, even though the corpus luteum continues to secrete estrogens. The mucus rapidly becomes impenetrable and hostile to sperm. Women can be taught to feel the change from the earlier, slippery 'ovulatory' mucus to the sticky mucus of the luteal phase. But before ovulation, WHO (1983) found 'a substantial' probability of pregnancy if intercourse occurs (even) in the presence of sticky mucus.

2.5 What other changes occur at the cervix during the cycle?

Continuing research into birth planning by methods of fertility awareness has shown that women can be taught to detect the changes occurring in the size of the external cervical os, and also in its position relative to the introitus. The cervix starts low and feels firm, then rises appreciably during the follicular phase, until around ovulation it reaches peak height from the introitus with maximum softness and sufficient dilation to admit a fingertip. The cervix then descends and narrows rapidly early in the luteal phase, becoming once more closed, firm and closer to the vulva. It is reported that daily autopalpation of these cervical changes can assist in the detection of the return of fertility towards the end of lactation (*see Q 2.36*).

2.6 What are the most important physiological facts about sperm that promote conception?

All of us whose work involves family planning rapidly develop an enormous respect for these little swimmers! There is great individual variation between men, and between individual sperm within the same man's ejaculate. Sperm counts and quality have fallen in some areas, attributed to estrogenic chemical pollutants in the environment: is Nature biting back, against the species that is multiplying like there were no tomorrow? (*see Chapter 1*).

Yet there is still an overkill of numbers produced by most men. From the point of view of preventing pregnancy we have to consider the very best sperm with regard to motility, survival and fertilizing ability, rather than those exhibiting average or lesser qualities.

2.7 How many sperm are present, and what are the implications?

Spermatogenesis proceeds in normal men at rates of the order of 1000 per second from each testicle! With a count of say 80 million/mL being not unrepresentative, it would not be unusual for there to be 350 million sperm in the 3–5 mL of a typical ejaculate. If each sperm could find an egg, this would be enough to populate most of North America! One per cent of this number (enough to people Costa Rica or New Zealand) might very well cause a pregnancy (*see Q 2.9*). Yet this would be contained in the hardly visible volume of less than 0.05 mL. This has obvious implications for coitus interruptus (*see Q 3.7*) and also for any lack of care when using the condom (*see Q 3.20*). In contraceptive terms, semen is a dangerous fluid!

2.8 What is the extreme limit of sperm survival in genital tract mucus, and what are the implications?

This has proved very difficult to study directly because the studies themselves are liable to alter what is being observed. It seems clear that sperm *normally* survive no more than about 6 h in the vagina, because its pH reverts to its normal low value after intercourse. However, motile sperm have been found even in the vagina up to 16 h after intercourse, and survival in the cervical, uterine and tubal fluids appears very variable. Survival depends on features of the sperm themselves, the seminal fluid and to what degree the estrogenic mucus approaches the ideal – in that woman or in that particular cycle.

In the past, most authorities talked in terms of average survival times of about 3–4 days. However, with so many millions ejaculated one must be concerned not with average sperm survival but 'lunatic fringe' sperm survival! It is the duration of the ability to fertilize of the first centile of the sperm (i.e. the most vigorous 3 million or so) that is the relevant figure. This is not known, but direct and indirect studies suggest that this can certainly reach 6 days. On some rare occasions in some rare couples, particularly where the woman produces good mucus for an unusually long time, it might even reach 7 days. Mucus assessment (*see Qs 2.4, 2.25*) should theoretically give more advance warning of ovulation than usual in those very cases, but it can fail to do so.

The main implication is the likely ineffectiveness, in long-term use by most couples, of the *first* phase of the so-called 'safe period' (*see Q 2.17*).

2.9   How can it be that 1% of a man's ejaculate (i.e. about 3 million sperm) could cause a pregnancy, when men with that number of sperm/mL are usually infertile?

This question implies a common misunderstanding of the nature of semen analysis in an infertility clinic. For a start, an excessively high count can actually be associated with male subfertility. Also, when there is a low count this might be acting as a marker for other much more important features of the sperm that are causing the subfertility, such as poor motility, frequent abnormal forms or the presence of antibodies. Paucity of sperm tends to go along with them being pretty poor individuals and this does not apply when 3 million good sperm from a fertile man are deposited at the cervix.

Evidence for the above comes from routine sperm counts in men having vasectomies who have fathered children. Counts less than 2 million/mL are not uncommon; and in a study of late recanalization reported from Oxford, it appeared that a man with counts of only 500 000 and 750 000/mL (with motility demonstrated) was responsible for his wife's pregnancy.

2.10   What are the relevant physiological facts about ova?

- More often than expected by many couples, ovulation occurs early. Many women claiming 28-day menstrual cycles really sometimes have 26-day cycles, and some can feature fertile cycles as short as 21 or 22 days in length (*see Q 2.15* for the implications).
- Ovum fertilizability is short – practically the only physiological fact so far discussed that helps contraception. From in vitro fertilization research, maximum ovum survival is believed to be 24 h but successful fertilization appears to be unlikely beyond 12 h. This means that if a pregnancy is desired, the best chance of successful fertilization is when that fragile ovum arrives at a tube that is already populated with adequate numbers of vigorous, motile sperm.

2.11   Can human females be like rabbits, ovulating on intercourse?

I think the answer to this question, which is often asked, can (fortunately) be a fairly definite 'no'. First, there is no need even to postulate any such mechanism when one adds together the data mentioned above concerning sperm survival and the frequent occurrence of ovulation earlier than usual. Intercourse can be fertile almost any time, not excluding during the menses, if sperm can survive for up to 7 days and ovulation can be unexpectedly early or late.

A second and more important reason for rejecting this hypothesis is the fact that, were it to be true, newly married women would have shorter menstrual cycles than women who were abstaining from intercourse (such as nuns). Such a shortening of the mean duration of menstrual cycles has not been observed.

2.12 After fertilization, how much preimplantation wastage occurs?

Here we have another fact that, fortunately, reduces the size of the contraceptive task. Assessments of total postfertilization wastage vary considerably but a good modern estimate would be around 40–50%. There are frequently chromosomal abnormalities, but local factors affecting the receptivity of the endometrium to the blastocyst are also important. These can be enhanced by contraceptive methods (*see Q 10.7*).

FERTILITY AWARENESS AND NATURAL FAMILY PLANNING: BACKGROUND AND MECHANISMS

2.13 Putting the above physiological facts together, how long is the fertile window in each cycle?

First, visit www.fertilityuk.org, which is an absolutely brilliant and non-sectarian website for the education of couples and (even) of their doctors, in this whole area.

Second, forget the traditional myth that fertility is 'midcycle'. Recent in vivo and in vitro studies, which form the basis of the physiology described in the last ten questions, clearly indicate that the fertile phase both starts and finishes earlier and is also longer than is often assumed. The latest work would imply that, under optimal conditions for sperm survival, the potentially fertile phase is not less than days 7–14 (i.e. the whole of the second week of a 4-week cycle). If ovulation takes place on day 14–15, a further 1-plus days needs to be added to allow for maximum ovum survival, i.e. in all there is a potential fertile window from day 7 to day 15 of a hypothetical, normal cycle. Given that the luteal phase is relatively fixed, such that ovulation occurs 12–16 days before the next menses starts, the start day of the fertile window alters if the cycle is longer or shorter than 28 days.

2.14 How was the classic Barrett and Marshall study designed? What is the risk of conception on each day of the cycle (*Fig. 2.1*)?

In brief, 241 previously fertile women who had been fully trained to keep basal body temperature (BBT) charts also kept a careful record of every act of intercourse. Whether conception took place in a given cycle was also known. Some were attempting to conceive, others to avoid pregnancy. All the data on 1898 cycles and 6015 acts of coitus were fed into a computer and, for each woman, the day of BBT shift, and hence presumed ovulation, was identified in a standard way for that cycle.

The analysis gave figures for the percentage risk of conception for intercourse on each day of the cycle relative to the BBT shift, and these

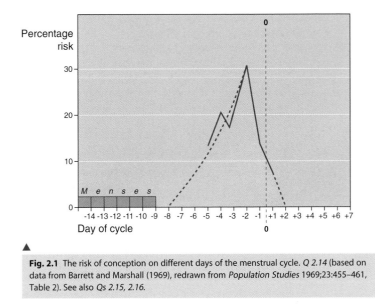

Fig. 2.1 The risk of conception on different days of the menstrual cycle. Q 2.14 (based on data from Barrett and Marshall (1969), redrawn from *Population Studies* 1969;23:455–461, Table 2). See also *Qs 2.15, 2.16*.

have been charted to produce *Fig. 2.1* (in which O represents the BBT shift). The continuous line joins the points for which the data were sufficient for an estimate of percentage risk of conception to be made; the dotted lines are approximate projections down to the horizontal axis.

2.15 What are the main observations from *Fig. 2.1*?

■ As just shown, the fertile window, when percentage risk of conception exceeds 0%, lasts in many fertile cycles for at least 8 days, 7 of which precede the moment of ovulation – as predicted from sperm and ovum survival studies (*see Q 2.13*). Later work by Wilcox et al [Timing of the "fertile window" in the menstrual cycle: day specific estimates from a prospective study. *British Medical Journal* 2000;321:1259–1262] suggests a slightly shorter fertile window of 7 days, but I prefer to retain the 1 day's extra margin. The congruence of this work with that of Barrett and Marshall in 1969 is remarkable.

■ Peak fecundability occurs well before ovum release, again congruent with the notion that it is best for the sperm to be waiting in the tubes in advance of ovulation.

■ The first 'infertile' phase of the cycle is shown to be short, even in a woman who never ovulates earlier than day 14. As it is well known that very many women do occasionally ovulate earlier in the cycle, in a 24-

day cycle intercourse any later than day 3 might, on the basis of these data, sometimes result in conception!

■ The good news from *Fig. 2.1* is that the second phase is potentially a very 'safe period', dependent only on the reliability of ovulation detection. There is, normally, only one ovum and it is fertilizable for a predictable, short time. This is quite unlike the first phase, which is beset by problems: the millions of sperm, the capriciousness with which enough of them might just survive on occasion for as much as a week, coupled with the possibility of a random, early ovulation. So far, no means have been devised of predicting ovulation accurately, far enough ahead, to eliminate the risk of sperm survival up to the point of fertilization.

2.16 And when in any given cycle will the fertile window occur?

In practice, no one knows – outside of research situations. Even women who believe they have 'regular cycles' can produce much shorter or longer ones 'out of the blue', perhaps every 2 years or so. Given the variability of the day of ovulation that this implies (14 ± 2 days before the unknown first day of the next menses), women need to understand that the 8-day fertile window can therefore 'move': it might start unpredictably even before the last days of a period, or contrariwise involve the whole of the third week should it be going to be a 5-week cycle.

Ideally, school sex and relationships education (SRE) should routinely include these 'new' facts. And clinicians need to note the implication that emergency contraception should very rarely be refused just because the exposure day was one of 'zero conception risk'.

2.17 How does the variable onset of the fertile window influence the efficacy of the two infertile phases identified in natural family planning (NFP)?

In my view, with any combination of present technologies, all users of NFP ought to be informed that the second infertile phase is the more effective of the two. Good results can be obtained by optimally trained and motivated couples when both phases are used. But, in my view, a woman who feels that she must avoid pregnancy should have otherwise unprotected sex only in the postovulatory ('green for go') phase. The first (or 'amber') phase is primarily suitable for those who are delaying a wanted pregnancy ('spacing'). The one exception to this recommendation might be a woman with very regular longish menstrual cycles (ideally not less than 28 days) who is good at detecting mucus and cervical changes. She should abstain in each cycle from the first day of detection of mucus or from 21 days before her shortest cycle would end, whichever comes earlier, to identify the first potentially fertile day (*see Q 2.18*).

However, the capriciousness of sperm survival under occasional optimal conditions still means that, whatever methodology based on fertility awareness is used, the preovulatory phase will always be 'in a different ballpark' of potential efficacy than the postovulatory phase.

2.18 Why have family planning specialists traditionally decried NFP methods? What should be their attitude now?

The bad reputation of these methods followed from the high failure rate of the old calendar/rhythm approach, coupled with a lack of awareness of the fundamental difference in effectiveness potential between the first and the second infertile phases, however they might be determined. That lack of awareness is still common today among both the opponents and the proponents of the methods.

The correct attitude today should be a very positive one to this choice for couples, with accurate information and advice about the appropriateness of the choice in each case. As already mentioned, the website www.fertilityuk.org is invaluable educationally and – along with www.fpa.org.uk – also provides the names of local teachers for potential NFP-users.

2.19 Although not recommended as the sole method, what calculations are required for the calendar/rhythm method?

1 The woman should define the shortest and longest menstrual cycle over the previous six (preferably 12) cycles.
2 She should subtract (preferably) 21 days from the length of the *shortest* cycle to derive the first day of the fertile phase. This allows 14, 15 or 16 days for the length of the luteal phase plus 7, 6 or 5 days for maximum sperm survival. Sadly, these durations might come to more than 21 days! Even so, in the identification of the start of the fertile phase, using 21 rather than 20 days in this calculation is an important additional safeguard (to the first appearance of any mucus, *see Q 2.28*).
3 Subtract 10 from the *longest* cycle observed to derive the last day of the fertile phase, so allowing 11 days for minimum length of a fertile luteal phase and 1 day for the duration of ovum fertilizability.

Even with 'perfect use' this method has a high failure rate (see *Table 1.2*, p. 14). Compliance is also difficult, because few women have regular menstrual cycles, so the amount of abstinence required becomes intolerable to many couples. The 'Standard Days' method (*see Q 2.38*) shortens this abstinence time at the price of a higher failure rate.

2.20 How are the phases of the fertility cycle defined (*Fig. 2.2*)?

- ■ The first infertile phase starts on day 1 of the menses and ends with the earliest time that any sperm could survive to cause a pregnancy. It varies in length, depending on the rapidity of the follicular response to the pituitary hormones.

- ■ The true fertile phase (or fertile window) extends from the end of phase 1 until that time following ovulation when the ovum is incapable of being fertilized. Its duration is therefore the sum of the maximum number of days of sperm survival (say 7 days) and the maximum duration of fertilizability of the ovum (say 24 h). In practice, the identified fertile phase tends to be longer than this, because the clinical indicators of fertility are not 100% accurate.

- ■ The second infertile phase extends from the end of the fertile phase until the onset of the next menstruation. This phase has a mean duration of 13 days with a range, in likely fertile cycles, of about 11–15 days. It is often called the 'absolute' infertile phase because significantly delayed

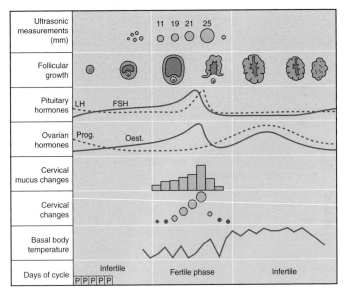

▲

Fig. 2.2 The relationship during the cycle of serial ultrasound measurements, hormonal control and clinical indicators of fertility. *Q 2.20* (reproduced courtesy of the late Dr A. Flynn, Birmingham Maternity Hospital, Queen Elizabeth Medical Centre, Birmingham).

superovulation almost 'never' occurs in the human. (If two or more eggs are released, this is nearly always within the same 24 h.) Provided ovulation is accurately determined and sufficient time is allowed for the ovum to succumb, conception is close to impossible in this phase.

2.21 How can the phases be determined, in practice?

We must distinguish carefully between:

1 The biological events that delineate the phases – these are clear-cut and defined in Q 2.20. But they are not the same as:
2 The biological *indicators* of the events, which can be further classified into:
   (a) biophysical methods (e.g. serial ultrasonic monitoring of follicular growth, changes in vaginal, ovarian or hand blood flow, etc.)
   (b) biochemical methods, which detect the change in concentration of the sex steroids or their metabolites in body fluids such as urine or saliva
   (c) clinical indicators, such as BBT, mucus and cervical changes. The accuracy of these indicators of the actual events at (1) varies, and must also be distinguished from:
3 The quality of the teaching of the couple, which results in the woman and her partner accurately detecting the indicator. And finally, after detection and recording of the indicator, we have to consider:
4 The compliance (with the requirement to abstain) of the woman and of her partner, which is a problem with **all** methods which require 'user' involvement.

The importance of (3) and (4) was well shown in a celebrated study, which apparently showed that the pregnancy rate was higher when charts of clinical indicators were interpreted by the woman's husband than when the woman decided when it was 'safe' to have intercourse!

2.22 What are the major clinical (patient-identifiable) indicators of fertility?

- Changes in the cervical mucus (*see Qs 2.4, 2.25*).
- Changes involving the cervix itself (*see Q 2.5*).
- Changes in the BBT (*see Q 2.23*).
- With the aid of technology, other indicators in body fluids (e.g. Persona).

2.23 How are the changes in the BBT used?

The biphasic nature of the temperature cycle is caused by metabolites of progesterone, hence this can only be used to detect the onset of the second infertile phase. A woman must measure her temperature under basal conditions after a period of sleep, without getting out of bed, having a drink or smoking a cigarette. The shift of temperature is small (0.2–0.4ºC), hence a special expanded-scale mercury thermometer should be used, or, better still, a modern, direct-reading, electronic version. The temperature may be taken orally or vaginally or in the auditory meatus, sticking to the same orifice for any given cycle.

The results are plotted daily on a special chart. To detect the shift a cover line is drawn 0.05ºC over the lower phase temperatures, of which there should be a minimum of six. The second infertile phase is held to begin on the morning of the third consecutive high temperature after the temperature shift; each being a minimum of 0.2ºC higher than those six earlier temperatures, covered by the line drawn as just described.

2.24 What are the difficulties of BBT assessment?

Some women have problems with using and reading thermometers, and with keeping interpretable charts. All should be taught to identify factors such as mild infection or drugs which can misleadingly raise the temperature prematurely before ovulation in what is actually going to be a relatively long cycle.

2.25 How are the mucus changes used to detect the fertile and infertile phases?

The woman is instructed to observe the quantity, colour, fluidity, glossiness, transparency and stretchiness of the mucus at every micturition. The most fertile characteristics of the mucus over the entire day are charted each night. The woman either fills in a colour (green for dry, yellow for mucus and red for bleeding) or writes in a description of the mucus seen.

The peak mucus day can only be identified retrospectively, and corresponds closely with the peak secretion of estrogen in the blood. This is the last day during which the mucus is clear, wet, slippery and with an elastic quality allowing it to be stretched for several centimetres before it breaks, like raw egg white. After ovulation, the rise in progesterone causes – within a day – a profound change in the amount and characteristics of the mucus. If present at all, it resembles the opaque, sticky and tacky postmenstrual type. The peak mucus day can hence be identified. Allowing 2–3 days for ovulation to be completed and 1 day for ovum fertilizability, the second infertile phase is defined as beginning on the evening of the *fourth* day after the peak mucus symptom.

Changes in the cervix itself (*see* Q 2.5) can be used to check on the other indicators, although this is not essential.

2.26 What practical problems can confuse mucus assessment?

■ The most frequent is the effect of intercourse, or of sexual excitement without intercourse. Both the fluid of sexual arousal and semen can mimic the sensations and the features of ovulatory mucus. Careful teaching can help the woman to distinguish the latter, but if in doubt she should presume possible fertility. Unprotected intercourse is usually only allowed on alternate days to allow mucus assessment. To identify the first potentially fertile day, the calculation at *Q 2.19* (shortest cycle less 21) must have priority over mucus observations. WHO (1983) has reported that in almost 20% of cycles no mucus at all was observed at the vulva until 3 days or less before the peak day. Therefore, mucus of any type must equate to potential fertility: sticky mucus is not reliably 'infertile'.

- Spermicidal jellies and lubricants can similarly cause confusion, particularly if the diaphragm is used during the fertile phase.
- Mucus assessment is impossible during bleeding – a problem in some short menstrual cycles.
- Vaginal infections and discharges can cause difficulty, notably thrush and its treatments, which tend to 'dry' the mucus.

2.27 What are the minor clinical indicators of fertility?

These tend to be specific to individual women or to occur only in some ovulatory cycles. When present they can be helpful in confirming the major signals. Among them are:

- Ovulation pain (Mittelschmerz): ultrasound scan studies show that this regular unilateral (rarely bilateral) pain occurs 24–48 h before ovulation, not at the event itself. It is probably caused as the ovarian tissue is stretched by the rapidly growing follicle.
- A midcycle 'show' of blood.
- The onset of breast symptoms, acne and other skin changes, and variations in mood and sexual desire.

The second infertile phase can be held to start 5 days after Mittelschmerz ends, provided this matches the findings on a woman's temperature/mucus chart (*see Q 2.28*).

2.28 Combining indicators is obviously more effective, but what should be done if different clinical indicators give variable results?

Basically, go on the 'safest' result. So, when identifying the second phase, for example, the woman should be instructed to act only on the *latest* of the signals being used. For example, if peak mucus plus 4 days would suggest that intercourse was 'safe' on a Thursday evening, but only two higher temperatures had been recorded, intercourse would be deferred until the third higher temperature was recorded the following (Friday) morning.

For those who are 'spacing' rather than limiting pregnancy, and therefore wish to rely on both infertile phases, the following summary rule is helpful:

■ The fertile time starts 21 days before the woman's shortest cycle would end or earlier when any secretions are detected.

■ It ends after at least three higher temperatures have been recorded, all *after* the peak mucus day.

2.29 What about Persona – the Unipath Personal Contraceptive System?

Charting mucus and temperatures and other symptoms is obviously rather a hassle. Persona is an innovative product, first marketed in 1996, consisting of a series of disposable test sticks and a handheld computerized monitor. As instructed by a yellow light on the monitor, the test sticks are dipped in the user's early morning urine samples and transferred to a slot in the device. There the levels of both estrone-3-glucuronide (E-3-G) and luteinizing hormone (LH) are measured by a patented immunochromatographic assay, utilizing an optical monitor (*Fig. 2.3*). As soon as the first significant rise in the E-3-G level is detected, the fertility status is changed to 'unsafe' and a red light replaces the green one on the monitor. After subsequent detection of the first significant rise of LH, the end of the fertile period is not signalled by a green light until four further

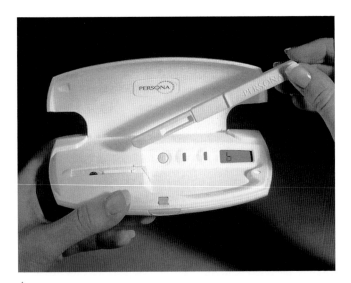

▲

Fig. 2.3 Persona (Unipath Personal Contraceptive System). *Q 2.29* (from Kubba et al 1999 *Contraception and office gynecology: choices in reproductive healthcare* p. 45. London, WB Saunders. With permission).

days have elapsed, to allow for the time to ovulation and then demise of the ovum.

The system initially requests 16 tests in the first cycle, dropping to eight thereafter. Utilizing data on the individual's previous six menstrual cycles as well as the current one, it is sensitive to cyclical changes, so that the number of 'red' days varies. In the first few months there are typically 12–15 red days, falling later (according to the manufacturer's brochure) to as low as 6 to 10 days among users with the most regular cycles but rising if urine tests are missed or subsequent to an unusually long or short cycle.

Given the facts about potential sperm survival (*see Q 2.8*), the group given only six infertile days must include some at a higher risk of follicular-phase method failures (*see also Qs 2.30, 2.31*).

2.30 Who can use Persona? And what are the short- and long-term contraindications?

Persona is usable if cycle lengths are between 23 and 35 days, and can accommodate variations of up to 10 days within this range. It should not be used:

- if the woman has experienced menopausal (vasomotor) symptoms
- while breastfeeding or soon after childbirth
- after recent use of any hormonal contraception, including all pills and injectables
- during a cycle in which tetracycline is used (itself, *not* any of its relatives, e.g. doxycycline) as this can result in an enhancement of the LH signal from the urine.

If the second and third bulleted points apply (including a single use of hormonal emergency contraception), the user is advised to wait for two natural consecutive cycles, each of 23–35 days, and initiate use of Persona only when the third menses start.

The main contraindication, of course, relates to suitability of the method to the lifestyle of the couple, and often too little thought is given to the man's views. If he is going to come home drunk on a Saturday night and (maybe only metaphorically) kick the Persona across the bedroom whatever light it shows, this is hardly the right method! Much attention also needs to be paid to explaining its known failure rate even with correct use (*see Q 2.31*).

2.31 What is the failure rate of Persona as currently marketed?

Efficacy information from the European trials by the manufacturer suggests a first-year failure rate in consistent users of around 6 per 100 woman-years. This is a best estimate, and is thought by Trussell (*see Q 1.18*) to be optimistic, for 'perfect use' of Persona.

The best results using multiple-index fertility awareness are as good as when Persona is used, so the main advantage of this device is just that of being more user-friendly. The device also usually signals a shorter fertile period than the 10–12 days' abstinence typically demanded by the multiple-index methods. However, a failure rate of 6% is considerably higher than would be acceptable to those accustomed to the efficacy, say, of the injectable or an implant.

Couples should be reminded that they might well themselves be among the (at least) 6% in whom the method fails in consistent use, and that this equates to a 1 in 17 chance of pregnancy in the next year.

2.32   What if that 1 in 17 risk of conception is not acceptable?

Then there is a useful combination option. Indeed, in my opinion this should always have been on offer – i.e. it should have been described in the instructions with this product. Given the higher in-built risk of intercourse before ovulation (because of those capricious sperm! *see Qs 2.8, 2.16*), I recommend the following combination method, for a monogamous couple wanting high efficacy:

- From day 1 until the red light first appears: *use condoms.* Consider this the 'amber for caution' phase.
- Throughout the 'red' phase: *abstain.*
- After the second 'green for go' phase starts: *unprotected sex is fine.*

I would confidently expect a low failure rate of 1–2% if this advice were followed accurately; and the scientists involved in the testing of Persona confirm that this was achieved in the trials by those who relied solely on the second (postovulatory) 'green' phase.

EFFECTIVENESS

2.33   What is the efficacy of multiple-index NFP or Persona?

If the second infertile phase only is relied on, provided during the fertile phase there is complete abstinence (*NOT* condom use, because condoms are often used inadequately!), a highly acceptable 'perfect use' method-failure rate of 1/100 woman-years is obtainable (see *Table 1.2*, p. 14). Moreover, similarly excellent 'perfect use' failure rates (up to 2% in the first year) have sometimes been reported for the use of multiple-index methods even where intercourse has been permitted in the first, preovulatory, phase. This is partly because of relative infertility in the successful users, which comes about because the most highly fertile couples tend to drop out of, or never enter, the studied population (through conceiving!).

As Trussell (*see Q 1.18*) has also pointed out, rates as low as 1–3/100 woman-years (*Table 1.2*) are not relevant for typical potential users of NFP. There is no doubt that it is *extremely unforgiving of less-than-perfect use*, which – let's face it – tends to be *normal* use of this, like any method, for most normal people. (Contrast the pill: most people forget pills from time to time but the difference is that they are much more likely to get away with it than are NFP-users.)

ADVANTAGES AND INDICATIONS

2.34   What are the advantages of methods based on fertility awareness?

- First and foremost, they are completely free from any known physical side-effects for the user.
- They are acceptable to many with certain religious and cultural views, not only Roman Catholics. According to strict interpretations, they are used rightly when the intention is family spacing, with the possibility of conceiving retained.
- The methods are under the couple's personal control (abstinence is always available!).
- The methods readily lend themselves, if the couple's scruples permit, to the additional use of an artificial method such as a barrier at the potentially fertile times – always with acceptance of that method's failure rate, which can never be as good as abstinence!
- Once established as efficient users, after proper teaching, no further expensive follow-up of the couple is necessary.
- Understanding of the methods can help any couple, with or without any subfertility, when they come to try to conceive.

PROBLEMS AND DISADVANTAGES

2.35   What are the problems of NFP methods?

- Interestingly enough, the majority of established users believe the method is helpful to their marriage/relationship, rather than a cause of stress – but the amount of abstaining required also causes frustration and conflicts. Indeed, whenever a woman suggests this option, *it is essential to ensure the partner is fully 'on board' with the decision.*
- Several studies, including the 1993 WHO study, have shown no hint of an increase in the incidence of birth defects among failures, due to ageing gametes, and this postulated risk can now be discounted.

BREASTFEEDING AS NATURAL BIRTH CONTROL

2.36 Can fertility awareness predict the return of fertility after lactation?

Full breastfeeding, in which the baby takes no fluids other than from its mother, is a highly efficient natural contraceptive. The most important factor is the frequency and duration of suckling. In practice, therefore, the return of fertility is a prolonged process, during which spurious attempts at follicular growth and ovulation occur over weeks or months before actual ovulation. Moreover, when breastfeeding ceases, the first ovulation often antedates the first vaginal bleed. The cervical mucus pattern at this time is not always sufficient to help the woman distinguish false alarms from genuine ovulation. If artificial contraception is acceptable to her, she will simply have to begin to use it from the very first mucus sign of ovarian follicular activity.

For those who wish to continue the natural methods, workers in Birmingham have found that marked changes in the cervix (i.e. softening in consistency, widening of the external os and elevation of position) occur only in the days immediately preceding the first true ovulation. The reliability of the cervix as an additional indicator at this time requires further testing (*see Q 2.5*).

There are similar problems in identifying the infrequent, yet still possibly fertile, ovulations of women approaching the menopause. *See Q 11.34.*

2.37 Can breastfeeding (lactational amenorrhoea method, LAM) alone be a satisfactory method?

Very much so, and no method could be more natural. A consensus statement from a conference in Bellagio, Italy, is summarized in *Fig. 2.4*. If all three facts apply – amenorrhoea since the lochia ceased, baby not yet 6 months old, and total breastfeeding (or very nearly so) – the risk of conception by 6 months is only 2%. This compares favourably with other accepted methods of birth control. Hence, it can be presented just like any other method to a woman – provided there is the usual caveat that she is never promised that she will not be one of those 2% for whom the method fails. Other considerations are:

■ Given that intentions to fully breastfeed may not be achievable – for even greater efficacy and peace of mind, many women will prefer to use the progestogen-only pill in addition to their breastfeeding (*see Qs 7.53, 7.54*).

■ Beware that there are several drugs that may be prescribed to the mother (e.g. lithium) which contraindicate breastfeeding and therefore

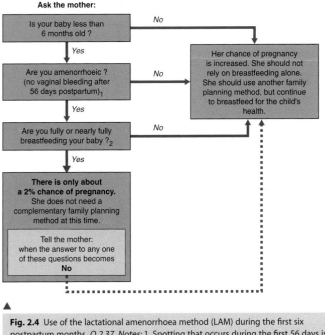

Ask the mother:

Is your baby less than 6 months old ? — *No*

Her chance of pregnancy is increased. She should not rely on breastfeeding alone. She should use another family planning method, but continue to breastfeed for the child's health.

Yes

Are you amenorrhoeic ? (no vaginal bleeding after 56 days postpartum)₁ — *No*

Yes

Are you fully or nearly fully breastfeeding your baby ?₂ — *No*

Yes

There is only about a 2% chance of pregnancy. She does not need a complementary family planning method at this time.

Tell the mother: when the answer to any one of these questions becomes **No**

▲

Fig. 2.4 Use of the lactational amenorrhoea method (LAM) during the first six postpartum months. *Q 2.37. Notes:* 1. Spotting that occurs during the first 56 days is not considered to be menses. 2. 'Nearly full' breastfeeding means (WHO definition) that *very* occasional liquid or food is given but more than three-fourths of all feeds are breast milk.

also the LAM method. A full list of these is in Appendix 5 of the current *British National Formulary* (www.bnf.org).

THE (NEAR) FUTURE

2.38 **What of the future? Are there any developments that could make fertility awareness methods more acceptable?**

Most of these are suggested in *Fig. 2.2*. One (Persona) has already arrived in the UK.

- *Ultrasound*: ultimately, the relative price of ultrasound machines might fall so low, and their user-friendliness increase to such a degree, that women could simply plug them in to their monitors. Follicular growth, rupture and corpus luteum formation could then be used as direct indicators of fertility, by the woman and her partner themselves!

■ *Home kits*: more realistically, a number of new home kits are being devised based on the cyclic changes in the hormones of the menstrual cycle, or their metabolites and other substances in body fluids. The most useful fluids are urine, saliva and breast milk; but biochemical changes in the mucus are also being studied.

■ *Other approaches*:

– *Standard Days Method* [Arevalo et al 2000 *Contraception* 60:357–360]: this is the calendar method reinvented for simplicity, using a ring of beads with different colours, one bead for each day of the cycle. Days 8–19 inclusive are those signalled for 'no unprotected sex'. Proponents claim that although no adjustments are made for cycles shorter or longer than 28 days (*see Q 2.19*) this is balanced by easier compliance. Hence this method should be as effective as calendar calculations would be in typical use: i.e. both would be expected, in any *typical* population, to have similarly higher failure rates than 'perfect users' would have (i.e. higher than the 1-year 'perfect use' failure rate reported as around 9 per 100 users, *Table 1.2*). This method should not be used by women who record two cycles outside the range of 26–32 days in any 1 year.

– The *Rovumeter*: this device simply measures the daily amount of cervicovaginal fluid aspirated from the posterior vaginal fornix by the woman into a sterile, disposable, calibrated, plastic aspirator. Volume changes are more objective than the usual mucus awareness approach, and can apparently be used for family planning purposes.

– New possibilities might arise by serendipity, such as occurred at King's College Medical School, London, where researchers studying Raynaud's phenomenon found that normal women (as well as those with Raynaud's) gave different measurements at different phases of their menstrual cycle. It appears that estrogen tends to increase the reactivity of the arteries of the hand and that progesterone tends to relax the vessels, producing a localized increase in blood volume. Appropriate daily measurements in the hand could – in theory – therefore be used both to predict and to detect the woman's fertile period. No device for possible home use has yet appeared, however.

Male methods of contraception

3

THE CONDOM: ADVANTAGES AND INDICATIONS

THE CONDOM: PROBLEMS AND DISADVANTAGES

THE CONDOM: PRESENT AND FUTURE DESIGNS

QUESTIONS FREQUENTLY ASKED BY USERS

PQ PATIENT QUESTIONS

COITUS INTERRUPTUS

3.1   What is coitus interruptus?

This is well described by its most common euphemism: 'withdrawal' (in time, before ejaculation, ensuring that all sperm are deposited outside the vagina). There are many other terms, notably 'being careful' and also local idioms such as 'getting off at Fratton instead of going through to Portsmouth' (used in Hampshire, but with many regional equivalents!). These have often misled interviewers into thinking that no contraceptive method is being used.

3.2   What is the history of the method? How is it viewed by religious groups?

Coitus interruptus is doubtless the earliest form of birth control. It is mentioned in Genesis, the only explicit mention of contraception in the Bible:

Then Judah said to Er's brother Onan, 'Go and sleep with your brother's widow. Fulfil your obligation to her as her husband's brother, so that your brother may have descendants.' But Onan knew that the children would not belong to him, so whenever he had intercourse with his brother's widow he let the semen spill on the ground, so that there would be no children for his brother. What he did displeased the Lord and the Lord killed him also. (Genesis 38:8–10)

Although this text is used to endorse the Vatican view that withdrawal is itself sinful, and by extension that other 'artificial' methods that prevent the sperm meeting the egg are also wrong, according to most commentators the sin was not in the method at all; it was Onan's failure to comply with the Levirate Law and perform his family duty that was sinful. (Even so, the penalty seems unbelievably excessive to modern eyes.)

Although Islamic societies and numerous Imams are often pronatalist, there are exceptions. The Koran describes a liberal attitude to withdrawal and, again, by inference, to other methods of contraception. In the *Tradition of the Prophet* we find:

A man said, 'O Prophet of God! I have a slave girl and I practise coitus interruptus with her. I dislike her becoming pregnant, yet I have the desires of men. The Jews believe that coitus interruptus constitutes killing a life in miniature form.' The Prophet (Mohammed) replied, 'The Jews are liars. If God wishes to create it, you can never change it.'

Iran is an Islamic country whose Shi-ite religious scholars have revisited the issue of contraception since the late 1980s. They then issued a number of *fatawa* which endorse any kind of contraception acting pre-fertilization (*see Qs 10.3, 10.4*), including withdrawal. Iran halved its total fertility rate – TFR, or 'average family size' – in 8 years, a success story for voluntary family planning.

Right up to the second half of the twentieth century, withdrawal remained a major and often the primary method of contraception. As late as 1947 the Royal Commission on Population in England found that amongst recently married couples with contraceptive experience, 43% used withdrawal as the sole method of birth control, the proportion rising to 65% in the lowest social class. Studies in developing countries showed its use, at least on some occasions, by more than half of all couples in Jamaica, Puerto Rico and Hungary in the 1960s.

3.3 What is the effectiveness of coitus interruptus?

High failure rates alleged by early family planners have been quoted and re-quoted by subsequent generations of writers. Yet the evidence contradicts that view. In 1949 the Royal Commission (see above) reported that:

No difference has been found between users of appliance and users of non-appliance methods as regards the average number of children.

Withdrawal was by far the most popular of the non-appliance methods and the pregnancy rate was found to be a creditable 8/100 woman-years of exposure. A study in Indianapolis revealed a Pearl failure rate of only 10, compared with an average rate of 12 for all other methods, and amongst high-income couples the rate was precisely the same as for the diaphragm.

Some older readers of this book may have met, as I have, couples with two well-spaced children both in their teens who claim that withdrawal has been their regular and sole method. So it obviously works for some.

3.4 What are the advantages of coitus interruptus?

Chiefly, that the method is free of charge, requires no prescription, is always available and cannot be left at home when the couple go on holiday. Moreover, it does not cause nausea or weight gain! Its use has been associated with some of the lowest birth rates in history, for example in Eastern Europe after the Second World War. It is obviously acceptable to many users.

3.5 What are the disadvantages?

Obviously, intercourse is incomplete, and many do find the method very unsatisfying to both partners. Yet no significant adverse effects have ever been demonstrated among those who do choose to use it. It seems to be assumed without discussion that there would be an inevitable lack of satisfaction of the woman, compounded by anxiety that her partner would not withdraw 'in time'. Psychological problems are assumed to follow. Yet in a survey of nearly 2000 British women questioned in 1967–68, only 31% of 311 who had discontinued use of the method did so because they found it unpleasant, and only 4% because they believed it harmful to health. By contrast, 54% of 381 former condom-users gave up the method because they found it unpleasant to use.

Even among those professionally engaged in family planning, withdrawal is unjustifiably overlooked, condemned or ridiculed. Marie Stopes stated that it was 'harmful to the nerves as well as unsafe'.

3.6   Why has the method been so neglected?

One reason, perhaps, is that it has no manufacturers to advertise its virtues. Also, because it has the reputation of being unsatisfying and ineffective, there is a feeling that it should certainly not be promoted. But it is unfortunate that many unplanned pregnancies among young people having intercourse unexpectedly are probably caused by the conventional teaching of doctors and nurses. Withdrawal is often not even attempted when it might have been, because the message that it is 'ineffective' has been so well conveyed. We must remember the old slogan of the twentieth century birth control pioneers:

Any method of family planning is better than no method, though some methods are better than others.

While encouraging the use of more modern methods, we should remember that – for many – this one works, and that it is a very great deal better than nothing 'in an emergency'.

3.7   Aren't there sperm in the pre-ejaculate?

Yes there are, sometimes. In 1931 Abraham Stone asked several medical friends to examine preorgasmic secretions for sperm. He finally collected 24 slides from 18 individuals. Two showed many sperm, two contained few, and one an occasional sperm. Stone correctly reported that the figures were 'insignificant for a definite conclusion'. The chances of such sperm causing fertilization must be low, although definitely not negligible (*see* Q 2.9).

A much more probable cause of failure results from the partial ejaculation of a larger quantity of semen which can occur a short while before the final male orgasm; or withdrawal during the latter rather than before it starts. Hence the suggestion for those who want to continue using the method that they might use a spermicide as well (*see* Qs 3.9, 3.18).

3.8   Should a couple always be discouraged from using coitus interruptus?

The answer has to be 'no'. We must remember the basic teaching of psychosexual medicine, that there are innumerable methods of giving and receiving sexual pleasure, which couples should feel free to devise for themselves. Why should they not be able to choose to use coitus interruptus, possibly along with oral sex and other forms of mutual pleasuring (most of which carry no conception risk), if that is their agreed choice and provides for them a mutually sexually satisfying life?

3.9 How do you counsel couples who volunteer that coitus interruptus is their usual method?

Clearly, other options should always be discussed. If, however, a couple finds all alternatives unacceptable, then I always just offer as an option the additional use of spermicide (a pessary, or contraceptive sponge if available). This should cope satisfactorily with any small deposit of sperm before withdrawal (but *see also Q 3.18*), though the couple should be warned it is likely to be inadequate to deal reliably with the whole ejaculate in fertile couples.

3.10 Your conclusion?

I end this section like Malcolm Potts (to whom I am indebted for much of this section), who, with Peter Diggory, wrote in his 1983 book *Textbook of Contraception Practice*:

Coitus interruptus is like . . . a buffalo cart; there are better methods of transport and better methods of contraception, but for a great many people it represents a practical solution to an everyday problem.

THE CONDOM: BACKGROUND AND MECHANISM

3.11 What is the male sheath/condom?

A condom is a closed-ended, expansile, tubular device designed to cover the erect penis and physically prevent the transmission of semen into the vagina. It is traditionally made of vulcanized latex rubber, which is as thin as possible while maintaining adequate strength, and often lubricated to minimize 'loss of sensitivity' during intercourse – which is perhaps the method's chief disadvantage. It is also a method for use by (often) the less well-motivated of the two partners: hence the renewed interest in female-controlled condoms, as well as more effective spermicide/virucides (*see Qs 4.55–4.58, 4.61*).

3.12 What is the method's history?

This apparently dates back to Roman times, when animal bladders were used, chiefly to prevent the spread of sexually transmitted disease. In folklore, the invention was much later, by Dr Condom, reputedly a physician at the court of Charles II. However, it is doubtful whether Dr C. even existed. Much more probably, the word 'condom' was derived from the Latin (*condus*: a receptacle), as a euphemism for an item already well known. The earliest published description is that of the Italian anatomist

Gabriel Fallopio, who in 1564 recommended a linen sheath moistened with lotion – again in order to protect against venereal infection. Only in the eighteenth century do we find condoms described specifically to prevent pregnancy. Condoms were then made from the caeca of sheep or other animals. Similar 'skin condoms' are still available, at a high price through the internet (http://www.shopinprivate.com/trojnatlamco.html), but they are *not recommended* for safer sex as they may fail to prevent virus transmission.

It was the process of vulcanization of rubber, first carried out by Hancock and Goodyear in 1844, that revolutionized the world's contraception, as well as its transport.

3.13 How acceptable and how frequently used is the condom method?

About 44 million couples used the condom worldwide in 2003 (UN estimate) but with striking geographical differences. Japan accounts for more than a quarter of all condom-users in the world. Seventy-five per cent of couples who use any contraceptive in that country use this method, generally purchased by the woman, and there has not been a major shift in usage since the (very late!) arrival in that country of 'the pill' in 1999. By contrast, and despite the massive problem of HIV/AIDS, use of condoms remains low in Africa, the Middle East and Latin America.

It was calculated in 2003 that if world condom usage for safer sex were at the appropriate level to control the HIV/AIDS epidemic, 24 000 million should be used each year; yet the estimated figure for condoms distributed that year was less than 10 000 million.

3.14 What is the acceptability and usage of the condom in the UK?

For many, 'spoilt' by modern non-intercourse-related alternatives, it must be admitted the method remains completely unacceptable for sustained use. There is an undeniable change of sensations reported, especially by men, although this sometimes has the benefit of prolonging intercourse.

In most recent surveys, approaching 20% of all couples use the condom. Estimates are always approximate because many couples use the condom as an occasional alternative to, or in addition with, other methods, but it continues to be the second most prevalent method within each 10-year cohort, during the reproductive years.

'Double Dutch', the shorthand phrase for using the condom to reduce infection risk at the same time as another more effective contraceptive, is believed to be increasing in prevalence: but to nowhere near the levels that would be appropriate to the epidemic of sexually transmitted infections (STIs) in general and *Chlamydia* in particular. . . .

3.15 How can the image of the condom as a method be improved?

In the past, condoms had a very poor image. AIDS has changed all that – or has it? There are still widespread misconceptions about efficacy and reduced sensitivity. For centuries, condoms were associated with prostitution and extramarital intercourse. Even today, as he purchases his condoms a married man might sense that the retailer assumes they surely cannot be for intercourse with his wife. Removal of this unfortunate image is unlikely as long as the media maintains double standards: there is widespread portrayal of intercourse on television, for example, yet it is still perceived as against morality or good taste to mention a condom in the storyline, leave alone actually to show the item on screen, in a matter-of-fact way.

THE CONDOM: EFFECTIVENESS

3.16 How effective is the condom method?

'Perfect use' method-failure rates can be less than 2 pregnancies/100 couple-years. These are based on selected populations where there has been no sexual contact whatever without the rubber intervening, the only failures being caused by condoms bursting due to a manufacturing defect (some bursts and most cases of condoms slipping off are user errors, see Q 3.20). As successful use depends so very much on the motivation and care taken by the couple, failure rates do vary widely: from a low of 0.4/100 woman-years in the north of England in 1973 to a high of no less than 32/100 woman-years in Puerto Rico in 1961. A large population-based US study of 'single' women in the 1980s documented between 8 and 11 failures per 100 woman-years. In four UK studies, the range was more relevant to the careful user, between 3.1 and 4.8/100 woman-years.

As usual, failures are more frequent with the young and inexperienced, and among couples who wish to delay rather than prevent pregnancy. Among such, average use leads to at least 10% conceptions in the course of 1 year: a one in ten chance (and we do such couples a disservice if this information is withheld from them). Older couples use the method better, perhaps because of diminished fertility and (though not always!) a lower frequency of intercourse, as well as more careful use. For example, in the Oxford/FPA study, a pregnancy rate of only 0.7/100 couple-years was reported among women aged 35 and older, as compared with a rate of 3.6/100 couple-years for women aged 25–34 (in both cases the partner having been before recruitment a condom-user for more than 4 years).

3.17 Why are so many men so bad at using condoms (at all, or well)?

Clearly, it has a lot to do with themselves not getting pregnant! A report from two university campuses in Georgia (published in the

Journal of the American Medical Association 1997;278:291–292) just about says it all:

Among 98 male students aged 18–29 (mean age 22.4 years) who participated in a standardized interview about their use of condoms, 50% reported ever experiencing condom breakage.

Among these 49 men, 15 (30%) had at some time failed to disclose knowledge of a broken condom to their female sex partner, nine of them many times! Overall, 13.2% of condom breakage episodes were never revealed to the partners! The reasons given were (*N* = number of individuals out of the 15):

- unwillingness to interrupt intercourse because orgasm was approaching (*N* = 6)
- wanting to avoid being blamed for the break (*N* = 5)
- desire to minimize anxiety of the partner about the break (*N* = 4).

I was quite speechless when I first learned of this study. Its implications, for example for emergency contraception, are devastating!

3.18 How important is the additional use of spermicide to condom-effectiveness?

Theoretically, this should increase contraceptive protection, but it has never been proved to do so. As the pregnancy rate among consistent users is already very low, it would require an enormous study to prove an extra degree of protection – a study that will never be done.

More importantly, the only such additional spermicide currently available in the UK is nonoxinol-9. This is an irritant to the vaginal mucosa (lesions have been shown colposcopically) and now a number of studies show that it increases rather than diminishes HIV transmission (*see Q 4.67* for the implications for female methods of contraception).

> The most common spermicide (nonoxinol-9 or nonoxinol-11) causes damage to the vaginal epithelium in very frequent use. This affects recommendations about virus transmission prevention but not those about routine contraception (*see Q 4.67*).

3.19 Are spermicidally lubricated condoms therefore yesterday's products?

Yes, indeed there are strong recommendations by WHO and other bodies to have nonoxinol-9 (N-9)-lubricated condoms removed from the market, along with N-9 vaginal lubricants (*see Q 4.67*). We badly need substitutes for this, ideally usable as regular microbicides as well as spermicides.

3.20 What common errors in condom use can result in pregnancy?

Particularly when the combined oral contraceptive (COC) has to be stopped after many years, and condoms are used as an alternative, most couples have no idea just how 'dangerous' a fluid semen will now become. It is important to stress that the 4–5 mL of an average man's ejaculate can easily contain 300 or 400 million sperm, and hence a minute proportion of this volume from a fertile man might cause a pregnancy. Common unrecognized errors include:

- ■ *Genital contact*: the condom is put on just before ejaculation – but often not in time to catch the first fraction of sperm.
- ■ *Loss of erection*: perhaps due to overexcitement or anxiety, so the condom slips off unnoticed before ejaculation. Another cause of slippage is mentioned in *Q 3.22*.
- ■ *Leakage on withdrawal*: when the penis is flaccid.
- ■ *Later genital contact*: with sperm already on the glans and in the urethra of the penis (from earlier intercourse) before a new condom is applied.
- ■ *Damage to the condom* (*see Q 3.21*).

3.21 What can cause condom breakage, aside from manufacturing defects?

- ■ *Mechanical damage*: e.g. by sharp fingernails, especially during attempts to force it on the wrong way, which result in rolling it up tighter rather than unrolling it (an easy mistake when excited!).
- ■ *Chemical action*: it is still not widely enough known that vegetable and mineral oil-based lubricants, and the bases for many prescribable vaginal products, can seriously damage and lead to rupture of rubber. Baby oil, for example, often suggested as part of sex play, destroys over 90% of a condom's strength after only 15 min of contact . . . a well-named substance, Baby oil! There are many common vaginal preparations that should be regarded as unsafe to use with condoms and diaphragms, and there might be others (*Table 3.1*). Here is a definite advantage of plastic condoms.

3.22 What instructions should be given to couples planning to use rubber male condoms?

- ■ *Use only good-quality condoms.*
- ■ *Avoid any chemical or physical damage*: do not use oil-based lubricants such as Vaseline or Baby oil. It is safest to avoid contact with all oily suntan lotions, but water-based and silicone lubricants are safe. Use jelly such as KY or Sensilube (*see Q 3.21*). Plastic condoms are unaffected by chemicals.
- ■ *Put the condom on the penis before any genital contact whatever*: if there is no teat, make room for the semen by pinching the end of the condom as it is applied. (Otherwise there is the theoretical risk of semen tracking

TABLE 3.1 Vaginal and rectal preparations that should be regarded as unsafe to use with latex condoms or diaphragms (but plastic appliances unaffected)

Arachis oil enema	Gyno-Pevaryl* (Pevaryl)
Baby oil	Nizoral ?OK
Canesten*/Clotrimazole*	Nystan cream*
Cyclogest*	Ortho-Gynest* (Ovestin ?OK)
Dalacin cream*	Petroleum jelly (Vaseline)
E45 (and similar)	Premarin cream ?OK
Ecostatin*	Witepsol-based products
Gyno-Daktarin*	

Note: Some suntan oils and creams, bath oils and massage oils are similarly not 'latex-condom-friendly'. But water-based products such as KY Jelly, also ethylene glycol, glycerol and silicones are not suspect.
*According to the BNF (March 2008).
?OK means caution, as the BNF states 'effect on latex . . . not yet known'.

up the shaft of the penis and either escaping or causing the condom to slip off.)

■ *After intercourse, withdraw the penis before it becomes too soft*: holding the base of the condom during withdrawal and taking care not to spill any semen.

■ *Use each condom once only*: inspect it for damage/possible leaks before disposal.

■ Most importantly, if the condom ruptures or slips off, on any potentially fertile day, obtain emergency (postcoital) contraception (*see Chapter 10*).

THE CONDOM: ADVANTAGES AND INDICATIONS

3.23 What are the advantages of the condom method?

The advantages are many:

■ Easily obtainable, relatively cheap or free from NHS clinics.
■ Free from medical risks.
■ Highly effective if used consistently and correctly.
■ No medical supervision required.
■ Protects against most STIs, including viruses.
■ Evidence of protection against cervical neoplasia and invasive carcinoma.
■ Offers visible proof of use (particularly to the woman, who has the greatest motivation to avoid pregnancy).

■ Involves the male in sharing contraceptive responsibility, although with some men this can be a definite disadvantage.

■ Can sometimes increase the woman's pleasure by prolonging intercourse.

■ Minimizes post-intercourse odour and messiness of vaginal semen, for those who perceive these as problems.

3.24 In what situations can the condom be particularly indicated?

■ Where couples are unable or unwilling to make use of formal family planning services.

■ During short-term contraception (e.g. while waiting to start oral contraceptives).

■ Where intercourse takes place only infrequently and unpredictably.

■ For protection against STIs, notably HIV.

■ With the agreement of the man (although this is not always obtainable) for the prevention of cervical neoplasia, particularly when this has already been treated (*see Q 3.26*).

The last two bulleted items are indications that might apply even if the main birth control method being used is an IUD, a hormone or sterilization (of either sex).

3.25 Against which STIs does the condom provide protection?

A major benefit from the woman's point of view is the reduced risk of upper genital tract disease (pelvic infection, with its serious threat to her future fertility). Consistent use of condoms is protective against gonorrhoea and *Trichomonas vaginalis*, the spirochaete of syphilis, *Chlamydia* and similar bacterial and protozoal organisms. It obviously provides little or no protection against infestations such as scabies and lice.

Most importantly, the rubber or plastic can provide a useful barrier – when intact – to viruses, including HIV, the far more infectious hepatitis viruses, herpes simplex types I and II and human papillomavirus (HPV).

Whereas fertilization is possible only during about 8 days per cycle, viruses can be transferred at any time. As we have seen, condom conceptions are not uncommon. So the method can only provide relative protection ('safer sex'). Bilateral (two-sided) monogamy has much going for it! (see my book for women, *The Pill* – details in Further Reading).

3.26 What evidence is there that the condom can be protective or even therapeutic against cervical cell abnormalities?

In a UK case–control study, the relative risk of developing severe cervical dysplasia decreased with duration of condom or diaphragm use, whereas it increased with duration of oral contraceptive (OC) use. After 10 years, the relative risk for women using any barrier method was 0.2, compared to 4.0 for the pill-users. Many other studies confirm their protective effect.

In a US study, as many as 136 out of 139 women with cervical cell abnormalities who received no treatment apart from their partners adopting use of the condom showed complete reversal of the condition. Unfortunately, there was no control group, and the findings need confirmation.

THE CONDOM: PROBLEMS AND DISADVANTAGES

3.27 What are the possible disadvantages of the method?

There are few, really, but they are enough to put many people off:

- Use is coitus-related and interrupts the spontaneity of intercourse.
- Decreased 'sensitivity', especially for the male (although this is now much less with modern products).
- Not uncommonly, especially in older men, the short time it takes to don the condom is enough for them to lose their erection sufficiently for penetration to fail. Failure can then lead to a vicious cycle of 'performance anxiety' and the outcome of a regular self-fulfilling prophecy of failure. In one case of my own, in his early 60s with a partner in her 30s for whom hormonal methods were contraindicated, the answer proved to be sildenafil (Viagra) to enhance erection and so enable this chosen contraceptive to be successfully used. These could be highly appropriate grounds, sometimes, for prescribing such phosphodiesterase-5 inhibitors (though not on the NHS).
- Perceived as acting as a barrier in psychological as well as physical terms.
- Perceived to be messy, rubber has a distinctive odour that is hard to mask (an advantage of plastic).
- They can slip off or rupture.
- Few users appreciate how small any leaks of semen can be, that cause a pregnancy (*see* Q 2.7).
- A high degree of motivation and extremely meticulous use are required for long-term avoidance of pregnancy; these characteristics are in fact possessed by a few men!

3.28 What are the medical unwanted effects of the condom?

Very few: it is difficult to imagine how death might occur – inhalation perhaps? . . .

- *Allergy*: some 'allergies' (in both sexes) are excuses, not real. But irritation is not uncommon and true allergy to residues left in the rubber after the manufacturing processes does exist. This is less of a problem with modern rubbers and there are special 'allergy' brands marketed, but the best solution is generally to transfer to a plastic condom (*see Q 3.32*).

■ The method obviously fails to protect against disorders linked to the normal/abnormal menstrual cycle, such as menorrhagia, premenstrual syndrome, functional ovarian cysts, endometriosis, and carcinoma of the ovary and endometrium. These can therefore be described not so much as side-effects of the condom, but more as 'side-effects of not using the pill' (*see Q 5.57*).

3.29 How can the disadvantages be minimized?

By using ultrathin and lubricated condoms, innovative materials, colours, scents, textures and shapes, and perhaps by involving the female more in the selection of specific brands and in their actual use. For example, if a condom (whether or not brightly coloured or ribbed) is applied by the woman as part of foreplay, this can counter the 'interruption' disadvantage, and even heighten eroticism. Or a female condom could be tried, say once a week, for variety. . . .

THE CONDOM: PRESENT AND FUTURE DESIGNS

3.30 Are there any condoms that are not recommended?

So-called American Tips, which are designed to fit only over the glans penis, have a bad reputation for slipping off during use. Also not approved are some 'fun' condoms available from sex shops, which do not conform to BSI kitemark specifications.

3.31 How are rubber condoms manufactured?

In a highly automated process, condom-shaped metal or glass moulds are dipped into latex solution, from where they pass to a drying oven. After a second immersion in latex, the moulds pass into another heated air chamber for drying and vulcanization. The finished product is usually rolled off the mould by nylon brushes and then subjected to quality control testing. Each of the millions produced is tested electronically for pinholes; and samples are put through a water test for holes and also now an air inflation test to bursting point. The international standard (ISO 4074) permits only 7/200 samples to rupture after inflation with 15 L of air.

3.32 Does the future perhaps lie with plastic condoms?

Very likely, in my view. They have no smell and are good heat conductors, non-allergenic and unaffected by any chemicals in common use. One version, Avanti, has been on the UK market since 1966. It is well lubricated and ultrathin, which many men find preferable. But despite using polyurethane, a material with good intrinsic strength, its thinness means it is at least as likely as (and, in one US study, more likely than) a good rubber condom to rupture in use.

A new polyurethane product is now CE-marked and has been on the market since 1998 in the Netherlands and California: Ez-on. It is the first baggy or loose-fit male condom. It has a patented soft flange at the open end, with which it is 'pulled on like a sock' (either way, it is 'bidirectional', unlike all rubber condoms there is no wrong way to put it on) over the erect penis – which it then firmly but comfortably grasps at its base. Importantly, the loose fit ensures that the major part of the shaft and all the glans of the penis feel free within the well-lubricated sac. In its present version it has only moderate tensile strength, which is odd because there is no need for its walls to be especially thin. Quotes from some acceptability trials suggest that it allows more 'normal' sensations during penetrative intercourse for the male partner and has 'no disadvantages compared with rubber condoms' for the female. However, in our own study at the Margaret Pyke Centre, it ruptured at least as often as the other two condoms with which it was compared (Avanti and Durex Gossamer) although it was the 'preferred' type by one-third of participants. No specific efficacy data are yet available.

Clients can be informed that Ez-on condoms are available by mail order from the manufacturer, Mayer Laboratories, through the internet: http://www.mayerlabs.com/orders/detail.asp?PRODID=00306.

PQ PATIENT QUESTIONS

QUESTIONS FREQUENTLY ASKED BY USERS

3.33   My main problem with condoms is that I am afraid I will get less hard while I am putting one on.

You are unusual in actually voicing what is a very common fear. It could well stop being a problem as you get more used to it and with your partner's involvement (maybe putting it on for you) and her being relaxed, reassuring and laid-back about it.

One possibility if this is a big problem to you is to request a prescription for Viagra or Cialis or Levitra, which are taken ahead of sex and help maintain your erection. This might then enable your chosen method to be used, especially where this is the only acceptable method to you both (*see Q 3.27*). (This would have to be a private prescription.)

3.34 The condoms keep breaking – why is this?

There are several possible explanations (*see Q 3.21*). Are you allowing any oily chemicals to come into contact with them? Sometimes you or your partner could be causing damage with fingernails while it is being put on. Waiting until she is more aroused and lubricated before penetration might help, or the use of KY Jelly or other lubricant from the chemist (check it won't damage the rubber). Otherwise you could try a different brand, larger and/or thicker – discuss with your pharmacist.

Perhaps surprisingly, none of the available plastic condoms has been shown to be any better with respect to rupture than the strongest rubber ones.

3.35 Do I have to use a spermicide with the condom?

No – indeed WHO is opposed to the main one (nonoxinol-9) being used at all. It might do more harm than good (*see Qs 3.18, 3.19*). If a condom fails, it is much more relevant to arrange emergency contraception (*see Chapter 10*) than to rely on any amount of spermicide in the vagina.

3.36 Some condoms have ribs, bumps and so on – are these contraceptives safe?

If they are tested to the standards of the BSI or DIN (the German equivalent), the answer is 'yes'. Beware of those that are not so approved.

3.37 If a condom breaks or slips off, is there anything you can do to avoid a possible pregnancy?

Yes, make sure you obtain emergency contraception – preferably in the next 24 h, next best within 72 h, and certainly within the next 5 days (*see Chapter 10*). Most chemists stock the tablet (the 'morning-after pill'), at a price, but clinics and surgeries should supply it free and also advise about whether the copper IUD might be better (*see Q 10.33*).

3.38 My partner gets very itchy and red, OR, I seem to be developing a rash every time we use the condom – could this be allergy and what can we do about it?

It is best for a doctor to examine your partner's vagina, OR, if you have the problem, your penis – in case, for example, the symptoms are being caused by something else, such as the infection called thrush (*Candida*).

If you are using a spermicidally lubricated condom, you could try one without the spermicide. Otherwise the best bet now would be plastic condoms such as Avanti or Ez-on (*see Q 3.32*).

3.39 Do condoms have a shelf-life?

Yes – it is usually stated to be a long one, of about 5 years, but it is important to realize that rubber condoms can deteriorate more rapidly in abnormal conditions, such as in the tropics – and anywhere if exposed to strong ultraviolet light (*see Q 3.21*).

3.40   Can I use the condom more than once?

This is not recommended – it was feasible with the old-style reusable types.

3.41   Why can't you get condoms free from your family doctor?

Why indeed? This is an excellent method of contraception and infection-protection that, in my view, should certainly be available from all GPs, as it is from clinics. Some surgeries do offer supplies, so it is well worth asking.

3.42   Can you throw a condom away down the toilet?

From the environmental point of view, it is better to wrap it in tissue and use a dustbin.

3.43   My partner feels very dry – is there a lubricant you can safely use with the condom?

Sometimes, dryness indicates a psychosexual problem you might need to address together, perhaps with help from a therapist (see websites p. 550).

3.44   I tend to put the condom on just before I 'come' – is this OK?

No! You are not alone in doing this, but it is probably the commonest reason that intact condoms 'fail'. *See Qs 2.6–2.9 and 3.7.*

Vaginal methods of contraception

4

THE (NEAR) FUTURE IN VAGINAL CONTRACEPTION

QUESTIONS ASKED BY USERS ABOUT VAGINAL CONTRACEPTION

PQ PATIENT QUESTIONS

OCCLUSIVE CAPS

4.1 Why should we try to avoid the terms 'female or vaginal barriers'?

Although these are convenient, ideally I wish we could find better terms to use. They should preferably be avoided in discussions with prospective users because sexual intercourse has to do with closeness, and one can reinforce wrong feelings and fantasies about the method being a 'barrier'.

4.2 What terminology will you be using? What types are available?

To avoid confusion, I will use the term 'occlusive caps' for all the standard female barriers. This has two subgroups, namely diaphragms and caps. The latter are either cervical or vault caps, with the vimule being here considered as a modified vault cap (*Fig. 4.1*). FemCap, a silicone cervical cap, is now also on the NHS Drug Tariff.

NB: Due to a sudden major shake-up in the market from Oct 2007 onwards all the non-diaphragm products (i.e. 'caps') – save one cervical cap (FemCap) – will cease to be available in the UK. They may remain on some clinic shelves for a while, so the text below in Q 4.27ff about vault caps and vimules is not yet entirely of historical interest – though it

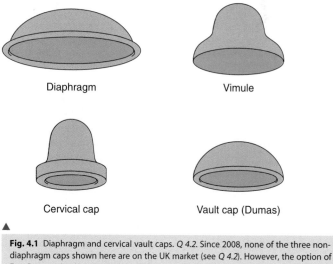

Diaphragm

Vimule

Cervical cap

Vault cap (Dumas)

▲

Fig. 4.1 Diaphragm and cervical vault caps. *Q 4.2.* Since 2008, none of the three non-diaphragm caps shown here are on the UK market (see *Q 4.2*). However, the option of FemCap remains (see *Q 4.76*).

probably soon will be. Fortunately, the great majority of users of this method in the past have opted for one of the diaphragms and it is understood that these, including the useful arcing type, will continue to be available.

4.3 What is the method's history?

It is a very ancient method, with descriptions dating back to 1850 BC; the Petri papyrus describes a spermicidal pessary made partly of crocodile dung. A section of the Talmud from the second century AD recommended a moistened sponge in the vagina before coitus. Rubber occlusive pessaries did not appear until the nineteenth century, in Germany, and the first diaphragm was popularized by Mensinga, the pseudonym of a German physician, Dr C. Hasse. The development of vulcanized rubber enabled him to produce a thinner and more pliable device, incorporating a flat watch spring in the rim. It became known as the Dutch cap because of the publicity given to it by the Dutch neo-Malthusians.

The occlusive pessary was referred to in the famous manual *The Wife's Handbook*, published in 1887; for mentioning it, the author – Arthur Allbutt – was struck off the British Medical Register. Because of this kind of opposition, occlusive pessaries became readily available only in the 1920s. Then, to quote Malcolm Potts, 'diaphragms and caps were to family planning what the steam locomotive was to transportation; they were the first in the field, brought emancipation to millions, and for a long time had no rivals'. Ultimately they were overtaken by a new technology; yet the methods have only two major problems: some lack of independence from intercourse and relative lack of effectiveness. If these could be overcome, there could be a large-scale return to vaginal methods.

4.4 How popular are vaginal methods worldwide?

The diaphragm reached the peak of its popularity around 1959, when it was reported that the method was used by about 12% of couples practising contraception in Britain. Usage declined rapidly with the advent of the pill, and now less than 1% of contracepting women use the method. In most developing countries, prevalence of use is too low to measure, and is likely to remain so unless vaginal 'barriers' are ever devised that do not require medical fitting or special training in use, do not pose storage and supply problems, and, above all, effectively prevent HIV transmission.

4.5 How important is medical attitude and training to the acceptability of vaginal methods?

Crucially, it has been well said that often the biggest 'barrier to the barriers' is the medical profession, and sometimes (although less so) the nursing profession. Many women introduced for the first time to the diaphragm at the age of 35–40 express surprise at its ease and convenience. They often complain that doctors and nurses had earlier damned the method with exceedingly faint praise.

This is a highly practical subject. The right attitude and skills can only be acquired by observing and being taught by unhurried and experienced professionals: in my experience, family planning trained nurses are usually best! (*see Qs 4.33–4.49*).

4.6 What is the mode of action of the diaphragm and cervical/vault caps?

The diaphragm lies diagonally across the cervix, the vaginal vault and much of the anterior vaginal wall. As the vagina is known to 'balloon' during intercourse (*see Q 2.3*), a sperm-tight fit between the diaphragm and the vaginal wall is impossible. On a theoretical basis, the main functions of the diaphragm are:

- acting as a carrier of the spermicide to the most important site, namely the external os, and preventing the spreading effect of intercourse (*see Q 2.3*)
- holding sperm away as a barrier from the receptive alkaline cervical mucus, long enough for them to die in the acid vagina
- preventing the mucus from entering the acid vagina and thereby providing a film within which the sperm can swim to the external os, and possibly
- preventing physical aspiration of sperm into the cervix and uterus.

Some authorities question the importance of the spermicide (*see Q. 4.7*).

Cervical/vault caps and FemCap are meant to stay in place by suction, which makes it possible that the barrier effect is more important to their contraceptive action than is the case with the diaphragm.

4.7 How important is the use of spermicide with occlusive caps?

This has been questioned, particularly in Australia, and especially for the cervical/vault caps, which act by suction. It is a fact that with no type of occlusive cap has there ever been a proper controlled trial. This should compare (preferably by random allocation) women who follow the full routine of instructions concerning the use of spermicide (*see Q 4.44*), in every detail, with women who use exactly the same method carefully and after the same fitting routine but without any spermicide at all. Such a study has been performed at the Margaret Pyke Centre and although the power of our study was not great enough to show statistical significance, the spermicide-using group did achieve better results. We do badly need better spermicides, however, without the tissue toxicity of nonoxinol-9 (*see Q 4.67*).

OCCLUSIVE CAPS: EFFECTIVENESS

4.8 How effective is the diaphragm?

See the Faculty of SRH Guidance *Female Barrier Methods* (www.fsrh.org) for an excellent review of these methods (106 references), including this issue of their efficacy.

Table 1.2 (p. 14) quotes a failure rate for the diaphragm with typical use of 16 and with consistent-and-correct use of 6 per 100 women after 1 year. Lower failure rates have been reported (*Table 4.1*) especially for older women, whose lowered fertility and heightened conscientiousness in regularly using the method efficiently are likely both to be important.

Professor Trussell of Princeton, NJ, has made a special study of contraceptive failure rates. The first-year pregnancy rates were much higher in parous women if they used the cervical cap (ranging up to over 25%, even with 'perfect use'!). Parous diaphragm 'perfect users' had similar rates to nulliparae, however, although still in the range of 4–8% in the first year. This, it should be noted, is an order of magnitude higher (less good) than the best rates obtainable by conscientious combined oral contraceptive (COC) use.

Table 4.1 relates the failure rates to an indicator of motivation recorded in the Oxford/FPA study, namely whether or not the woman considered her family to be complete. As clearly shown, the failure rate tended to be higher when the family was not felt to be complete, implying less careful use of the diaphragm when another baby would be acceptable (i.e. 'spacers').

4.9 Are the diaphragm failure rates of the Oxford/FPA study a good indication of the rates to be expected in routine family planning practice?

No.

TABLE 4.1 Diaphragm failure rates per 100 woman-years according to age, duration of use and completeness of family

Duration of use	Age 25–34			Age 35+		
	<2 years	2–4 years	>4 years	<2 years	2–4 years	>4 years
Family complete	6.1	3.5	2.3	2.1	1.6	0.7
Family not complete	5.3	4.3	2.4	4.5	2.0	1.3

Source: Oxford/FPA Study, 1982. Q 4.9

■ At recruitment, every woman was aged 25–39 years, married, a white British subject, and had to be already a current user of the diaphragm of at least 5 months' standing.

■ The women were basically 'middle class' and were probably unusually well motivated and careful.

■ Younger and more fertile women having intercourse more frequently must be expected to have a higher failure rate, even if the method were properly fitted and always used.

The most important factor is the recruitment in the Oxford/FPA study of established users only. By 5 months, the most fertile and least careful women, along with those with anatomical problems interfering with the effectiveness of the method, would not have been available for recruitment – by virtue of already becoming pregnant! All studies show the highest failure rates in the first few months of use. Even using the data of *Table 4.1*, faced with an 'Oxford/FPA-type' woman under 35 one can only quote a likely failure rate of around 5–6/100 woman-years for the first year of use. This is about the best to be expected, with a rate of around 10 expected for most young unmarried women of average motivation.

4.10   What failure rates can be given for cervical caps?

These are considered later (*see Qs 4.27–4.32*). Available effectiveness data are sparse, but Trussell's data in *Table 1.2* (p. 14) give a best estimate of 9% at 1 year of use for nulliparous 'perfect users'. This might possibly be acceptable for 'delayers' or 'spacers' of pregnancy. His quoted rate of 26% for parous women suggests to me that this is no longer a method to be recommended for most in that group of potential users. The failure rate for FemCap in consistent users (pre-marketing trial) was reported to be 10.5/100 woman-years.

4.11   In summary, what factors promote the effectiveness of the diaphragm and similar vaginal methods?

The following questions need to be asked:

■ Is she an established user or starting the method from scratch?

■ What is her age?

■ What is her frequency of intercourse?

■ What is her motivation for obsessionally careful and regular use? In particular, is she really trying to avoid a pregnancy or just to delay one?

■ Is she at all uncomfortable about handling her own genitalia? This important factor is not at all linked with intelligence.

■ Are there any anatomical problems on examination? (*see Qs 4.22, 4.30, 4.31, 4.35*).

■ During initial training, is she good at inserting the device and particularly at checking that the cervix is covered?

4.12 What common errors in the use of occlusive caps can result in pregnancy?

The most common is *failure to use* at all, on one or more occasions in the cycle of conception. Women often report minor errors in use of the spermicide. It is not at all clear how important these are, especially as they are frequently reported also in non-conception cycles.

During use, the most important error is failure to make a secondary check after insertion that the cervix is correctly covered.

Clinicians' errors include: wrong selection of users, poor fitting (with regard to size, choice of flat-, coil- or arcing-spring diaphragm or other cap) and poor teaching.

OCCLUSIVE CAPS: ADVANTAGES AND BENEFICIAL EFFECTS

4.13 What are the advantages of occlusive caps?

- Effective if used with care by older women, similar to those recruited in the study documented in *Table 4.1*.
- Much more independent of intercourse than the male condom (*see Q 4.14*).
- In general, neither partner suffers any loss of feeling.
- The method is under a woman's control and needs only to be used when required.
- Aesthetically useful for intercourse during light uterine bleeding but not for too long at a time (*see Qs 4.73, 4.83*).
- No proven systemic effects.
- Some definite non-contraceptive benefits (*see Q 4.15*).

4.14 Are occlusive caps necessarily intercourse-related methods?

No. In counselling, this is a most important point to explain. It is perfectly in order to insert any rubber or silicone barrier many hours ahead of intercourse. Beyond 3 h it is advisable to add extra spermicide before intercourse (*see Qs 4.44, 4.49*), but, certainly, not having to insert the cap itself just before sex helps compliance.

4.15 What are the beneficial medical effects?

- Protection against some sexually transmitted infections (STIs), including the agents causing pelvic inflammatory disease. However, though it remains entirely acceptable for use in appropriately selected diaphragm- or cap-users, in some circumstances the nonoxinol spermicide may *increase* the risk of HIV transmission (*see Q 4.67*).
- Reduction in the risk of cervical intraepithelial neoplasia (CIN; *see Q 4.17*).

4.16 How are occlusive caps protective against STIs?

In two ways:

- Partly by providing a mechanical barrier that reduces the chance of organisms reaching the cervix and upper genital tract. However, this will not fully protect against the viruses or non-viral diseases (e.g. syphilis) that can form lesions of the vagina or vulva.
- The associated spermicide is also relevant. Spermicides tend also to be 'germicides', though with respect to HIV transmission this potential benefit is unfortunately not realized, for a different (vaginal) reason (*see Qs 4.66, 4.67*).

4.17 What is the evidence for at least some protective effect against cervical neoplasia?

In the Oxford/FPA study, the rate per 100 woman-years for oral contraceptive (OC)-users was 0.95 and for intrauterine device (IUD)-users 0.87. For diaphragm-users, however, the rate was 0.23 after adjustment for age at first coitus, number of partners and smoking patterns. Another Oxford study showed a steady decline in the relative risk of severe cervical neoplasia for users of all types of barrier method, from 1 down to 0.2 after 10 years. This benefit is believed to be mainly because of reduced transmission of the oncogenic types of human papillomavirus (HPV). However, diaphragm-users might also be protected by their own sexual lifestyle and that of their partners.

OCCLUSIVE CAPS: MAIN PROBLEMS AND DISADVANTAGES

4.18 What are the disadvantages of occlusive caps?

- Although not necessarily coitus-related, they involve a woman handling her genitalia, some forward planning and a slight loss of spontaneity.
- Loss of cervical and some vaginal sensation (unnoticed by most).
- Can occasionally be felt in use by the woman's partner, although not by her if properly fitted.
- Require fitting by trained personnel and (except FemCap, *see Q 4.76*) a period of training in use, usually 1 week, during which another method must be used.
- Definitely less effective than hormonal contraception or the IUD, especially under age 35 (see *Table 4.1*).
- Perceived as being 'messy' due to the spermicide.
- Capable of producing some local adverse medical effects (*see Q 4.19*).

4.19 What are the possible adverse medical effects?

- Increased risk of urinary tract infections and symptoms. This problem seems to apply specifically to the (size of) diaphragm (*see Q 4.51*), and is not a problem of the caps.
- A small minority of women develop vaginal irritation and allergy due either to the rubber (not FemCap), or to the spermicide, or to a coincidental infection such as thrush.
- Pressure effects due to the rim of the occlusive cap itself, leading very rarely to vaginal abrasions or ulcers (*see Q 4.54*).

As a list of adverse effects, this is remarkably short. . . . But there are also a few unresolved safety issues, considered later (*see Qs 4.67–4.74*).

OCCLUSIVE CAPS: SELECTION OF USERS AND DEVICES

4.20 What are the conditions for the successful use of occlusive caps?

In the main, the answer depends on favourable answers to the questions about the woman herself, listed at *Q 4.11*. In addition, experience plus a positive attitude by the providers, ideally both a doctor and a nurse, are of paramount importance. Skilful fitting, knowledge of when to suggest a cervical/vault cap instead, and, above all, really satisfactory teaching of the woman, are vital factors.

4.21 What are the indications for use of occlusive caps?

- The woman's choice – usually an older woman, preferably monogamous (and at low risk of HIV), who might be less fertile through her age, but primarily if she can accept a possible conception due to the method failing.
- As an alternative to a medical method (hormones, IUDs) in return for getting rid of any side-effects she has with the medical method.
- For some, the need for contraception on an intermittent yet predictable basis.
- For protection against pelvic infection or recurrence of cervical neoplasia. This can be worth suggesting even if another method is in use as the main contraceptive. But *see Q 4.67* regarding spermicide use and the implications for HIV/AIDS.

4.22 What are the contraindications to the diaphragm, or a cap?

For many women, the most important item is the relatively high failure rate, which needs to be highlighted.

Otherwise these include:

■ Aversion to touching the genital area.
■ Congenital abnormalities such as a septate vagina.
■ Most forms of uterovaginal prolapse.
■ Inadequate retropubic ledge on examination – not a problem with cervical caps.
■ Poor vaginal or perineal muscle tone – cervical cap such as FemCap usable.
■ Inability to learn the insertion technique.
■ Lack of hygiene or privacy for insertion, removal and care of the cap.
■ Acute vaginitis – treat first.
■ Recurrent urinary infections – which often indicate a vault or cervical cap such as FemCap.
■ Past history of cap-induced vaginal trauma.
■ True allergy to rubber – use a silicone product.
■ Past history of toxic shock syndrome (TSS)? No link has been proved with diaphragms or caps. This is, however, a relevant consideration for contraceptive sponges (see *Table 4.2*, p. 90), which should not (pending more data) be in situ for more than 24 + 6 h.
■ *Virgo intacta* – condom use is commonly advised first, until the vagina is 'ready'. But well-motivated tampon-users can receive a small diaphragm, with refitting planned to follow after, say, 1 month's regular use.

4.23 What is the structure of a diaphragm?

This is the most commonly used occlusive cap. It consists of a thin latex rubber hemisphere, the rim of which is reinforced by a flexible flat or coiled metal spring (*Fig. 4.2*). The sizes, measuring the external diameter, range from 55 to 95 mm in steps of 5 mm.

4.24 What types of diaphragm are available?

■ *The flat-spring diaphragm*: has a firm watch spring and is easily fitted, remaining in the horizontal plane on compression. It is suitable for the normal vagina and is often tried first.
■ *The coil-spring diaphragm*: has a spiral coiled spring. This makes it softer than the flat-spring type.
■ *The arcing-spring diaphragm*: combines features of both the above and consists of a rubber dome with a firm double metal spring. It exerts strong pressure on the vaginal walls but its main characteristic is that when compressed it forms an arc, directing the posterior part of the diaphragm downwards and away from the cervix during insertion. This can be an advantage (*see Q 4.26*).

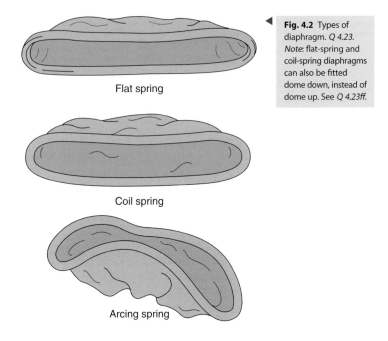

Flat spring

Coil spring

Arcing spring

◀ **Fig. 4.2** Types of diaphragm. *Q 4.23. Note*: flat-spring and coil-spring diaphragms can also be fitted dome down, instead of dome up. See *Q 4.23ff.*

The coil-spring and arcing-spring diaphragms are available in hypoallergenic silicone as well as rubber.

4.25 What are the indications for the coil-spring diaphragm?

Because it exerts slightly less pressure, it can be more comfortable for some women than the flat-spring type. The reduced pressure makes it seem to the woman about a half-size smaller than the equivalent flat-spring diaphragm.

4.26 For whom might the arcing-spring diaphragm be indicated?

This is the most widely used type of diaphragm in some countries. Some women find it more difficult to handle during insertion because of its non-horizontal shape when squeezed.

Its main positive indication is in cases where the length or direction of the cervix, or the woman's own technique, are resulting in a tendency to squeeze the diaphragm into the anterior fornix (*see Q 4.40 (7)*).

4.27 What types of cervical/vault caps are available?

NB: See here (and in relation to all *Qs 4.28–4.32* below), the important note at *Q 4.2* regarding UK availability. They are now mainly of historical interest.

■ *The cervical cap*: this is shaped like a thimble (see *Fig. 4.1*, p. 63) and is designed to fit snugly over the cervix. The most common variety is the cavity rim cap with an integral thickened rim incorporating a small groove. This is intended to increase suction to the sides of the cervix. The available internal diameters of the upper rim are 22, 25, 28 and 31 mm. *FemCap* is a silicone rubber cervical cap with a unique brim (see *Fig. 4.6*, p. 94).

■ *The vault or Dumas cap*: this rubber cap is shaped like a bowl with a thinner dome through which the cervix can be palpated. It covers, but does not fit closely to, the cervix. Five sizes (1–5) are available, ranging from 55 to 75 mm in 5-mm steps.

■ *The vimule*: this is a variation of the vault cap, with a hat-shaped prolongation of the dome to accommodate longer cervices. There are three sizes (1–3): small (45 mm), medium (48 mm) and large (51 mm).

4.28 What is the mode of action of cervical/vault caps?

They all operate by suction, not by spring tension like the diaphragm. Otherwise the mode of action – and the uncertainties about spermicides – are the same as for the diaphragm (*see Qs 4.6, 4.7*).

4.29 What indications and advantages do the cervical/vault caps share?

■ They share the advantages of the diaphragm but are in addition suitable for patients with poorer muscle tone and some cases of uterovaginal prolapse.

■ They are generally not felt by the male partner.

■ There is no reduction of vaginal sensation.

■ They are unlikely to produce urinary symptoms.

■ Fitting is unaffected by the changes in the size of the vagina, either during intercourse or as a result of changes in body weight.

4.30 What are the conditions necessary to fit a cervical cap?

■ The cervix must be easily felt.

■ The cervix must be healthy, not torn.

■ The cervix must ideally point down the axis of the vagina.

■ The cervix must be straight-sided.

4.31 What conditions are necessary for fitting a vault cap?

■ The cervix must be easily felt.

■ The cervix must be fairly short, although it can be quite bulky if it does not protrude too much into the vaginal vault.

4.32 In what circumstances would you recommend a trial of the FemCap or, if available, vault or vimule caps?

These can be useful where there are contraindications to the diaphragm (*see Q 4.22*), particularly absence of the retropubic ledge, poor muscle tone and a history of recurrent cystitis.

Where there is a free choice, I would recommend a trial of the vault cap or, for longer cervices, the FemCap (*see Q 4.76*). The vimule was never much used.

OCCLUSIVE CAPS: INITIAL FITTING, TRAINING AND FOLLOW-UP ARRANGEMENTS

4.33 What aspects are important in the initial counselling?

The factors in *Qs 4.9 and 4.11* should be explored very carefully with the woman, particularly determining that the method is socially and psychologically acceptable to her, and in particular that she will be a regular conscientious user. She must also, in fairness, be told that the method has a moderately high failure rate despite ideal fitting, even if she follows every detail of the instructions as for its use.

4.34 How is the fitting performed?

In a sensitive and unhurried way. The practical aspects cannot be learnt from books. Apprenticeship is necessary in two aspects: fitting technique and instruction of the woman.

4.35 What points are noted in the initial examination?

- The apparent health and direction of the uterus and cervix. Tenderness must be absent.
- The type of retropubic ledge. This can be more fully assessed with a practice diaphragm in position.
- Assessment of the vaginal musculature and tone, including the perineal muscles.
- If the diaphragm is chosen, the distance from the posterior fornix to the posterior aspect of the symphysis is measured, as shown in *Fig. 4.3*.

Cervical cytology and other screening procedures are performed according to local practice.

4.36 Successful fitting of the diaphragm – what are the steps?

1 The woman should have emptied her bladder and an initial choice of diaphragm to be used (only) for practice is made, based on the distance measured at the first examination (*Fig. 4.3*).

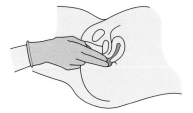

To measure for diaphragm size

Hold index and middle fingers together and insert into vagina up to the posterior fornix. Raise hand to bring surface of index finger to contact with pubic arch. Use tip of thumb to mark the point directly beneath the inferior margin of the pubic bone and withdraw fingers in this position.

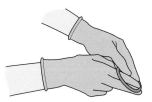

To determine diaphragm size

Place one end of rim of fitting diaphragm or ring on tip of middle finger. The opposite end should lie just in front of the thumb tip. This is the approximate diameter of the diaphragm needed.

▲

Fig. 4.3 Procedure for estimating the size of diaphragm to be tried. *Q 4.35* (reproduced courtesy of Janssen Cilag Pharmaceutical Ltd, Diaphragm Teaching Aid). See *Q 4.35ff.*

2 With the index finger inside the rim, compress the practice diaphragm between the thumb and remaining fingers. Separate the labia and insert the diaphragm downwards and backwards to the posterior fornix, tucking the anterior rim behind the symphysis pubis.

3 Check that the cervix is covered.

4 Insert a fingertip between the anterior rim of the cap and the symphysis:

(a) if the diaphragm is too small, a wider-than-fingertip gap will be felt, or the whole diaphragm might be found to be in the anterior fornix

(b) if the diaphragm is too large, it projects anteriorly/inferiorly and might cause immediate discomfort (or become uncomfortable or distorted later, after wearing).

4.37 Which way up should diaphragms be fitted?

Usually dome upwards. It is slightly easier to remove a flat-spring type if it is inserted dome upwards and the patient is instructed to hook her index finger under the anterior rim. However, this is a non-problem anyway if she simply uses both index and middle fingers to grasp the rim. The arcing diaphragm forms the correct shape (with its leading edge pointing downwards) readily if it is initially held dome upwards. This requires careful demonstration.

4.38 What are the important points when teaching the prospective user?

Generating confidence in the user is essential for success. A three-dimensional plastic model helps, but a short video is better still. Unless the doctor is a woman, a female nurse usually takes over at this stage (if she did not do the initial fitting). She must be very encouraging and able, without embarrassment on either side, and in secure privacy, to supervise closely all aspects of the learning process.

4.39 Successful teaching – how important is the position the woman should adopt?

This is crucial but often overlooked by the trainer. Unless instructed to the contrary, many women automatically adopt a half-standing, half-squatting position when inserting the diaphragm or when checking that it is correctly located over the cervix. This should be discouraged, as it makes it almost impossible for the fingers to reach the cervix. It might explain some 'cap failures', caused solely because the woman was unable to check that the device was correctly positioned. The two best positions are:

- Standing with one foot resting on a chair – a right-handed woman should raise her left leg and vice versa (*Fig. 4.4*).
- Squatting right down on the ground.

Other positions are possible according to the woman's choice.

4.40 Successful teaching (diaphragm) – what are the steps?

1 In her own preferred position (as just described in Q 4.39), teach the woman to locate her cervix. Most women prefer to use one finger, but it is an error to insist on this. Even 'short-fingered' women can learn to feel their cervix if taught to use both index and middle fingers.

2 The instructor then inserts the diaphragm for the patient, allowing her to feel her cervix covered with thin rubber.

3 The patient then removes the diaphragm for herself, either by hooking it out or by the use of two fingers each side of the anterior rim. If this is

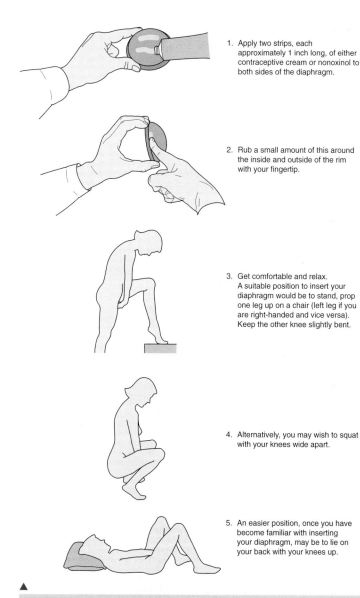

1. Apply two strips, each approximately 1 inch long, of either contraceptive cream or nonoxinol to both sides of the diaphragm.

2. Rub a small amount of this around the inside and outside of the rim with your fingertip.

3. Get comfortable and relax. A suitable position to insert your diaphragm would be to stand, prop one leg up on a chair (left leg if you are right-handed and vice versa). Keep the other knee slightly bent.

4. Alternatively, you may wish to squat with your knees wide apart.

5. An easier position, once you have become familiar with inserting your diaphragm, may be to lie on your back with your knees up.

Fig. 4.4 Instructions for prospective users of the diaphragm. *Q 4.39* (images reproduced courtesy of Janssen Cilag Pharmaceutical Ltd, Diaphragm Teaching Aid; associated text updated by author in 2008). *Qs 4.39, 4.40.*

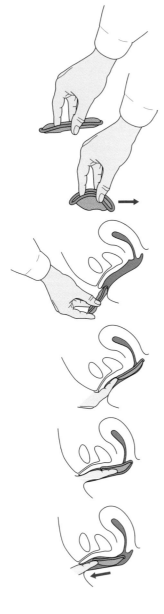

6. To insert your diaphragm fold it in half by pressing the middle of the opposite sides together between the thumb and forefinger of one hand. You may find it helpful to place your index finger in the dome between your thumb and fingers to help prevent it springing away.

If you have been given an arcing-spring diaphragm hold it with the arc pointing downwards to ensure that the cervix will be covered.

7. Hold the lips of your vagina apart with your other hand. Gently slide the folded diaphragm into your vagina, placing your index finger on the rim to guide it. Aim towards the small of the back as if inserting a tampon. You may feel the rim pass over the cervix.

8. Use the index finger to push the front rim up behind the pubic bone.

9. To check if the diaphragm is in place insert your index finger into your vagina and touch the dome. You should feel the cervix underneath. Move your index finger to the front of the diaphragm and make sure it is firmly in place behind the pubic bone. Finally check that the back rim is behind the cervix.

10. Do not remove your diaphragm for 6 hours after intercourse. Put your index finger in your vagina and hook it behind the rim of the diaphragm under your pubic bone. Gently pull the diaphragm down and out. You may find it useful to bear down slightly especially if it is well tucked up behind the pubic bone. The latex diaphragm should not be left in place for more than 24 hours (plus the usual 6 hours to ensure sperm non-viability). Silicone types may be left for longer.

Fig. 4.4—cont'd

found difficult, practising with a slightly too large diaphragm might be all that is necessary to boost confidence.

4 The woman should feel again for the cervix to emphasize the different feel when it is uncovered.

5 She should then be taught to insert the diaphragm as described above and shown in steps 6–8 of *Fig. 4.4*. The instructor should emphasize that the direction of insertion is similar to that for a tampon – primarily backwards.

6 The woman should then examine herself to check that the cervix is covered by the soft rubber dome. It is absolutely vital to explain that *the fact that a diaphragm fits snugly behind the symphysis and feels comfortable is no guarantee of correct insertion.*

7 If the woman repeatedly inserts the diaphragm into her anterior fornix, the following useful tips come from our Sister-in-Charge (as in the 1980s she was called) at the Margaret Pyke Centre:

(a) the woman lies on her back and holds the diaphragm in her left hand (if right-handed). She then uses her right hand to separate the labia and guide insertion, vertically. Alternatively, and in any convenient position (*see Q 4.39*), she inserts the diaphragm halfway only, then the half that is still outside is pressed towards the symphysis while completing the insertion.

(b) the use of an arcing diaphragm. When held dome down, compression between middle finger and thumb, with the index finger between to steady it, produces a downwards bend (see *Fig. 4.2* and *Q 4.26*). This helps the posterior rim to pass below the cervix and so into the posterior rather than the anterior fornix.

Occasionally, with either diaphragm design, the woman's partner might be able to learn to insert it for her.

4.41 How are cervical and vault caps fitted?

NB: See the important note regarding UK availability at *Q 4.2*.

1 The correct size allows the rim of the chosen cap to touch the fornices with no gap, comfortably accommodating the cervix (the cervical cap and FemCap being the only ones that truly fit it) and giving evidence of a suction effect.

2 To insert the chosen cap, the rim is compressed between thumb and first two fingers and guided along the posterior vaginal wall towards the cervix. The cap is allowed to open by removing the thumb, and then is pushed over the cervix with the fingertips. A final check is made to ensure that the cervix is palpable through the cap and that there is no gap at the top between the rim and the vaginal vault (the fornices).

3 Cervical and vault caps are removed by inserting a fingertip above the rim and then easing the cap downwards, before removal with the index and middle fingers. FemCap has a useful removal strap (see *Fig. 4.6*).

4.42 Successful teaching – what instructions for vault and cervical caps?

Feeling for the cervix, insertion and removal are taught as just described for the fitting. The important point is that if the right sort of woman has been chosen for these caps (which are definitely more tricky to use than the diaphragm), she rapidly develops her own technique both for insertion and removal.

Further practical details about fitting these smaller suction caps are best learnt in the practical, clinical situation, aided by the relevant fpa leaflet and manufacturer's leaflet.

4.43 Successful teaching – what is the training 'timetable' for any type of occlusive cap?

It is usual and preferable to provide the woman with a cap to practise with for the first week, during which she should use an alternative contraceptive. This enables her to increase her confidence in the techniques of insertion and removal, and to test whether the method is comfortable during all normal activities. She should be informed, with the aid of the most recent edition of the fpa's leaflet, of all the 'rules' (*see Q 4.44*) before she leaves after the first visit. The same points should again be run through at the return visit, before she starts to rely on the method.

4.44 Successful teaching – what actual instructions are given at the first visit?

See *Fig. 4.4*.

The wording that follows is addressed to a particular woman and relates specifically to the diaphragm (*see also Qs 4.46, 4.49*):

■ Always use the spermicidal nonoxinol. Apply two strips, each approximately 2.5 cm (1 inch) in length, to each side of the diaphragm. It is unnecessary to smear the surfaces too much, but you might also want to put some on the leading part of the rim.

■ Put your diaphragm in place (see *Fig. 4.4*), using the position and technique you found most comfortable when you were fitted. This could be at any convenient time before lovemaking.

■ If you are having a bath, you should put your diaphragm in after rather than before it (*see Q 4.85*).

■ Most important: check the position of your diaphragm (or cap) with either your index finger or with index and middle finger, as you prefer.

The important thing is that you check that the diaphragm covers your cervix. This feels a bit like a rounded nose with a single nostril (or dimple if you have not yet had a baby), upwards and backwards somewhere near the top of your vagina. You should get used to the particular way your cervix points, which could be forwards, backwards or straight downwards. Check that the rubber on your diaphragm actually covers the cervix – do not rely just on it feeling comfortable.

■ Should lovemaking take place more than 3 h after you put the diaphragm or cap in, either insert more nonoxinol with an applicator, or use a spermicidal pessary pushed well up with the finger. You need to allow about 10 min for pessaries to disperse in the vagina before your partner actually deposits semen there.

■ If you have intercourse more than once, more spermicide should be added beforehand, leaving the diaphragm or cap in place.

■ You should leave your diaphragm or cap in place for at least 6 h after the last intercourse. It can be kept in longer, but should be removed once a day for cleaning. FemCap is licensed to be retained continuously for 48 h.

■ It is no problem if your period starts while the diaphragm or cap is in place. Also it is quite possible to get pregnant during your period. So continue to use your method for any intercourse, especially towards the end or just after a period, when many people think they can get away without using it.

■ After removal, the diaphragm or cap can be washed in warm water with mild toilet soap. It should then be dried and stored in its box in a cool dry place. Do not use heat, solvents, disinfectants, detergents or any mineral- or vegetable-oil-containing oils or lubricants (*see Q 3.21*) on rubber products. However, the silicone of FemCap and some diaphragms allows autoclaving and is resistant to chemical attack.

■ Inspect your cap regularly for holes by holding it up to the light.

Although you have been given the cap with spermicide, everything is just for practice during the first week. Wear it during the day to make sure it stays in place. You should not be able to feel it if it is the right size and in the right position. Report any discomfort or other problems when, after 1 week, you return to the clinic or surgery. You should come with it in position so that the doctor or nurse can do a proper check.

4.45 What should take place at the second visit?

■ Any discomfort or problems should be identified.

■ If there are problems, a change in the size of the cap or use of a different spermicide might be recommended.

■ Repetition of the instructions above is important, before the woman actually begins to rely on her method.

■ A final warning about the danger of risk-taking might be useful: coupled with a reminder about the availability, if ever needed, of postcoital contraception (*see Chapter 10*).

4.46 What extra instructions are given for users of cervical/vault caps?

■ A usual recommendation is to one-third fill the bowl of cervical, vault or vimule caps with spermicidal cream. None is used on the rim for fear of impairing suction.

■ With these caps, an extra measure of spermicidal cream or a pessary should be added on the vaginal side before the first as well as subsequent acts of intercourse after insertion.

4.47 What arrangements are made for routine subsequent follow-up?

None! After the first visit (FemCap, *see Q 4.76*) or two visits (diaphragm), this is no longer advised for users of this method (or indeed any method except injectables). What is crucial is that each should feel free to return more frequently if she has any problem, question or concern.

Reassessment of the fitting is particularly required:

■ after full-term delivery
■ after any unplanned pregnancy, whether ending in a termination or miscarriage (chiefly to assess possible improvements in fitting or the user's technique – or discuss a different method)
■ after having vaginal surgery
■ after the woman loses or gains more than 3 kg in weight.

4.48 What is the scientific basis for the rules and regulations about use of occlusive caps, as in *Qs 4.44–4.47* above?

Weak! Many assumptions, some of them fundamental ones, have never been tested in proper controlled trials, namely (in quotes below):

■ 'Spermicides add significantly to the effectiveness of occlusive caps.' Actually, this has now been tested with a good study design at the Margaret Pyke Centre, but the statistical power was insufficient for a conclusive result (*see Q 4.7*). In practice, spermicide use is advised with all the products, including newer ones like FemCap.

■ 'Fitting the largest diaphragm that the woman finds comfortable will improve its effectiveness.'

- 'Extra spermicide should be used at each intercourse.'
- 'Extra spermicide should be used if intercourse is delayed for more than 3 h after placement of the cap.'
- 'The spermicide should be applied both to the top and under surface of the diaphragm.'
- 'The shortest safe time after intercourse that any occlusive cap can be removed is 6 h' (though this is based on some data, on the spermicidal effects of the acid vagina).
- 'Gain or loss of as little as 3 kg in weight might influence the effectiveness of the diaphragm.'

4.49 What variations in the instructions given to patients are worth considering?

Numerous variations are accepted practice in different countries around the world. In Australia, use of spermicide at all with occlusive caps is often left to the patient's choice. The rationale for this is the high rate of user-failure in that country and the belief that increased compliance is likely when 'messy' spermicides are avoided. This view, however, is a minority one. Pending more data, most authorities feel that spermicides should continue to be used. In addition, two variants seem reasonable, both with respect to the diaphragm:

- Application of spermicide to the superior surface only of the diaphragm. This is the norm in the US and is also becoming more usual in the UK (about an 8-cm [3-inch] strip of nonoxinol cream from the tube being applied).
- Increasing to 6 h the interval after placement of the diaphragm and before intercourse after which further spermicide is advised.

Other minor variations are also permitted by various family planning authorities.

OCCLUSIVE CAPS: MANAGEMENT OF SIDE-EFFECTS AND COMPLICATIONS

4.50 What should be done if the partner can feel the diaphragm during intercourse?

- Check the size – a larger or smaller variety might be needed.
- Re-teach the patient. The couple might already have decided not to use certain positions (e.g. for rear entry vaginal intercourse they might use the condom instead).
- Change from a flat-spring to a coil-spring diaphragm.

- Change to a vault or perhaps a cervical cap.
- Change the method.

4.51 Why are urinary tract infections more common in diaphragm-users, and how should they be managed?

- The fact that urinary tract infections develop more frequently is believed to be caused mainly by the pressure of the rim on the urethra and bladder base, predisposing to urethritis and cystitis.
- Some work has also suggested that use of the diaphragm and other occlusive caps with spermicide alters the vaginal flora so as to promote infections. Vaginal cultures from cap-users grow *Escherichia coli* more often than those from relevant controls.

It would appear that the first explanation is the more important, because the following actions usually help, especially the second one:

- change to a smaller size of diaphragm – i.e. the first was too large
- change to FemCap.

4.52 What are the possible causes of the complaint of 'vaginal soreness'?

- There might be an incidental infection such as thrush (or urethritis, *see Q 4.51*).
- Inflammatory reactions, abrasions or even frank ulcers can also be caused by local pressure.
- Allergy is possible though rare, either to the spermicide or to chemicals in the rubber. Silicone products are non-allergenic.

4.53 How should vaginal soreness be managed?

- *Examine the patient*: particularly her vulva and the whole vaginal surface. If there is widespread erythema and multiple vesicles or scaling, suspect allergy. Allergy cannot easily be treated by change of spermicide since only one is now marketed (nonoxinol as Ortho-Creme)! For true rubber allergy, the polyurethane female condom or FemCap are good options, or a polyurethane male condom such as Avanti.
- *Take swabs for possible infections*: if there is a discharge with a slightly fishy odour, it is useful to test the pH, using test paper with a pH range of 4–6. A result >4.5 suggests either bacterial vaginosis (BV) or infection with *Trichomonas vaginalis* (TV), both of which are treatable with metronidazole. For BV, clindamycin (Dalacin) 2% can also be used – but beware its known adverse effects on rubber (*see Q 3.21*).

4.54 What should be done if actual abrasions or ulcers are seen?

I have personally seen only one severe case, in an arcing-diaphragm user, but they have been described in users of other diaphragms, vimules and cervical caps.

In our case the ulcers were posterolateral on each side, 2–3 cm long and about 0.5 cm wide and deep, and very indurated. At first, a carcinoma of the vagina was suspected! However, complete recovery followed non-use of the diaphragm (which was size 85 and fitted correctly) and abstinence from intercourse for 3 weeks. No other treatment was required.

The woman concerned had met a new partner and intercourse had been unusually vigorous and frequent, with the diaphragm left in place for long periods of time. Cases reported from the US had similarly worn the diaphragm or vimule cap for three or more days in succession. This rare complication is also said to be more likely if the diaphragm is too large, and might be related to variations in individual anatomy (*see Q. 4.84*).

Regrettably, the Today and Protectaid contraceptive sponges – products that were found to be very user-friendly, popular and useful for women whose fertility could be expected to be low, such as perimenopausal women and some breastfeeders – were removed from the UK market (solely for commercial reasons). But there are plans to reintroduce one of these, possibly (but do not hold your breath!) during 2009 or 2010.

FEMALE CONDOMS

4.55 What is the female condom, first marketed during 1992?

Various designs have been proposed, including the bikini condom with its integral latex pouch, from the US, and, more recently, the Janesway panty condom, with a latex pouch attached to frilly knickers! Neither of these has reached the market to date.

The most successful and still available product is Femidom (Reality in the US), which was first devised in Denmark. Made of polyurethane and preloaded with an efficient silicone lubricant, the currently marketed version is 17 cm long. There is a large-diameter (70 mm) outer ring attached at the opening, designed to prevent it advancing beyond the vulva. A 60-mm diameter loose ring at the inner closed end aids its retention

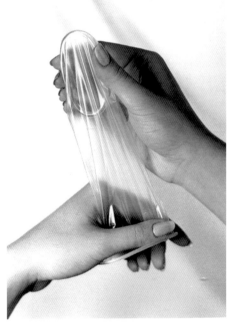

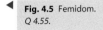
Fig. 4.5 Femidom.
Q 4.55.

within the vagina and is also squeezed like a diaphragm for insertion. The whole device thus forms a well-lubricated secondary vagina (*Fig. 4.5*).

4.56 What advantages are claimed for female condoms?

■ Over-the-counter method, not requiring fitting by any outsider.

■ Under the woman's control.

■ Insertable before intercourse, like the diaphragm.

■ Does not require an erect penis at outset.

■ Male sensations are usually reported as feeling more normal than for intercourse with a (tight-fitting) male rubber condom.

■ Odour-free.

■ A better barrier against STIs, including viruses, than any intravaginal method can provide.

■ Worth suggesting if local soreness makes sex uncomfortable or during menses or postpartum lochia.

■ Shown to be less likely than the male condom to rupture in use.

■ Not damaged by any common chemicals.

■ Virtually without risk of causing allergic reactions in either partner.

Its use-effectiveness (13.5 conceptions per 100 women at 6 months in one US trial) is probably broadly similar to the male condom (see *Table 1.2*, p. 14).

4.57 Are there any problems?

Users of the female condom report a few, of varying importance:

- It may seem rather in the way during foreplay.
- There is the potential for the penis to become wrongly positioned (between the sac and the vaginal wall). Users should be warned about this very real risk.
- Some say it is 'noisy' . . . 'So what,' I say, 'sex itself can be noisy! You could always have some music on . . .'.

4.58 What is the place of Femidom in the range of methods?

Reports about its acceptability are mixed. It was given qualified approval as a method by about half the users in the first study by the Margaret Pyke Centre. Among 106 volunteers of the same Centre's trial of Femidom as the sole contraceptive, more than half found it unacceptable. However, 9 of the 11 users who continued for 1 year, and most of 20 who had to stop using it solely because supplies ran out, would have wished to continue long term. As the first female-controlled method with high potential for preventing HIV transmission, it must surely be welcomed to the range of contraceptive options. Further development of new variants will hopefully make it more acceptable and use-effective.

Trials in developing countries have confirmed that female condoms are definitely reusable if:

- washed, then
- 'sterilized' by drying in the ultraviolet light of strong sunshine, then
- used again along with a simple lubricant.

A proportion of UK condom-users have elected to ring the changes between female and male condoms according to choice, i.e. having 'his' nights followed by a 'her' night!

SPERMICIDES

4.59 What are spermicides?

These substances chemically immobilize or destroy sperm. They are one of the oldest and simplest forms of fertility control and make a useful contribution, chiefly to increase the efficacy of other methods.

4.60 What is the mode of action of spermicides?

They have two main components: a relatively inert base and an active spermicidal agent. Hence they operate both physically and biochemically, forming a partial barrier and also immobilizing sperm. The base materials vary in their physical characteristics, the best being water-soluble. The active ingredients are of five main types:

- Surface-active agents, of which the most widely used worldwide is nonoxinol-9. Indeed, due to commercial pressures, this has now become the only spermicide still on the UK market – resulting in real difficulties for users of occlusive caps who develop soreness or irritation (*see Q 4.67*) or a true allergy.
- Enzyme inhibitors.
- Bactericides.
- Acids.
- Local anaesthetics and other membrane-active agents.

4.61 What is actually available?

In previous editions of this book there could be a table showing a variety of these. Regrettably there is now very little choice: Ortho-Creme alone was on the UK market till the end of 2007 and Gygel (a clear jelly similar to the earlier and very popular product Gynol II) replaced it, in early 2008. The return of the contraceptive sponge now seems also to be further delayed (see p. 85). However, a spermicidal film termed VCF Film (which can be used as spermicide on the top of diaphragms or FemCap) and VCF Foam (equivalent to the old Delfen foam) are options that *may* become available, through the Durbin company.

Given the HIV/AIDS problem, neglect of this field by a generation of scientists seems unforgivable: far too little research has been done, so far, to devise better substances, more effective and safer not only as spermicides but also potentially as microbicides (*see Qs 4.66, 4.67*).

4.62 How are spermicides used?

To be effective, the products should disperse quickly yet remain in sufficient concentration at the cervix to exert their action at the end of intercourse. The cream, like the old Delfen foam, may be inserted by applicator just before intercourse; but pessaries (and the foaming tablets available outside the UK) should be inserted at least 10 min before ejaculation, to allow sufficient time for dispersal.

4.63 How effective are spermicides used alone?
(*See also Q 2.3*)

Spermicides are far more effective in vitro than they ever prove to be in vivo. There are greater variations in reported effectiveness for spermicides than for almost any other birth control method. The limits in studies of different populations range from less than 1 to over 30 pregnancies/100 woman-years! In a study of almost 3000 well-motivated women attending six family planning clinics in the US, who received the proper instructions and follow-up, Bernstein documented a pregnancy rate of only 4/100 woman-years. Trussell indicates a 'perfect use' rate of 18% in the first year.

4.64 Are spermicides recommended for use alone as contraceptives?

General teaching in the UK has been that spermicides are not effective enough for use alone. Where available, contraceptive foam and spermicide-impregnated sponges such as Today are believed to be more effective than the other presentations. They are user-friendly, non-greasy and essentially unobtrusive, non-coitally-related. Hence they can be a very useful choice under certain conditions, mainly where reduced fertility and good compliance are both expected:

■ Women's natural fertility can be low because of:
   - *Age*: fertility declines, most steeply after the age of 45 but less so in those with continued regular cycling (*see Qs 11.33, 11.34*). Hence spermicides can be very appropriate, as well as acceptable, for use from the age of 45 if irregular cycles are occurring along with definite vasomotor symptoms (and even more so after 50), through until 1 year after the menopause. This may be especially acceptable as an alternative to condoms during cyclical HRT, which alone is not adequately contraceptive.
   - *Lactation*: the method could be used to supplement natural hypofertility. This is hardly necessary while all the LAM criteria apply (*see Q 2.37*), but, in the real world, plans for full breastfeeding may not always be achieved.
   - *Secondary amenorrhoea* (*see Q 5.66*): although if the woman is hypo-estrogenic, HRT might need to be added, or both might be substituted by the COC.
■ Spermicide may also be used as an adjunct to other methods of birth control, such as coitus interruptus.
■ It can also be used for those who are planning their first child fairly soon, or who are spacing their family.
■ It would certainly be better than nothing, for women who are unable or unwilling to use any other more effective method.

> **TABLE 4.2 Advantages and disadvantages of spermicides**
>
> | Advantages | Disadvantages |
> |---|---|
> | ■ Easy availability | ■ Perceived to be messy |
> | ■ Freedom from major health risks | ■ Not highly effective in general use |
> | ■ No medical intervention/ supervision necessary | ■ Coitus-dependent and thus inconvenient to use |
> | ■ Need only be used when required | ■ Waiting period of 10 min before some products (e.g. pessaries) effective |
> | ■ Allow the female to be in control of contraception | ■ Not effective if inserted too far ahead |
> | ■ Some forms provide extra genital lubrication | ■ Can cause local heat (foaming tablets), irritation or allergy |
> | ■ Are a valuable adjunct to other methods, including LAM (see *Q 2.37*) and during perimenopausal hypofertility | ■ Evidence of damage by nonoxinol to the vaginal mucosa and *increased* risk of HIV transmission, in frequent use. This makes nonoxinol useful primarily for monogamous couples using the diaphragm or one of the caps (see *Qs 3.19, 4.67*) and greatly increases the urgency to develop a better product |
> | ■ Possible protection against some sexually transmitted diseases – and research proceeds to enhance this benefit through innovative microbicidal compounds released vaginally | ■ Issue of toxic shock syndrome arises with contraceptive sponges due to their similarity to tampons. Each should be used for no more than 24 h |

4.65 What are the advantages and disadvantages of spermicides?

These are summarized in *Table 4.2*. Note the point that it is advised, pending more data, not to use contraceptive sponges for more than 24 h.

4.66 Do spermicides protect against STIs?

In vitro studies have shown that most spermicides can kill sexually transmitted pathogens as well as sperm. Nonoxinol has some activity against the organisms causing gonorrhoea, *Chlamydia*, *Trichomonas vaginalis*, genital herpes and even HIV.

However, in vivo, none of this promise has been confirmed with respect to the risk of HIV/AIDS virus transmission, and the virucidal effect is completely nullified by tissue toxicity affecting the vaginal mucosa (*see Q 4.67*).

There is at last some innovative research in progress to produce vaginal microbicides that would be active against HIV and other STIs (*see Q 4.75*).

VAGINAL CONTRACEPTION: UNRESOLVED SAFETY ISSUES

4.67 Is it true that nonoxinol is capable of damaging the vaginal epithelium? How might this affect HIV transmission?

The answers are 'yes' and 'adversely', respectively. An early study in Nairobi prostitutes of nonoxinol-9 (N-9)-containing spermicides as a possible aid to safer sex reported 'soreness' as a frequent complaint. This was at first thought to be linked in part with trauma from very frequent coitus, but subsequent studies have shown that frequent use of the product itself is the main factor. When used on average four times a day for 14 days, N-9 released from pessaries caused erythema and colposcopic evidence of minor damage to the vaginal skin. Worse than that, Van Damme et al in 2002 found, in a randomly controlled trial, a higher incidence of HIV in users of N-9 than in placebo-using controls. This study and others reviewed and referenced by Wilkinson et al [*The Lancet Infectious Diseases* 2002;2:613–617] prompted the WHO to issue new recommendations (www.who.int), including:

- ■ N-9 should **not** be used for STI or HIV prevention.
- ■ Women at high risk of HIV should not use N-9 at all.
- ■ Women who have multiple daily acts of intercourse should be advised against N-9 use.
- ■ Women at low risk of HIV and having sex at a 'normal contraceptive frequency' may use N-9, e.g. with the female barrier methods.
- ■ Condoms should in future not be lubricated with N-9-containing lubricants (*see Qs 3.18, 3.19*).

Pending the development of more alternatives, for the time being it is considered good practice to continue to recommend nonoxinol-containing products for normal contraceptive use (at a frequency not defined by WHO but clearly less than four times a day!), whether alone or with diaphragms or cervical caps.

4.68 Are spermicides absorbed and is there therefore a risk of systemic effects?

Most substances in the vagina can be absorbed into the circulation. Hence it is impossible to say that a method that uses a spermicide is entirely free of the risk of systemic harmful effects. There have been some reports suggesting an association with unwanted effects following spermicide absorption (*see Qs 4.69, 4.70*), but the overall picture remains a reassuring one.

4.69 What is the evidence that standard spermicides might have toxic effects after absorption?

In 1979 it was suggested from animal experiments that N-9 might have hepatotoxic effects and cause changes in serum lipids. However, controlled studies of the blood chemistry of women using spermicides have not demonstrated any significant changes. Certainly no obvious harm has ever been reported among long-term users of vaginal contraceptives.

4.70 What is the evidence about teratogenesis?

Exposure to the spermicide early in pregnancy, or fertilization of an ovum by a sperm damaged by the spermicide, might in theory increase the rate of malformations. In 1981, one study reported an increase in various unrelated fetal abnormalities among the children of women who could have used spermicides around the time they became pregnant. This has been criticized because of flaws in the study design, and more recent studies have completely failed to show the risk. Present opinion is that the teratogenic effect of spermicides is either negligible or nil.

4.71 Are there reports of an increase of neoplasia in women using vaginal contraception?

No – neither as a consequence of systemic absorption, nor because of any effect of spermicide or rubber on the vaginal or cervical epithelium. A few women who are sensitive to spermicides might develop hyperkeratosis of the cervix or vagina. This has not been shown to result in neoplasia. Moreover, it is very likely that barrier methods are protective against cervical neoplasia (*see Q 4.17*).

4.72 Can vaginal contraception promote infection?

Concern arises from the above story concerning HIV transmission (*Q 4.67*) coupled with evidence that *Staphylococcus aureus*, some streptococci and *E. coli* tend to proliferate in the presence of a diaphragm or a cervical cap, at the expense of the usual protective lactobacilli: which indeed can be adversely affected by the nonoxinol spermicide. This could promote bacterial vaginosis and has already been mentioned as a possible factor in the increased risk of urinary infections. Once again, a low frequency of N-9 use appears to be advantageous.

4.73 Can the diaphragm or other caps cause toxic shock syndrome?

Possibly yes. There is some positive evidence from Schwartz et al [*Reviews of Infectious Diseases* 1989;11 Suppl 1:S43–S88]. However, any added risk is probably greater (though still tiny) from any use of tampons by those diaphragm-users.

4.74 What is the overall safety of vaginal contraceptives?

Even allowing for the unresolved safety issues above, potential users can be told that all these methods are still believed to be medically safer than the hormonal methods. However, honesty dictates that it would be wrong to say that any method that uses an absorbable spermicide is completely free from systemic effects.

In assessing safety it is also important to remember that unwanted pregnancies are more frequent among users of any of these methods. One then has to consider the potential health hazard to the mother of the resulting unwanted pregnancies.

THE (NEAR) FUTURE IN VAGINAL CONTRACEPTION

4.75 What innovative spermicides and microbicides are being studied?

Inhibitors of the sperm's own enzymes, principally acrosin, show promise, and several surprising drugs (like propranolol) that are normally used for non-contraceptive indications have aroused interest because of their effect on the sperm membrane and motility. Derivatives of natural products such as gossypol have also been screened. Another approach is to develop agents that directly alter cervical mucus both chemically and physically.

However, there is special interest in microbicides for preventing vaginal transmission of all kinds of STIs but especially HIV. These might or might not be also spermicidal and were well reviewed by Stone [*Nature Reviews* 2002;1:977–984]. Progress is slow to identify candidate compounds which, unlike N-9, are non-irritant to the vaginal epithelium. More research is also urgently required into better carrier (base) materials and systems.

4.76 What is new among occlusive caps?

- *Disposable spermicide-coated diaphragms*: designed to overcome the perceived 'messiness' of any vaginal contraceptive that requires separate application of the spermicide. No further progress has been reported.
- *New sponges*: with different spermicides, or combinations of spermicide with microbicides: these might well be useful, judging by the high acceptability of the sponge method in the trial by the Margaret Pyke Centre (*see Q 4.64*).
- *New cervical caps*: there was great interest back in the 1980s in the so-called custom-fitted cervical cap, made from a mould of the user's cervix. Although trials of this Contracap gave a quite unacceptable failure rate, the objective remains attractive – of a non-coitally-related appliance designed to be left in place in the upper vagina for long periods of time.
- However, FemCap is now marketed and from 2008 in the UK will become more important in the absence of alternative cervical caps. It is a

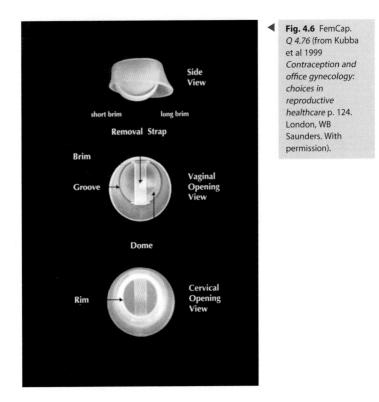

Fig. 4.6 FemCap. *Q 4.76* (from Kubba et al 1999 *Contraception and office gynecology: choices in reproductive healthcare* p. 124. London, WB Saunders. With permission).

small reusable cap of distinctive design (*Fig. 4.6*) made of silicone rubber, available from Durbin (see MIMS). It is available on the NHS Drug Tariff in sizes 22, 26 and 30 mm diameter. Initial fitting by a doctor or nurse is desirable, but not essential, and there is no requirement for future follow-up visits. FemCap must be used with a spermicide (e.g. Gygel jelly or the expected new spermicidal film, *see Q 4.61*), and may be worn continuously for up to 48 h in all, including 6 h after the last intercourse. The manufacturer's stated pregnancy rate of 10.5 per 100 women for 1 year of use in US trials requires independent confirmation.

PQ PATIENT QUESTIONS

QUESTIONS ASKED BY USERS ABOUT VAGINAL CONTRACEPTION

4.77 Can I use some kind of cap if my womb tilts backwards?

It is a myth that this makes it impossible to use the method. Some positions of your cervix (entrance to the womb) can make it preferable for you to be given an arcing diaphragm and could result in rejection of a cervical cap, but the method is not ruled out if you wish to use it.

4.78 How do I know where my cervix is?

It is absolutely essential that you feel confident that you can find your cervix, whatever the kind of occlusive cap you are going to use. It is often helpful to ask your doctor or the nurse to tell you in which direction its opening points. You might also find it easier to feel if you use two fingers rather than one.

4.79 How much nonoxinol cream should I use with my diaphragm?

A common error is to use too much (*see* Q 4.44 for the standard instructions). If you find messiness a particular problem but still want to use the method, ask your doctor or nurse about putting spermicide only on the top when it is first inserted (but continue to follow all the other rules you were taught).

4.80 What if, after lovemaking, I find that I have put my diaphragm in the wrong place, like in front of my cervix? Or it just fell out afterwards when I went to the toilet?

If either of these things happens, consider postcoital contraception (*see Chapter 10*). Moreover, if your diaphragm or other cap comes out, it might be that you have a prolapse, or the wrong size, or are not inserting it correctly. So you should also make an early appointment to discuss things with the doctor or nurse.

4.81 Can caps and diaphragms be fitted with strings to help removal? I have difficulty in getting mine out.

There are no longer any marketed with strings. You might have been taught to use just one finger to hook out the diaphragm, and the solution to your problem could well just be to use two fingers, one each side of the front rim. FemCap has a special removal strap.

4.82 How do I check the diaphragm is in good condition? Its dome has become much softer and floppier and it has lost its new whiteness – do these changes matter?

You should hold your diaphragm up to the light and stretch it, being careful not to damage the rubber with your fingernails. If no holes are seen, and if the rim can readily be restored to a reasonable shape, then all is well. The change in colour and texture of the rubber is quite normal.

4.83 Can I leave the cap in during my periods?

The US Food and Drug Administration (FDA) advises against this because of a completely unproven extra risk of the rare TSS. It can be used short term to reduce messiness if you fancy lovemaking during any bleeding, but a better solution might be Femidom (*see* Q 4.55).

4.84 I have heard you can leave the cap in all the time – is this right?

If you follow the rules, yes – almost! It can be in position most of the time if your love-life is unpredictable and frequent. The important thing is to remove it at least once in 24 h (48 h if you have a FemCap), always 6 h after the last intercourse, wash it in mild soap and rinse it thoroughly, after which it can be reinserted. Continuous use without giving your vaginal wall an occasional rest seems a bad thing, however (*see Q 4.54*).

4.85 Can I have a bath or go swimming with the cap in place?

Yes – although it would be ideal to wait until 6 h after the last intercourse, in case the water helps the sperm to escape the action of the spermicide. And if you make love after bathing with the diaphragm in, put some extra spermicide in first.

4.86 I've had a baby – can I go back to using my old diaphragm or cap?

Quite possibly not. It is certainly important to get the fitting rechecked for size, and maybe take the opportunity to re-discuss *all* your contraceptive options. (*See also Q 4.47.*)

4.87 How often should I change the diaphragm or cap for a new one?

Only when your inspection (*see Q 4.82*) shows damage. Successful regular use of the same one for 2 years is common. Remember too that if you lose it, you should be able to buy the right size at any good pharmacy.

4.88 Is Femidom a recommended method?

Yes. Follow the instructions that come with it carefully, every time. As long as you are careful to avoid wrong positioning of the penis (*see Q 4.57*), and the sperm are caught completely within the Femidom, it is comparable to a male condom both as a contraceptive and for safer sex.

4.89 Can I use a homemade barrier 'in an emergency'?

Improvised barriers can be made. Probably the best is a suitable piece of sponge or plug of cloth, soaked either in vinegar–water solution diluted 1 in 20 or in a lemon juice or soap solution.

4.90 Do you recommend the 'honeycap', which my friend uses?

Definitely not. Available from some doctors in private practice in London, this is really only a size 60 arcing-spring diaphragm that is first soaked in honey for 7 days and then used without spermicide for up to a week at a time. The honey is meant to reduce the risk of vaginal infection or odour, but even this is unproven – and its effectiveness has also not been properly tested.

All in all, it is highly likely to have the same failure rate as in a 1982 Marie Stopes Centre study of the 'non-spermicide, fit-free diaphragm' (of the same 60-mm size), which amounted to a risk, in the first year, that one in every four users would become pregnant!

The combined oral contraceptive – selection and eligibility

5

DRUG INTERACTIONS AFFECTING THE COC

SELECTION OF USERS AND FORMULATIONS: CHOOSING THE 'SAFER WOMEN' AND THE 'SAFER PILLS'

THE PROS AND CONS OF PHASIC PILLS

BACKGROUND: EFFICACY AND MECHANISMS

5.1 What is the definition of oral contraception?

An orally administered substance or combination that prevents pregnancy. Specifically, at the present time, such substances are only for use by women. Although steroids and other potential systemic contraceptives can also be given by non-oral routes (*see Qs 6.81–6.84* and *Chapters 8 and 11*), in this chapter I will consider only the combined oral contraceptive (COC), which is a combination of estrogen and progestogen. Unless qualified, the word 'pill' refers to the COC. The progestogen-only pill (POP) is considered in Chapter 7.

5.2 What is the history of oral contraception?

This is discussed in more detail elsewhere (see my book *The Pill*, details in Further Reading). In brief, it was shown by the early 1900s that the corpus luteum of pregnancy stops further ovulation. In 1921, Haberlandt transplanted ovaries into female rabbits, which rendered them infertile for several months. He suggested that extracts from ovaries might be used as oral contraceptives. In 1941, Marker used diosgenin, from the Mexican yam, as the raw material for sex steroids. This led to the synthesis of norethisterone (known as norethindrone in the US) by Djerassi and his colleagues in 1950. Frank Colton independently produced norethynodrel, which – with mestranol – was the first marketed oral contraceptive. Margaret Sanger, supported by her wealthy friend Catherine McCormack, financed the studies of the biologists Gregory Pincus and M.C. Chang, together with the obstetrician John Rock. After systematic experiments in animals, the first human trials in North America were reported in 1956. In the Puerto Rico field-trial that followed, the intention appears to have been to use progestogen alone, but there was contamination with mestranol. Thus, the invention of the 'combined pill' – which was shown later to give much better cycle control than any progestogen-only method – owes a definite debt to chance.

The regular pill-free interval inducing hormone-withdrawal bleeds was, as we shall see later, arguably a mistake. It made the method more likely to fail, for both pharmacological and compliance reasons, and greatly complicated the advice if pills were missed. There was a strong assumption – since shown to be not necessarily so – that women would welcome the monthly bleeds for reassurance that they had not conceived. Moreover, John Rock, a Roman Catholic, hoped that through appearing more like the natural menstrual cycle the pill method might be seen by the Vatican hierarchy as acceptably 'natural' family planning. Tragically, for millions of Catholic couples since, especially in poor countries, this was not to be.

In 1964, Pope Paul VI created a Papal Commission on Population and Birth Control with two components: one consisting of 64 lay persons, the other of 15 clerics including a Polish cardinal, Karol Wojtyla, who later became Pope John Paul II. After 2 years of intense study, the Commission concluded that, while it was not possible to make any change without undermining papal authority, the Church should make the change anyway because it was the right thing to do. Both parts of the Commission voted in favour of change: the lay members by 60 votes to 4 and the clerics by 9 to 6. However, a minority report, co-authored by the future Pope, set forth the exact opposite, that if it should be declared that contraception is not evil in itself, then in the context of earlier papal pronouncements papal infallibility would be unacceptably undermined. It was this report that was finally accepted.

The combined pill became available in the US in June 1960 and in the UK during 1961. In 1963, the Wyeth Company achieved the total synthesis of norgestrel.

The first case report of venous thromboembolism (VTE) was reported in *The Lancet* in 1961 by an astute British GP. Subsequently, there have been numerous case–control studies, three main prospective (cohort) studies and, in recent years, several which utilize large practice databases, researching both the adverse and beneficial effects. Much more money has been spent on testing than on originally developing the method.

5.3 What is the usage of the pill, worldwide and in the UK?

Currently well over 100 million women rely on the pill. There is enormous variation between countries, and within countries, according to age groups. The differences have more to do with medical politics, religion and the inertia of institutions than with the acceptability or otherwise of the method to potential consumers. Estimated overall usage varies between less than 10% of married women in Japan through to about 50% in Western Europe.

In several recent surveys, around 95% of sexually active UK women under the age of 30 reported use of oral contraceptives at some time.

5.4 What are the main mechanisms of contraceptive action of the combined pill?

These are summarized in *Table 5.1*. Without exception, all steroidal methods operate by some combination of the mechanisms there described. The COC has a very similar primary action in most women, namely the

TABLE 5.1 Various progestogen delivery systems

	COC	Evra	POP (old type)	DMPA	Cerazette	Implanon
Active component	EE + one of 7 progestogens	Norelgestromin: active metabolite of norgestimate	One of 2 progestogens ('2nd generation')	Medroxyprogesterone acetate	Desogestrel	Etonogestrel: active metabolite of desogestrel
Administration	Oral	Transdermal	Oral	Intramuscular	Oral	Subdermal
Frequency	Daily	7-day patches	Daily	3-monthly	Daily	3-yearly
Estrogen dose	Low	Low	Nil	Nil	Nil	Nil
Progestogen dose	Low	Low	Ultra-low	High	Low	Ultra-low
Blood levels	Daily peaks & troughs	Steady	Daily peaks & troughs	Initial peak then decline	Daily peaks & troughs	Steady
First pass through liver	Yes	No	Yes	No	Yes	No
Major mechanisms						
Ovary: ↓ ovulation	+++	+++	+	+++	+++	+++
Cervical mucus: ↓ sperm penetrability	Yes	Yes	Yes	Yes	Yes	Yes
Minor mechanism						
Endometrium: ↓ receptivity to blastocyst (a weak effect, usually never utilized (see Q 5.4)	Yes	Yes	Yes	Yes	Yes	Yes

TABLE 5.1—cont'd

	COC	Evra	POP (old type)	DMPA	Cerazette	Implanon
Percentage, among consistent/correct users, conceiving in 1st year of use	0.3	0.3	0.3	0.3	<0.2	<0.1
Menstrual pattern	Regular	Regular	Often irregular	Very irregular	Often irregular	Often irregular
Amenorrhoea during use	Rare	Rare	Occasional	Very common	Common	Common
Reversibility						
Immediate termination possible?	Yes	Yes	Yes	No	Yes	Yes
By woman herself at any time?	Yes	Yes	Yes	No	Yes	No
Median time to conception from first omitted dose/removal	c. 3 months	c. 3 months	c. 2 months	c. 6 months	c. 2 months	c. 2 months

Notes:
1 For more details regarding efficacy issues, see *Table 1.2* (p. 14). Regarding Cerazette, see *Q 7.11* and footnote to *Table 7.2*.
2 NuvaRing: when available, this combined contraceptive vaginal ring will have similar features to Evra (see *Q 6.83*).

prevention of ovulation – both by lack of follicular maturation and by abolition of the estrogen-mediated positive feedback that leads to the luteinizing hormone (LH) surge. Of the other mechanisms shown in the table – reduction in sperm penetrability of cervical mucus (*see Q 7.17*) and possibly of the receptivity to the blastocyst of the endometrium – the first, interfering in sperm transport (most probably through the uterine fluids as well), is the prime back-up mechanism for the COC. It is also of great relevance to the effectiveness of the estrogen-free hormonal methods of Chapters 7–9.

The two pre-fertilization mechanisms are so strong in 'perfect users' of the pill that *the weak anti-implantation effect – even if potentially available – should NEVER need to be utilized.* This fact needs stressing to some prospective COC-users, who have an ethical view that would reject any method that might, however rarely, operate post fertilization. For even greater security, an option for them is to 'tricycle' the pill along with a shortened (4-day) pill-free interval (*see Q 5.32*); or even to take the COC continuously on a 365/365 basis (*see Q 5.34*).

5.5 What are the types of COC?

Current COCs are either fixed-dose or phasic; both types contain estrogen and progestogen. The ratio of the two is not fixed, however, but changed in a stepwise fashion, either once (biphasic pills) or twice (triphasic pills) in each 21-day course. They are discussed in more detail below (*see Qs 5.181–5.186*). We should note here, however, that – like all COCs – the phasic types remove the menstrual cycle, but these pills attempt to replace it with cyclical variations, chiefly in the progestogen dose. There is as yet no proof that this has important health benefits (aside, that is, from the giving of a low dose of each hormone).

5.6 What are 'everyday' (ED) varieties of COC? Do they have advantages?

These are regimens that include, usually, 7 days of placebo tablets. They have the advantage of simplicity, a tablet a day for 365 days per year – and a reduction in the risk that the user will fail to restart her next packet on time. This is one of the most common times to miss and a potent cause of pill failure (*see Q 5.19*) especially as so many women do not seek advice for 'late restarting' as they don't see that as missing pills, at all!

For a variety of unscientific reasons, placebo packaging has never been popular in the UK – or in most of Europe. Yet it is the norm in most countries, in all the other continents. Microgynon ED has been available since the UK's first-choice pill Microgynon itself was first marketed, and is at present actually priced slightly cheaper.

For these reasons, my own practice in recent years is to *offer* Microgynon ED as the first-choice product to all new pill starters – or restarters. But no pressure, it's their choice. *See Q 5.8.*

5.7 What are the disadvantages of ED packaging?

- The starting routine in the first cycle can appear slightly complicated (but *see Q 5.8*).
- Some women dislike the implication that they are too unintelligent to remember when to stop and restart treatment.
- Some women think that the dummy lactose (sugar) pills might be fattening or otherwise bad for them! Perhaps the placebos should be made of bran, as everyone knows that bran is good for you!
- More relevantly, but also easily dealt with: if pills are missed in the final week of the 3-week cycle, one has to make it clear that the woman should miss out the seven inactive tablets and go directly to the first active pill of a new pack (*see Q 5.20*).

5.8 If a woman chooses Microgynon ED, what is your way of explaining the starting routine?

I strongly recommend that you obtain and study a packet of this product and its PIL. You will notice that the tablet blisters in each pack are unlabelled, but there is a separate thin card with seven removable stickers bearing the days of the week, each one starting with a different day. Using a first day of period starting routine, the woman is instructed to apply the sticker starting with that day of the week to the top of the pack, beside the first of the three rows of seven active (yellow) tablets and fourth single row of larger white placebos. This establishes the days that each tablet should be taken.

My own practice is to advise the woman to discard all but the Sunday start stickers, applying one to the first pack (and in due course all subsequent packs). In the first cycle, she should take her first active pill on the first Sunday after whatever day her period starts and abstain or use condoms until she has taken seven yellow active tablets – i.e. for a maximum of 13 days.

The advantages of this practice are as follows:

- An easier starting-routine to explain and to understand
- Retaining the primary advantage of never having to stop and restart pill-taking
- Finishing active pills each fourth Saturday means never having a bleed at weekends.

> Even with the non-ED pills, have you ever thought that three out of
> every seven pill-takers are regularly bleeding on at least one night
> during one weekend in four – for the sole reason that (maybe 10
> years earlier) in their starting cycle, their period happened to start on
> a Thursday, Friday or Saturday?! This means, in each packet, their last
> pill being taken on a Wednesday, Thursday or Friday – with bleeding
> starting about 2 days after that.
>
> If this applies, it is extremely easy to shift the bleed: by advising
> the woman (just once) to start her next packet early, on a Sunday or
> a Monday, after a shortened pill-free time (see Qs 5.52, 6.87).

5.9 What modified regimens would you like to see marketed?

■ Given that the pill-free interval (PFI) is 'the Achilles' heel' of the COC's
efficacy, there would be particular merit in returning across the board
to an earlier scheme of 22 active pills with six placebos. Indeed, even
without placebos this might help compliance because the 'finishing day'
is then the same day of the week as the 'starting day'.

■ ED packets of ultra-low-dose monophasic brands with four placebo
tablets are at last beginning to be marketed. With the PFI so shortened,
new products for general use can safely offer even lower doses of both
hormones than are currently viable. Such products (e.g. Minesse or
Meliane Light; other names are on the IPPF website: www.ippf.org.uk)
are already marketed in some countries. Minesse is an effective
anovulant despite containing only 15 µg of ethinylestradiol (EE) plus
60 µg of gestodene, given as 24 tablets followed by just four hormone-
free days.

■ Tricycling (*see* Q 5.32) with a shortened PFI where extra efficacy is
required and 365/365 pill-taking (*see* Q 5.34) are other useful regimens
which either can be constructed by the prescriber or are, increasingly,
being packaged (as in Seasonale, Seasonique and Lybrel).

5.10 What about other estrogen–progestogen agents (especially sequential pills and regimens of HRT)?

High-estrogen sequential pills were shown to double the risk of
endometrial carcinoma and have rightly been consigned to history.

Older women may be given for HRT a similar regimen of estrogen
alone for up to 16 days, followed by estrogen plus progestogen for 12 days.
The estrogen is, of course, a natural estrogen, in doses that have a far
smaller effect on the endometrium. There is evidence that these regimens
do not significantly increase the risk of endometrial cancer, but they are
not safely contraceptive.

The continuous combined HRT regimens (including tibolone) would almost certainly be contraceptive – but are not recommended while there is any residual fertility (only because they might cause irregular bleeding if so used). *See Chapter 11.*

5.11 What link is there between the COC cycle and the menstrual cycle?

Very little, but endless confusion is caused by the fact that women consider their hormone-withdrawal bleeds as the same thing as 'periods'. In reality, of course, the normal menstrual cycle is removed during use of the COC. The ovaries show no follicular activity during pill-taking (contrast the situation between packets, *see Q 5.16*) and hence produce minimal endogenous estrogen. Withdrawal bleeding (WTB) is an end-organ response to withdrawal of the artificial hormones and is irrelevant to events elsewhere in the body, and specifically at the pituitary and the ovaries. In physiological terms, everywhere except at the endometrium, the pill causes secondary amenorrhoea for as long as the woman takes it.

Absence of WTB is totally irrelevant to future fertility, although a pregnancy test is indicated after two WTBs have been missed: sooner if there are good reasons to suspect pill failure. Aside from pregnancy testing, it is pointless to investigate this.

Breakthrough bleeding (BTB) is likewise a purely endometrial response but it might be heavy enough to simulate a 'period' to the woman. This also needs explaining in advance as a reason to continue taking her daily pills with extra diligence (until an early appointment), rather than stopping.

Lack of adequate instruction about WTB and BTB commonly causes avoidable 'iatrogenic' pregnancies (*see Qs 11.13, 11.18*).

5.12 What is the importance of the pill-free interval (PFI)?

Enormous – yet it is still not fully explained in most pill leaflets or by many prescribers. It influences all the following issues:

- The efficacy of the COC, in that lengthening the PFI risks ovulation whereas mid-packet pill omissions are unimportant
- The recommendations once pills are omitted or vomited
- Short- or long-term use of interacting drugs or use of the pill if past 'breakthrough pregnancies' have occurred.

EFFECTIVENESS OF THE COC – CIRCUMSTANCES IN WHICH IT CAN BE REDUCED

5.13 What is the efficacy of the COC?

There is no simple answer to this question because efficacy is so user-dependent. According to Trussell, with 'perfect use' only 0.3% of women in the US will experience a pregnancy during the first year of use, but in 'typical' use he gives an amazingly high figure of 8% (see *Table 1.2*, p. 14).

The 'perfect use' effectiveness approaches (but, because of individual variation in absorption/metabolism, will never reach) 100% – partly because of the adjunctive mechanisms mentioned above (*see Q 5.4*). However, it appears that for some women the modern (less than 50 µg estrogen) pills are only just sufficient for efficacy, particularly if omitted tablets lead to the slightest lengthening of the pill-free week. Minor errors of compliance are extremely common and most pill-takers (through, it has to be said, provider failure) are uninformed about the importance of the pill-free time; or the specific risk of being a 'late restarter' with the next packet after the PFI (*see Qs 5.16–5.29*).

NB: *See Q 6.92* regarding how to minimize the effect of flying through time zones on pill efficacy.

5.14   What is the effect of increasing age on efficacy?

The Oxford/FPA study shows the expected decline in pregnancy rate with increasing age, due mainly to declining fertility and also some reduction in the frequency of intercourse (see *Table 1.2*, columns 4 and 5, and *Q 1.19*). The latter effect does not of course apply to older couples in new relationships, which are becoming more common.

5.15   Are overweight women more likely to conceive while taking modern ultra-low-dose COCs?

Maybe yes; it might be expected intuitively because an 80-kg woman receives exactly the same dose in normal pill-taking as her 40-kg friend. Moreover, there is a definite weight influence on the efficacy of some never-marketed progestogen-only methods (*see Q 7.14*) and also of the skin patch Evra (*see Q 6.81*). However, this has only been shown for the COC in one study [Holt VL et al 2002 *Obstetrics and Gynaecology* 99:820–827]. Using absolute weights, a cut-off of 75 kg was the upper limit beyond which conception risk rose significantly and it doubled at 86 kg. This was for all conceptions – through ALL causes, including missed pills etc. Moreover, the research design was unorthodox, a retrospective cohort study of the controls from a case–control study primarily researching functional ovarian cysts. So whether the finding represents a true risk for 'perfect users' – due to increased metabolism or more likely a dilution effect (of the same dose in a larger volume of body water) – remains to be confirmed.

Clinical implications

■ The combined pill is contraceptively such a strong anovulant, along with its back-up actions especially on the cervical mucus, that in practice it usually has sufficient margin to cope with women of any weight. This is believed to be the case also with Cerazette (*see Qs 7.15, 7.16*).

■ Other factors like 'late restarting' will affect efficacy far more (relatively) than body mass.

■ Given the obesity epidemic in western countries, this paper (pending confirmation) lends weight to NOT offering the COC at all to very overweight women, now because of added uncertainty about efficacy on top of the established circulatory reasons. If she were of average UK height (1.63 m), the BMI of the 86-kg woman in Holt's study with doubled overall failure rate would be 32.5. As we shall note later (*Q 5.122*) a BMI of 30–39 is classified WHO 3 for the COC because of VTE risk – and this *always* implies first discussing an alternative option to the requested method.

5.16 As it is the contraceptive-free part of the pill-taking cycle, does the PFI have efficacy implications?

When you think about it, we have here a bizarre contraceptive: one that we providers actually instruct the users not to use – for 25% of the time. See *Fig. 5.1*. Any systemic contraceptive must be at its lowest ebb when it is longest since it was actually ingested. Hardly surprisingly, biochemical and ultrasound data demonstrate varying degrees of return of pituitary and ovarian follicular activity during the PFI.

Fig. 5.2 shows the findings from a 1979 study based on patients attending the Margaret Pyke Centre. It is the rapid and sustained decline in the artificial hormones at the start of the PFI (top half of *Fig. 5.2*) that leads to the WTB. More importantly in this context, the figure shows the resulting slight average increase in (natural) estradiol, implying regular return of ovarian follicular activity during the pill-free week. Wide standard deviations are also shown, meaning that in a subgroup the levels are high – indeed, as high as has been observed well into the follicular phase of spontaneous menstrual cycles.

In a further study by the Margaret Pyke Centre, apparently preovulatory-type follicles of diameter 10 mm or more were present on the seventh pill-free day in 23% of 120 pill-takers; in three women the follicle was 16–19 mm in diameter (i.e. potentially only 1–2 days from fertile ovulation). In the other women there was no important change, suggesting continuing quiescence of their ovaries.

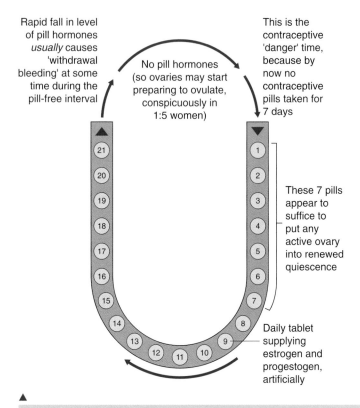

Rapid fall in level of pill hormones *usually* causes 'withdrawal bleeding' at some time during the pill-free interval

No pill hormones (so ovaries may start preparing to ovulate, conspicuously in 1:5 women)

This is the contraceptive 'danger' time, because by now no contraceptive pills taken for 7 days

These 7 pills appear to suffice to put any active ovary into renewed quiescence

Daily tablet supplying estrogen and progestogen, artificially

Fig. 5.1 The pill cycle displayed as a horseshoe. *Q 5.16. Note:* a horseshoe is a symmetrical object and thus the pill-free interval (PFI) can be lengthened (resulting in the risk of conception) either side of the horseshoe – by forgetting pills at the beginning or at the end of the packet. See also *Fig. 5.4* (and *Qs 5.31, 5.32, 5.34*) with respect to the issue of patient choice: arranging to have far fewer PFIs and therefore bleeds.

However, for the purpose of maintaining contraception we have to be concerned about the extreme cases. Among them, breakthrough ovulation is most likely to follow any lengthening of the PFI. Most important, such lengthening can result from the following, involving pills *either at the start or at the end of a packet*:

■ omissions
■ malabsorption due to vomiting (an advantage of the new non-oral combined products Evra and NuvaRing)
■ relevant drug interaction.

The pill-free week

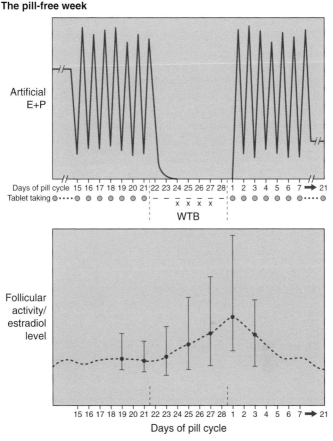

▲

Fig. 5.2 The hormone changes of the pill-free week. *Q 5.16.* Changes through the pill-taking cycle in the blood levels of both the ingested artificial hormones (estrogen (E) and progestogen (P)) and in follicular activity as demonstrated by growth of the dominant follicle by ultrasound. Note the rapid return to low ovarian activity during the first 7 days of pill-taking. The bottom half of the figure is from a study of patients attending the Margaret Pyke Centre. WTB, withdrawal bleeding.

See the legend to *Fig. 5.1*: pill-taking is depicted as a horseshoe because a horseshoe is a symmetrical object whose 'gap' can be enlarged either side.

Clearly, the old advice that is still sometimes given to a woman – to take extra precautions to the end of her packet – is wrong: it fails to allow for ovarian activity returning in the pill-free time.

5.17 So how would you summarize the scientific basis of the advice we should give a woman who has missed pills for any reason?

In 1986, in a fascinating study of previously regular pill-takers [Smith SK et al *Contraception* 34:513–522] it was shown that if only 14, or even as few as seven, pills had been taken since the last PFI, no women ovulated after seven pills were subsequently missed! (One woman in the seven-pills-then-seven-missed-pills group got very close, producing progesterone – albeit at non-fertile levels.) This and much other work was comprehensively reviewed in 1995 [Korver T et al *British Journal of Obstetrics and Gynaecology* 102:601–607], and more recently by the WHO *Selected Practice Recommendations for Contraceptive Use* (WHOSPR) and the UK Faculty of Sexual and Reproductive Healthcare.

Though there is continuing disagreement between authorities as to the best wording of advice for pill-takers in the UK context, everyone appears to accept the following summary propositions:

- Seven consecutive pills are enough to 'shut the door' on the ovaries.
- Thereafter, pills 8–21 in a packet, or many more if the woman tricycles, simply maintain the ovaries in quiescence ('keep the door shut').
- Seven pills can be omitted without ovulation, as indeed is regularly the case in the pill-free week.
- More than seven pills missed (in total) risks ovulation.

5.18 So what do you now (2008) recommend for missed COCs?

Fig. 5.3 and the Box on page 122 answer this question. It has to be a personal answer since the recommendations keep changing!

In my view it is very unfortunate that the latest (2005) WHOSPR – on which Faculty (UKMEC) and fpa leaflet advice is based – issued instructions (against my advice) which differ according to the estrogen dose in the particular pill. I argue this is illogical, given that individual variation in blood levels and response to contraceptive hormones is so great. Even with the 30–35-µg brands, ovulation has been demonstrated occasionally if the PFI is lengthened to only 8 or 9 days [Guillebaud J 2005 *Journal of Family Planning and Reproductive Health Care* 31:252].

Therefore we should use a simple-to-explain single set of instructions that err on the side of caution. Based on WHO's ≤20-µg pill advice we should give the same advice regardless of the formulation – to cater for those (unknown) individuals who are regularly most close-to-ovulating.

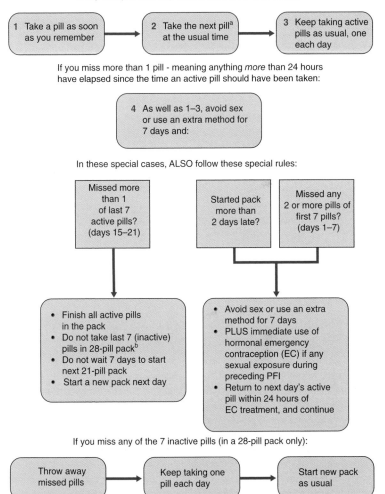

Every time you miss any one pill (late by up to 24 hours):

1 Take a pill as soon as you remember → 2 Take the next pill[a] at the usual time → 3 Keep taking active pills as usual, one each day

If you miss more than 1 pill - meaning anything *more* than 24 hours have elapsed since the time an active pill should have been taken:

4 As well as 1–3, avoid sex or use an extra method for 7 days and:

In these special cases, ALSO follow these special rules:

Missed more than 1 of last 7 active pills? (days 15–21)

Started pack more than 2 days late?

Missed any 2 or more pills of first 7 pills? (days 1–7)

- Finish all active pills in the pack
- Do not take last 7 (inactive) pills in 28-pill pack[b]
- Do not wait 7 days to start next 21-pill pack
- Start a new pack next day

- Avoid sex or use an extra method for 7 days
- PLUS immediate use of hormonal emergency contraception (EC) if any sexual exposure during preceding PFI
- Return to next day's active pill within 24 hours of EC treatment, and continue

If you miss any of the 7 inactive pills (in a 28-pill pack only):

Throw away missed pills → Keep taking one pill each day → Start new pack as usual

Fig. 5.3 What to do if you miss one or more pills. *Q 5.18ff* (from Informa Healthcare).
[a]This can mean taking two pills at once, both when you would normally take the second. (But if it is any later, see the 'more than 1 pill' advice)
[b]28-pill (ED) packs can obviously help some pill-takers not to forget to restart after each PFI (the contraception-losing interval). Even with triphasic pills, you should go straight to (the first phase of) the same brand. You may bleed a bit but you will still strengthen your contraception.

Summary of instructions for 'missed pills'

1 'ONE tablet up to 24 h late': aside from taking the delayed pill and the next one on time, *no special action* is needed. This applies up to the time that two tablets would need to be taken at once, 'to catch up'.
'ANYTHING MORE THAN ONE tablet missed' (i.e. a second tablet is also late, by ≥1 h): *use CONDOMS as well, for the next 7 days*

Plus (*i.e. as well*)

2 If this happened **in the third active pill-week,** *at the end of pack RUN ON to the next pack (skipping seven placebos if present)*

And (*as well as the condom advice*):

3 **In the first pill week,** EMERGENCY CONTRACEPTION *is usually advisable* IF, with sexual exposure since the last pack, the COC-user:

■ is a '*late restarter*' by more than 2 days (9-day PFI) or more than two of pills 1–7 are missed, or

■ she had a >9-day PFI through missed pills at *end of last pack*.
This should be followed, next day, by taking the appropriate day's tablet and continuing her pack to its end.

Finally, all women should be asked to return for the exclusion of pregnancy if they have no bleeding in the *next* PFI.

Note in this Box that the definition of what constitutes 'missed pill(s)' has changed (i.e. the trigger for the pill-taker – or rather now non-taker! – to take a specified action other than just getting back to pill-taking). The WHO Scientific Working Group (WHOSPR) judged from available data in 2001 that the number of women who might conceive by a less demanding definition – away from the previous 'more than 12 h late' – would be negligible.

Note too that in 'late restarters' or those missing any two or more pills in the first week, the 7 days of added contraception are logical in view of the first bulleted point in the Box in Q 5.17. This is because if there is already some follicular activity – which applies (almost) only at *the start of the packet after the PFI* and then only to just around one-fifth to one-quarter (23%) of a pill-taking population – seven tablets seem to be capable of putting any ovary back into a quiescent state. Moreover, if it has been too late to stop ovulation, this is likely to occur during the same 7 days of condom use: therefore hopefully without conception, as after ovulation the egg quickly ceases to be fertilizable.

5.19 **It is easy to see from *Figs 5.1* and *5.2* that missing pills at the start of a packet, lengthening the contraception-losing time to more than 7 days, could well be 'bad news', but what about omitted pills in the middle of a packet?**

Tablets *omitted following on prior tablet-taking for 7 or more days*, and not followed by a PFI, are very low risk omissions for breakthrough ovulation. Once seven tablets have been taken, many pills may be missed mid-packet with impunity (the Smith study quoted in *Q 5.17* suggests up to *seven!*).

The condom advice above in *Q 5.18* and *Fig. 5.3* is actually unnecessary for both pill-days 8–14 and, actually, for days 15–21 as well *(see Q 5.20)*. WHO and UKMEC and the fpa are united in the view that it is preferable to make this a 'blanket' instruction, rather than focusing it where it is truly relevant (days 1–7).

Unless we prescribers re-educate them, patients worry most about missed pills when it matters least, as their initial thought is bound to be that the 'worst' pills to miss would be in the middle of a packet (i.e. they use the wrong analogy with the middle of a normal cycle). ALL prospective COC-users deserve some simple teaching about this (*Q 5.22*). Otherwise the present unsatisfactory situation will just continue, in which they will rarely even seek advice when pill omissions or a stomach upset have led to a lengthening of the pill-free time, or (at the end of a pack) will now be going on to lead to a similar lengthening.

A 'triple whammy'

In summary, being a 'late restarter', which is timing one's missed pills to be the first after the PFI, is:

- ■ The time that it is MOST RISKY to miss pills (affecting BOTH ovulation risk and the mucus effect, *see Q 5.27*)
- ■ The time that it is, in practice, MOST COMMON to miss pills *and*
- ■ The time when it is SO OFTEN UNRECOGNIZED by users that pills early in the next pack ARE missed pills at all: 'I just started my pack a bit late!' Moreover, women are *falsely* reassured by their maybe ongoing hormone-withdrawal bleed. . . .

5.20 **What are the implications of late-packet pill omissions?**

If a woman omits a number of tablets in the last week of her preceding packet and simply recommences the next packet on her *usual* starting day (something she is sure to do, unless otherwise instructed), there will be an ovulation risk at the end of the thereby lengthened pill-free time, after what is a falsely reassuring withdrawal bleed. She will doubtless remember, as many do, to use condoms for the next 7 days, but on its own that advice is almost useless. If you think about it, *she will stop using condoms just as she is on the point of ovulating!*

Indeed, if she missed active pills in the last week and it has already happened that she followed this by her usual PFI, during which she has had unprotected sex, this would indicate emergency contraception plus the usual 7 days of an additional method. See end of Box in Q 5.17. And, interestingly, if she is not seen until MUCH later, perhaps in the antenatal clinic, any questioning about missed pills must include asking about tablets she might have missed *before* the last 'menstrual period' (LMP).

If she is properly taught, however, and follows the scheme in *Fig. 5.3*, going straight on to the next packet (or missing the seven white placebos with Microgynon ED), she will actually be more protected than usual, due to having a shorter PFI than the usual 7 days! So, for her, emergency contraception is never indicated: even if she missed the lot, all seven pills allocated to days 15–21.

5.21 Should this advice for late tablet omissions (*Q 5.20*) be different if the woman is on a triphasic pill brand?

No; at the end of the packet she should start immediately with the first-phase (lower-dose) tablets (*see 5.176–5.181*). She will probably have a 'withdrawal-type' bleed, but contraceptive efficacy will nevertheless still be increased. This is a different situation from postponing 'periods' as described at Q 5.181.

5.22 Clearly it would be better if there emerged a new generation of pill-takers who understood this pill physiology ahead of time!

And it could happen, with our help as providers. In my opinion, every new pill-taker has the right to know the basics of the 'contraception-losing' PFI, which I find takes no more than 4–5 min to explain in lay terms, based on *Fig. 5.1*, the horseshoe image. See Box below.

Explaining 'missed pills' advice

- Would you expect your pill to still work well when you haven't taken it – or have taken 'blanks' – for a whole 7 days? *(No).* Yet we tell you to do that!
- Some women (one in five, and we can't be sure you're not one of them) have an ovary that is close to 'waking up' just before the first active (day 1) pill is swallowed. Not a problem though, if you DO start your next pack on the dot and so put your ovary back to sleep.

■ You can have sex any time, so long as you DON'T start your next packet late. Your 'safety' in the days between packs depends on your *next* packet being started on time. So, by the way: make a note for the future that if you ever take a break from the pill you are NOT safe for any days, certainly not 7 days, before you have to start to use condoms – see no. 18 within Q *11.17*.

■ If one day you are late restarting, your 'period' may just have happened, but in pill-takers that's not reassuring, it's got nothing to do with when egg release might happen.

■ All in all, here's a good thing for you to keep saying over to yourself as a kind of 'mantra', if you like, now you're on the pill:

'I must never be a "late-restarter" . . . I must never be a "late-restarter". . . I must . . .'

■ Now, suppose you missed pills or had a bad stomach upset for days near the end of a packet. This would be like letting your ovary start waking up early, wouldn't it? *(Yes)*. So wouldn't it be a bit silly to add on the regular pill-free break on top? *(Yes)*. So that's why we say you should skip the white sugar pills and start your first active pill straight after the last one.

Let's face it, current advice regarding missed pills seems a bit strange to most users, especially the 'run on' component. However, when this bit of simple explaining in the Box is done (whether by a nurse or a doctor), in my experience, missed-pills advice becomes understandable and remembering it and complying with it much more probable.

5.23 What if the pill-taker has actually or effectively missed five or more pills?

It might be worth asking her the question (in addition to sorting her immediate problems) whether, after missing that many pills, she considers that she is really a (suitable person to be a) pill-taker! It is very logical to offer her one of the 'more forgettable' LARCs (long-acting reversible contraceptives) in future, such as an implant or IUD/IUS.

As explained above (Qs *5.17*, *5.20*), once seven tablets are 'on board', there is evidence that seven tablets can be missed with impunity. However, those who forget so many pills may also have forgotten that they have also forgotten other ones recently! Though probably actually needed only in very rare cases, if five or more pills really are omitted in mid-packet (pill days 8–14) it will do no harm to advise:

■ hormonal emergency contraception and

■ for the next 7 days to use an additional method, such as condoms, and

- to restart pill-taking 'today' with a brand new packet of pills, maybe of the ED kind (*Q 5.6ff*), and in future (if not – preferably! – switching to an LARC)
- to set her mobile phone reminder alarm for each daily pill!

5.24 What other now outdated 'rules' for missed pills are there that a pill-taker might have read or been taught?

- The 'take precautions from now to the end-of-packet' rule is probably commonest and is delightfully *simple*; but sadly (*see Q 5.20*) it is also dangerously *wrong* for missed pills near the end of a pack.
- The 'take precautions for the next 14 days, whatever happens' advice is acceptable; since the *second 7* days of the fortnight does cover the time of ovulation risk at the end of a PFI that has been lengthened by missed pills just before it (i.e. near the end of a pack). But because it is so counterintuitive, many men as well as women see use of the unpopular sheath method as pointless, especially just after what they (falsely) see as a reassuring 'period'.

We however know that the ovary can be ovulating in synchrony with the endometrium bleeding, since that happens only because of exogenous hormone withdrawal.

5.25 What about emergency contraception for the *extremely* late pill restarter who is continuing to be sexually active?

To minimize the chance of disturbing an implanted pregnancy, which in present UK law is only legal if the terms of the Abortion Act are complied with, my view is that (with continuing sexual exposure) any intervention should perhaps not normally be later than day 14 of any such greatly lengthened PFI: i.e. after a week of missed pills, which could of course have happened either before or after it. This calculation assumes that the very earliest likely ovulation might occur after 9 completed days that are pill-free, to which are added 5 days for the usual expected interval between ovulation/fertilization and implantation. Copper IUD insertion would be the preferred method of emergency contraception in such a case (*see Chapter 10*).

But the main message from this section, *Qs 5.13–5.25*, is that for almost all mid-packet and late-packet (days 8–21) pill omissions, postcoital treatment would be over-treatment.

5.26 What advice for vomiting and diarrhoea?

If vomiting began over 2 h after a pill was taken, it can be assumed to have been absorbed. If it started less than 2 h after a pill was swallowed, another active tablet should be taken. If the replacement tablet (e.g. taken in emergency from the end of a pack) and a second one 25–26 h or more later both fail to stay down – i.e. once more than one pill has been effectively missed, as defined in Q 5.18 – the actions described in Fig 5.3 should be triggered, depending as usual on the phase of the pill cycle.

In a long illness with vomiting of consecutive pills sufficient to produce lengthening of the PFI, extra contraceptive precautions should be continued for 7 days after it ends; if a subsequent PFI would be lengthened by the tablets 'missed', it should be omitted, once again as indicated by Fig. 5.3. Warn that BTB is now likely.

NB: Diarrhoea alone is not a problem, unless it is of cholera-like severity!

5.27 Surely the above discussion of the PFI takes too little account of the adjunctive contraceptive effects (see Q 5.4)?

Actually, these do not change the argument about the PFI. The most important extra effect is probably the progestogenic reduction in sperm penetrability of cervical mucus. But this too will be at its lowest ebb at the end of any PFI which has been lengthened: obviously, since it is then as long as is possible since progestogen was last ingested.

Once tablet taking is resumed, however, the pills in the next pack should be able to operate usefully, both by the mucus effect and by their anti-implantation effect on the endometrium.

5.28 Pending the marketing of packets with a shortened PFI, what is the best regimen for women who have had a previous combined-pill failure?

Some of these women claim perfect compliance but most will admit to the complete omission of no more than one pill. Most women admit to missing tablets from time to time (in one NOP survey the modal number missed per year was eight!), yet very few conceive. One can therefore argue that the ability to do so after missing only one tablet selects out those who are likely to have ovaries with above average return to activity in the PFI.

Therefore, all women in this group should, in my view, be advised to take two or more packets in a row, the so-called bicycle or tricycle regimens (see Q 5.32 and Fig. 5.4), followed by a shortened PFI. Often 6 days is a good choice in these cases because it is easy to remember, with each PFI start-day now being identical to the finish-day – but the gap can be shortened even further in a 'high-risk' case (see Q 5.38, also Q 5.34).

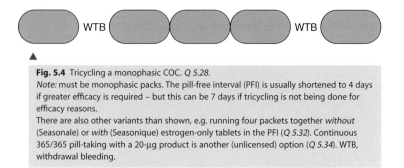

▲

Fig. 5.4 Tricycling a monophasic COC. *Q 5.28.*
Note: must be monophasic packs. The pill-free interval (PFI) is usually shortened to 4 days if greater efficacy is required – but this can be 7 days if tricycling is not being done for efficacy reasons.
There are also other variants than shown, e.g. running four packets together *without* (Seasonale) or *with* (Seasonique) estrogen-only tablets in the PFI (*Q 5.32*). Continuous 365/365 pill-taking with a 20-µg product is another (unlicensed) option (*Q 5.34*). WTB, withdrawal bleeding.

Tricycling or continuous 365/365 pill-taking (*see 5.34*) is surely more logical than the reaction of many doctors after a woman conceives on the pill, a summary of which is 'read her the Riot Act about better pill-taking and give her the same one as before'! Even giving her a stronger formulation might be of less relevance than eliminating plus shortening the PFIs.

5.29   Aren't there other disadvantages to taking a PFI?

Yes: in summary, the 'cons' of the PFI are:

■ It makes the COC method less effective.
■ The withdrawal bleeds can be heavy/painful; or even when not so are increasingly perceived, by many women now, as an avoidable nuisance.
■ In some women, migraines or other types of headache occur during the PFI, triggered by hormone withdrawal.
■ On theoretical grounds, compared with the normal cycle, it is 'unphysiological' to have a whole week with almost no estrogen circulating (in the majority with quiescent ovaries, that is, not the 23% who start producing their own).

5.30   With all these snags, why do we continue to recommend the PFI to anyone?

Because one can list quite a few potential 'pros' of the PFI as well, though most of them are theoretical:

■ Many women like monthly bleeds to reassure 'that all is normal', and that they are not pregnant, more frequently than every 10–13 weeks or longer. Others just hate the bleeding, however, and explaining pill physiology can overcome this objection in cases where continuous use is indicated or preferred.
■ Avoids the complaint of bloatedness, which some experience through the last weeks of an extended cycle.

■ Can avoid the breakthrough spotting that sometimes occurs, especially during the last packet of a tricycle sequence.

■ Tricycle regimens do entail taking more tablets per year: 15–16 packets rather than the 13 when a regular PFI is taken. This increase in the hormone dose taken runs counter to the general philosophy of giving the lowest dose of both hormones for the desired effect of contraception. Yet there is no increase in annual dose if an exceptionally low-dose brand pill is substituted for a 30-μg brand (*see Q 5.34*).

■ One has to remember that all data generated from epidemiological studies about the (great) safety and the (remarkable) reversibility of the COC have been gained from women who were taking regular monthly breaks.

■ In one study, high-density lipoprotein–cholesterol (HDL-C) suppression (*see Q 5.100*) by the COC brand in use was restored towards normal by the end of the PFI. In a major RCT now being analysed at the Margaret Pyke Centre, this phenomenon has been confirmed for other important substances, including coagulation factors. No one knows whether this is an important safety feature, it is entirely theoretical.

5.31 What do you conclude, given the advantages of the PFI?

■ First, it can be useful to point out to a woman who actually wants to continue with the method but 'someone has suggested' that she ought to 'take a break' from the pill after (say) 10 years' use, that she has already taken 130 breaks. Or, put another way, she has really only taken it for $7^1/_2$ years!

■ Secondly, most women will still probably prefer not to cut out the gap between packets unless there are indications – although one of these can certainly be the woman's own choice (*Table 5.2*). In the short term this can be done upon request if the woman wishes to avoid a 'period' on a special occasion like her honeymoon (*see Q 5.186* and *Fig. 5.15* for the procedure if a phasic brand is in use).

There are also longer-term indications for eliminating the PFI, as in *Table 5.2* and *Q 5.32*.

5.32 When is the tricycle pill regimen (or one of its variants) indicated? And what are Seasonale and Seasonique?

The regimen has nothing to do with triphasic pills. Indeed, it necessitates use of monophasic pills, which are simply run together – three or four packets in a row – followed by a PFI of the selected length (7 days, or less if the indication is to increase the efficacy of the method) (see *Fig. 5.4*).

Seasonale is a brand in the USA that uses dedicated packaging to provide four packets of the exact equivalent of Microgynon 30 in a row

---

TABLE 5.2 Indications for the tricycle regimen or one of its variants, using a monophasic pill

1 At the woman's choice
2 Headaches, including migraine with non-focal aura, and other bothersome symptoms occurring regularly in the withdrawal week (see Q 5.29)
3 Unacceptable heavy or painful withdrawal bleeds
4 Paradoxically, to help women who are concerned about absent withdrawal bleeds (this concern and the nuisance of pregnancy testing therefore arising less often!)
5 Premenstrual syndrome – tricycling can help if COCs used to treat PMS
6 Endometriosis: a progestogen-dominant monophasic pill can be tricycled, for maintenance treatment after primary therapy
7 Epilepsy: this condition benefits from relatively more sustained levels of the administered hormones (see *box at Q 5.38*), and moreover is often treated with an enzyme-inducer see (8)
8 Any enzyme-inducer therapy
9 Suspicion of decreased efficacy (see Q 5.28) for any other reason

---

Notes:
1 This modified pill-taking usually means more hormone is ingested per year, so one of these indications should normally apply. However, if a 20-μg brand is used (even absolutely continuously, see Q 5.34) this is less estrogen per year than a 30-μg product taken along with the usual pill-free intervals (PFIs). See also *Appendix A* 'named-patient use' because so far none of the continuous regimens are licensed for long-term use.
2 During tricycling, in circumstances (8) and (9) in the table the PFI after every three (or four) packets should be *shortened*, usually to 4 days. For none of the other indications is there a special need to shorten any PFIs that are taken.

---

followed by a 7-day PFI. Seasonique provides 10 μg of EE in the 3-monthly pill-free week but is otherwise identical. Both are intended to produce four WTBs per year, i.e. seasonally! If, as intended, they come to the UK, many women will welcome this choice, provided they also accept the implications of three extra packets of hormone per year. If the indication is pill-withdrawal headaches, they should get only four bad headaches per year – instead of the usual 13! *Table 5.2* summarizes the indications for tricycling.

5.33 What is the significance of BTB or spotting after the first pack during 'tricycling'? And how may it be managed?

If it occurs during the second or third packet in a woman who had no BTB problems with 21-day pill-taking, and if none of the explanations in *Table 5.15 (see Q 5.170)* applies, then it is most likely to be an 'end-organ' effect. In other words, the current formulation is proving to be incapable of maintaining this woman's endometrium beyond a certain duration of continuous pill-taking, i.e. without the 'physiological curettage' of a WTB. Although we lack data, it is my belief that this type of BTB – in the course of *continuous* pill-taking of three to four packs (or more, *see Q 5.34*) – is less likely to be due to low blood levels of the contraceptive steroids than when they are taken cyclically and BTB occurs on the 'wrong days'. The latter is discussed in *Qs 5.163–5.178*.

Therefore, the first step, if this is a problem to the woman, is to try a shorter continuous sequence of pills, e.g. by 'bicycling' (two packets in a row) – rather than to use a stronger pill. Another option during annoyingly prolonged BTB is to simply take a bleeding-triggered pill-free break of 3–7 days and restart. This is always contraceptively safe, provided at least seven pills have been taken since the last PFI.

5.34 Why have any PFIs at all? How about totally continuous 365/365 combined-pill-taking?

There have been promising studies of this in the USA using 20-μg EE pills, specifically Loette (EE 20 μg with levonorgestrel 100 μg, a formulation that might be called 'Microgynon 20' if it were marketed in the UK), but also with our existing Loestrin 20 (see *Table 5.13*, p. 208). With either formulation, the tablets were taken every day for up to a year with no periodic breaks at all. Counter-intuitively for such low doses, the studies [Miller L et al 2003 *Obstetrics and Gynecology* 101:653–661 and Edelman A et al 2006 *Obstetrics and Gynecology* 107:657–665] demonstrated very acceptable bleeding patterns for most users. In Miller's randomized comparison with 'Microgynon 20' taken in the usual 21/7 manner, irregular spotting (usually, rather than bleeding) was common in early cycles, but in 88% of the continuous-user group bleeding had ceased by 12 cycles.

Reassuringly, since 20-μg formulations are used, this continuous regimen means that *less* artificial estrogen is taken per completed year (a total of 7.3 mg) than with Microgynon 30 or Loestrin 30 taken the ordinary way (total 8.19 mg).

Lybrel (licensed packaging of a product very similar to Loette, namely EE 20 μg with levonorgestrel 90 μg taken continuously 365/365) is already marketed in some countries and expected shortly in the UK, though probably with a different name. Therefore, even now, *on a 'named-patient' basis* (see *Appendix A*), patients who wish to do so may try taking continuously the UK-marketed product Loestrin 20 or indeed one of the other 20-μg COCs. See Boxes on facing page for more details.

We shall certainly be hearing more in future about this approach to correcting the 'mistake' made by the early researchers of the pill (*see Q 5.2*).

Likely advantages of 365/365 pill-taking with a ≤20-μg COC

■ For most women there would be fewer total days, though occurring more erratically, of bleeding or spotting per year: a convenience advantage for many, but the unpredictability would put off some

■ More days likely to be available for sex . . .

■ *Greater* efficacy despite low doses, because there are no 'contraceptively dangerous' pill-free intervals at all, along with complete elimination of the 'triple whammy' of Q 5.19

■ If pills missed, much less confusing 'rules', which would very rarely be needed (see Box below)

■ Fewer cyclical symptoms, including:
  – premenstrual syndrome (minimized by the steadier hormone levels)
  – headaches, which so commonly occur in the pill-free interval
  – 'functional cysts'

■ Expected maintenance or improvement in non-contraceptive benefits, e.g.:
  – cancers of ovary and endometrium
  – endometriosis
  – less anaemia

Practical aspects of 365/365 pill-taking with a ≤20-μg COC

■ Suitable for women for whom the COC is not contraindicated and who after discussion want the advantages in the above Box. This might well include teenagers because of the simplicity of the regimen and the expected greater efficacy

■ They should understand that very unpredictable bleeding and particularly spotting is common and could take more than 6 months to settle: usually to nil, or just occasional spotting, but in the Miller (2003) trial above there was also a subset of about 18% who dropped out for unacceptable bleeding

■ Balancing that, what they will NOT get of course each year is 39 days or more of 'scheduled' predictable bleeding for which some sanitary protection would likely be required (occurring for about 3 days every cycle for 13 cycles)

■ They should also know that if there should be an episode of bleeding/spotting that lasts much longer than desired, it will usually help to then take a pill-free break of between 3 and 7 days (*see* Q 5.33). This 'tailored' pill-taking depends on what might be seen as having a periodic 'pharmacological curettage' (*see* Q 8.47)

Missed pills: with any 20-μg pill used continuously, the simple advice to use condoms for 7 days would only be triggered if the user had omitted seven pills! (After all, once continuous pill-taking is established, i.e. after the first seven tablets, the slogan on p. 120 means that as many as seven tablets may be missed with impunity.) This might change to, say, five tablets if <20-μg EE products are marketed

DRUG INTERACTIONS AFFECTING THE COC

5.35 What is the enterohepatic cycle?

After pill ingestion, the progestogens are 80–100% bioavailable from the upper small bowel, but EE is subject to extensive 'first-pass' metabolism, chiefly by being conjugated with sulphate in the gut wall (*Fig. 5.5*). After absorption, the artificial estrogen and progestogen are carried in the hepatic portal vein to the liver. Liver metabolism then or later (after the steroids have been transported around the body) creates metabolites of both steroids. The liver mostly forms glucuronides. Once these conjugates re-enter the lumen of the bowel, the bowel flora (chiefly *Clostridium*

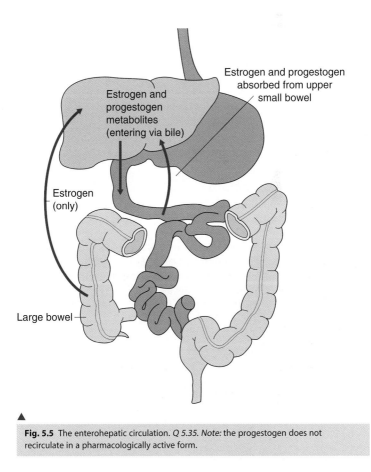

Fig. 5.5 The enterohepatic circulation. *Q 5.35. Note:* the progestogen does not recirculate in a pharmacologically active form.

species) remove the sulphate and glucuronide groups. This restores some EE for reabsorption and, in some women, can help to maintain its level in the circulation.

However, in the case of all the artificial progestogens in current use, the progestogenic metabolite that is reabsorbed after the action of the bowel organisms is biologically inactive. This has the important implication that non-enzyme-inducing antibiotics can have no effect on the efficacy of the progestogen-only pill (POP) or indeed any progestogen-only method.

Moreover, according to researchers in Liverpool, both studies in women with an ileostomy and formal studies with antibiotics suggest that, in the vast majority of COC-takers, even the recycling of the estrogen seems to be unimportant for maintaining efficacy. There is some detectable reduction of the area under the curve (AUC) for EE in a few women when antibiotics are co-administered, but ovulation has not been shown. It is generally agreed, however, that because we do not know which few individuals might be affected by any antibiotics that destroy the relevant bowel flora, it is medico-legally best to play safe, as described in *Q 5.37*.

5.36 What is the effect on pill efficacy of drug interactions linked with the enterohepatic cycle?

These can reduce the pill's efficacy in two main ways, both related to the pharmacology of *Fig. 5.5*:

1 The first and by far the more important mechanism is by **induction of liver enzymes,** which leads to increased metabolism and thus elimination in the bile of both estrogen and progestogen. Various drugs are involved, as detailed in *Table 5.3*. The main ones of clinical importance are rifampicin and its relatives, some antiretroviral drugs used in the treatment of HIV, griseofulvin and a number of antiepileptic drugs. Among the latter, note that valproate, clonazepam, clobazam and all other relatively recent antiepileptics (except for topiramate in dosage above 200 mg daily) are *not* enzyme-inducers.

2 Alternatively, **disturbance by antibiotics of the gut flora** that normally split estrogen metabolites arriving in the bowel can reduce the reabsorption of reactivated estrogen in a very small (but unknown) minority of women. Note the following:

   (a) This problem does not relate to any of the drugs used to prevent or treat malaria, except one – doxycycline – which has recently acquired that indication; nor (probably) to trimethoprim; nor, certainly, because they actually somewhat *inhibit* hepatic metabolism, to co-trimoxazole, sulfonamides and erythromycin (*Table 5.3*).

   (b) The effect applies only to short-term antibiotic treatment or, in long-term therapy, at the time of change to a new antibiotic. This is

TABLE 5.3 The more important drug interactions affecting blood levels of oral contraceptives

Class of drug	Approved names	Main action	Clinical implications for COC use
Drug that can reduce COC efficacy			
Anticonvulsants	Barbiturates (esp. phenobarbital) phenytoin, primidone, carbamazepine, oxcarbazepine, topiramate (≥200 mg daily)	Induction of liver enzymes, increasing their ability to metabolize *both* COC steroids	DMPA or LNG-IUS preferred. Otherwise tricycling with shortened PFI using 50 μg or 60 μg estrogen (2 tablets). *Sodium valproate, vigabatrin, lamotrigine* and *clonazepam* are among anticonvulsants *without* this effect (see Q 5.36)
Other drugs			
(a) Antitubercle	Rifamycins (e.g. rifampicin, rifabutin)	Marked induction of liver enzymes	Short term, see text Long term, use of alternative contraception is advised e.g. DMPA (see Q 8.11) or LNG-IUS
(b) Antifungal	Griseofulvin Ritonavir, nevirapine, and others	Induction of liver enzymes	As for anticonvulsants
(c) Most protease inhibitors and other antiretroviral agents		Induction of liver enzymes	Do not use COCs – DMPA or LNG-IUS are often good choice (+ continuing use of condoms). For all antiretroviral drugs, details available from www.hiv-druginteractions.org
(d) Miscellaneous	Tacrolimus, modafinil	Induction of liver enzymes	As for anticonvulsants
(e) Other antibiotics	For simplicity, act as if all antimicrobials might (rarely) cause this problem – except those in text at (2) in Q 5.36	Change in bowel flora, reducing enterohepatic recirculation of ethinylestradiol (EE) only, after hydrolysis of its conjugates	Short courses – see Q 5.37 Long-term low-dose tetracycline for acne – no apparent problem, probably because resistant organisms develop, within about 2 weeks. POP is unaffected by this type of interaction NB: doxycycline now in use as antimalarial prophylaxis

TABLE 5.3—cont'd

Class of drug	Approved names	Main action	Clinical implications for COC use
Drugs that can increase COC blood levels			
	Paracetamol	Competition in bowel wall for conjugation to sulphate. Therefore, possibly more EE available for absorption	No effect on the progestogen. Advise: at least 2 h separation of the analgesic from the time of pill-taking. Similar advice applies for the ingestion of grapefruit juice (see Q 5.45)
	Co-trimoxazole	Inhibits (weakly) EE metabolism in liver	None, if short course given to user of low-dose COC
	Erythromycin, ketoconazole	Potent inhibitors of EE metabolism	See Q 5.36

Notes:

1 St John's Wort, widely used as 'Nature's Prozac', is an enzyme-inducer. Because its potency in different batches is marked and can vary up to 50-fold, it is unsuitable for use by COC- or POP-takers (CSM warning notice issued). However, it might be being taken by a woman requesting emergency contraception, see Q 11.30.

2 Tretinoin, isotretinoin, miconazole and lansoprazole, despite rumours to the contrary, do not pose a clinical problem.

3 See Q 5.46 for interactions potentially altering actions of other drugs.

because the bowel flora rapidly develop antibiotic resistance, in under 2 weeks.

Antibiotic-related diarrhoea is unlikely to be a problem because any diarrhoea has to be 'cholera-like' before absorption is affected.

5.37 What should be advised during short-term use of any interacting drug?

■ *Enzyme-inducers*: if, for example, griseofulvin is to be used (up to say 6 weeks – if longer, *see Q 5.42*) in the treatment of a cutaneous fungal infection, extra contraceptive precautions are advised for the duration of the treatment. These should be continued for a further 7 days, with omission of the next PFI if the last potentially ineffective pill was taken in the last 7 days of the current pack. Rifampicin is such a powerful enzyme-inducer that even if it is given only for 2 days (as, for instance, to eliminate carriage of meningococcus), increased elimination by the liver must be assumed for 4 weeks thereafter. Extra contraception with elimination of the relevant one or two PFIs should be recommended to cover that time. This advice applies also to a relative of rifampicin, rifabutin.

■ *Other antibiotics*: the large-bowel flora responsible for recycling estrogens are reconstituted with resistant organisms in about 2 weeks. In practice, therefore, if the COC is commenced in a woman who has been taking, say, a tetracycline long term (e.g. for acne or as malaria prophylaxis), there is no need to advise extra contraceptive precautions. There is a potential problem only – although this is now believed to pose a small risk – when the antibiotic is changed or first introduced in the treatment of a long-term pill-taker. Even then, extra precautions need to be sustained only for the first 2 weeks, but plus the usual 7 days (i.e. 3 weeks in all), with elimination of the next PFI, if the first 2 weeks of antibiotic use extended into the last 7 days of a pack.

5.38 Given that because of antibiotic resistance no action is required with long-term use of non-enzyme-inducing antibiotics, what should be done if long-term use of an enzyme-inducer is required?

Note first, this situation is 'WHO 3' for all hormonal methods (UKMEC) and implies 'use another method' wherever possible (*see Q 5.121*). The obvious alternative for many is now depot medroxyprogesterone acetate (DMPA – *see Q 8.11*).

■ *Rifampicin/rifabutin*: these are such potent enzyme-inducers that in some women a fivefold increase in the rate of metabolism of the COC was observed by the researchers in Liverpool, who recommend alternative methods of contraception for long-term users of rifampicin, i.e. avoiding the COC altogether, even in the higher-dose tricycling regimen described below. Fortunately, the main COC hormone affected is EE, so the injectable progestogen DMPA (*see* Q *8.11*) is a good option.

■ *Long-term use of other enzyme-inducers*: mainly anticonvulsant therapies. This too is a WHO 3 situation (*see* Q *5.121*), so an alternative contraceptive option is definitely preferred, such as ideally an intrauterine method (IUD or IUS – *see* Q *9.147*) or DMPA (*see* Q *8.11*).

What if, after counselling, the woman *insists* on continuing the COC? See Box below.

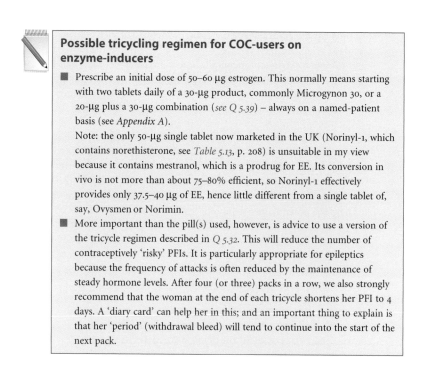

Possible tricycling regimen for COC-users on enzyme-inducers

■ Prescribe an initial dose of 50–60 µg estrogen. This normally means starting with two tablets daily of a 30-µg product, commonly Microgynon 30, or a 20-µg plus a 30-µg combination (*see* Q *5.39*) – always on a named-patient basis (see *Appendix A*).
Note: the only 50-µg single tablet now marketed in the UK (Norinyl-1, which contains norethisterone, see *Table 5.13*, p. 208) is unsuitable in my view because it contains mestranol, which is a prodrug for EE. Its conversion in vivo is not more than about 75–80% efficient, so Norinyl-1 effectively provides only 37.5–40 µg of EE, hence little different from a single tablet of, say, Ovysmen or Norimin.

■ More important than the pill(s) used, however, is advice to use a version of the tricycle regimen described in Q *5.32*. This will reduce the number of contraceptively 'risky' PFIs. It is particularly appropriate for epileptics because the frequency of attacks is often reduced by the maintenance of steady hormone levels. After four (or three) packs in a row, we also strongly recommend that the woman at the end of each tricycle shortens her PFI to 4 days. A 'diary card' can help her in this; and an important thing to explain is that her 'period' (withdrawal bleed) will tend to continue into the start of the next pack.

5.39 What if it seems more appropriate to use a gestodene-, desogestrel- or norgestimate-containing COC for a pill-taker needing treatment long term with an enzyme-inducer?

In selected cases I would again prescribe two sub-50-µg pills a day, e.g. one Marvelon plus one Mercilon-20 with desogestrel as the progestogen (*see Q 5.131*). But whenever two or more are prescribed daily, the grounds – as here – must be solid and record-keeping must be meticulous (named-patient use, see *Appendix A*), because the manufacturer will not accept product liability should a serious problem arise.

5.40 What could signal the need to consider a new drug interaction – or the need to take action during tricycling for an established drug interaction?

BTB is sometimes the first clue to a drug interaction in the first place (e.g. when a woman decides to take St John's wort). It could also be used as an indication to advise a complete change of method.

If the user of an enzyme-inducing drug develops BTB while tricycling the COC, once again exclude another cause (*see Q 5.170*). The next step is to try taking an early break (of 4 days in this case) and thereafter fewer packs in a row – e.g. 'bicycling' (*see Q 5.33*).

If the problem persists, a change of method will nearly always be preferable. The alternative of trying an even higher dose, combining pills to a total estrogen content of, say, 80–90 μg in an attempt to increase the blood levels of both hormones to above the threshold for bleeding, is NOT now recommended. This might produce an unacceptable risk of VTE, despite the enzyme induction.

5.41 How can one explain this increased dosage to a woman, i.e. that she is not receiving a 'dangerously' strong pill regimen?

The risk of this policy, given that BTB is not a fully accurate measure of blood levels (*see Qs 5.162–5.170*), must be assessed carefully by the prescriber, especially if the woman has any risk factor for arterial or venous disease. Thereafter it can be explained that, as described more fully in *Qs 5.164–5.170*, one is only attempting to give the minimum dose of both hormones to finish just above the threshold for bleeding. Reassure her that she is metaphorically 'climbing a down escalator so as to stay at the right level'. Her increased liver metabolism means that her body should still only be receiving a normal low-dose regimen, despite taking a 50–60-μg dose. She is exposed to more metabolites but this is not believed to be harmful.

5.42 Can a woman go straight back to the normal dose and regimen as soon as the enzyme-inducers are stopped?

No: it could be 4 weeks or more before the liver's level of excretory function reverts to normal. Hence, if any enzyme-inducer has been used for 6 weeks or more (or at all in the case of rifampicin), Professors Michael Orme and David Back of Liverpool recommend a delay of about 4 weeks before the woman returns to the standard low-dose pill regimen. This delay should be increased to 8 weeks after more prolonged use of established enzyme-inducers. And logically there should then be no gap between the higher- and the low-dose packets (see *Table 5.4*, p. 145).

Compared with the complexities described in the last five questions, how much simpler for a woman just to use DMPA or have an IUD or IUS fitted . . . . *See Q 5.38*.

5.43   What are the implications of long-term and possibly changing antibiotic treatments in women suffering from acne or (for example) cystic fibrosis?

■ *On long-term antibiotics and then first starting oral contraception*: no problem (*see Qs 5.36, 5.37*).

■ *On oral contraception either when first starting antibiotics or at each switch to a new broad-spectrum antibiotic*: here the counsel of perfection would be to use an additional method such as the condom for the first 3 weeks (also missing out any PFIs that are due), to permit antibiotic resistance to develop (*see Q 5.37*).

5.44   What drugs can increase the bioavailability of EE? Does a high intake of vitamin C do this?

■ New research on the vitamin C interaction shows no increase in circulating levels of EE and no rebound on discontinuation, refuting earlier concerns.

■ Any effect of paracetamol – in competing for EE conjugation and therefore raising EE blood levels – is probably clinically unimportant. However, in the absence of a definitive (negative) study, it is still best to advise separating pill-taking from the paracetamol by a couple of hours.

■ Co-trimoxazole, erythromycin, clarithromycin, itraconazole and the interferons inhibit liver CYP 3A4 enzymes and so also tend to increase the bioavailability of the COC.

Dose adjustment of the COC or the other drug does not seem to be clinically necessary for any of the above.

5.45   Is the rumour about an interaction between the pill and grapefruit juice founded on fact?

Yes, this one is, although not the one that it might make the pill fail; it is the other way round. Grapefruit is a rich source of flavonoids, which compete for the enzymes that metabolize EE, so increasing bioavailability (and blood levels). But even in high consumers of grapefruit this is unlikely to cause any significant added prothrombotic risk from the pill. If concerned, the simple solution is to ensure grapefruit juice is always quaffed at least 2 h after the time of pill-taking.

5.46 Are any of the interactions in which COCs affect the metabolism of other drugs of any clinical significance?

Yes. The clinically significant effects relate to lamotrigine, ciclosporin and warfarin.

1 *Lamotrigine* (new since the last edition): though this antiepileptic is not an enzyme-inducer and so poses no COC-efficacy-reducing problem, blood levels of the lamotrigine itself can be *lowered* by COCs. Therefore:

■ Starting a COC in a patient already taking this drug may result in poorer control of her epilepsy. Awareness of this possibility and a small increment in the dose of lamotrigine is all that is required. Moreover, be aware of the same *possibility* with all progestogen-only methods also (but there are no good data).

■ There is no problem in giving lamotrigine to patients already taking a COC, because the dose of antiepileptic drug is simply titrated to the patient's needs, as usual.

However, the lamotrigine dose may need to be lowered to reduce toxicity risk when the COC is discontinued.

2 Oral contraceptive (OC) steroids are themselves weak inhibitors of hepatic microsomal enzymes. So they may lower the clearance of ciclosporin, diazepam, tricyclic antidepressants, prednisolone, and some other drugs – including, according to some reports (but not others), alcohol. Most of these interactions are unimportant clinically, but exceptions are:

■ *Ciclosporin* levels can **definitely** be *raised* by COC hormones: the risk of toxic effects means blood levels should be monitored with added care in pill-takers.

■ There is evidence that COCs (and progestogens alone, including the levonorgestrel-only emergency contraceptive Q 10.6) inhibit the metabolism of *warfarin* to a variable extent, potentially raising its blood levels and therefore the international normalized ratio (INR). Also, independently, the COC alters clotting factors.

Thus, their interaction is unpredictable and the combination is usually best avoided. However, in specific individuals it is nevertheless sometimes used, on a WHO 3 basis. After a venous thrombosis, for example, the contraindication to the COC only becomes WHO 4 (absolute) after anticoagulation ceases. Moreover, COCs are, rarely, the only acceptable contraceptive method for a few women on long-term warfarin due to structural heart disease and atrial fibrillation risk (*see* Q 5.141). In all such cases the warfarin needs careful monitoring by more frequent INRs, at least initially.

Pharmacodynamic interactions:

3   *Potassium-sparing diuretics*: there is **already** a tendency to *hyperkalaemia* with drospirenone, the progestogen in Yasmin, so these diuretics should not be used (WHO 4) with that **particular brand of COC.**

4   As COCs tend to impair glucose tolerance, sometimes cause depression and can raise BP, they naturally tend to oppose the actions of antidiabetic, antidepressant and antihypertensive treatments, respectively. With respect to hypertension, see the important point in Q 6.9; but otherwise this type of effect is fairly easily compensated for clinically by monitoring the dose/response of the other drug.

5.47   What else, apart from treating my patient, should I do if I suspect a drug interaction of any type?

Practitioners who do detect possible drug interactions are asked to continue the practice of completing a yellow card for the Committee on Safety of Medicines (CSM).

5.48   Should women with an ileostomy or colostomy avoid hormonal contraception for fear of absorption problems, or be given a stronger brand than usual?

Despite the interference in the enterohepatic cycle after an **ileostomy,** the bioavailability of EE, as well as levonorgestrel, was not detectably altered [Grimmer SF et al 1986 *Contraception* 33:51–59]. Efficacy would not be expected to be impaired unless there was associated significant small-bowel disease and malabsorption.

   Yet, because of anecdotes of unexpected conceptions, due presumably to reduced reabsorption of EE from the large bowel (*see Qs 5.35, 5.36*) in apparently compliant women with an ileostomy, I would now recommend added precautions or a regimen with fewer and shorter PFIs in such women (*see Q 5.32*). But I would not advise increasing the COC dose solely on these grounds.

Colostomy, however, does not (and would not be expected to) have any effect on the enterohepatic circulation of estrogen.

5.49   Does coeliac disease impair absorption of the COC?

No. Paradoxically, while this disease is active the diminished function of the gut wall leads to less conjugation of absorbed EE. So more bioactive EE is absorbed than usual! Once coeliac disease is successfully treated, absorption is normal.

STARTING ROUTINES WITH THE COC

5.50 What factors need consideration in devising starting routines for the COC?

■ First and foremost, women with short cycles can ovulate very early in the second week of the menstrual cycle. Hence the value of the day 1 (or 2) start, to ensure seven tablets are taken in time (*see Q 5.17*) and with no need for additional contraception from the outset. Yet Sunday starting, *with added contraception till seven active pills have been taken,* also has advantages (*see Q 5.8*).

■ First-timers can usefully be warned that their first 'period' might come on after only about 23 days. Also that each new pack should start after no more than 7 days and this will always be on the same day of the week (*see Qs 5.51, 5.52*).

■ There are studies, especially from Israel, showing that the older routine of a day 5 start has one advantage: less BTB and spotting in the first cycle. This is therefore well worth considering, and the 1998 Tel Aviv study showed a higher rate of early discontinuations for bleeding in the group that started on day 1. If this is preferred, extra precautions until seven active pills have been taken are always advisable.

■ **'Quick starts'** are pill-starts even later in the cycle. This is perfectly acceptable if any earlier intercourse is judged to have been adequately protected, or in selected cases immediately after emergency contraception – once again with 7 days of extra precautions. It is my practice also to advise the latter whenever the first tablet of the first pack is taken later than day 2 (see *Table 5.4*), though UKMEC is less cautious.

■ After a first-trimester pregnancy has ended, the earliest fertile ovulation seems to occur no earlier than about day 10.

■ After a full-term pregnancy (in the absence of breastfeeding) the earliest possible fertile ovulation has been shown biochemically at around day 28. However, starting too early has to be avoided because of evidence that the estrogen in the combined pill can increase the risk of puerperal thromboembolism. The coagulation factor changes of pregnancy are largely reversed by 2 weeks. So, for most, a start date of day 21 is appropriate. Starting the COC should be further delayed in those at highest risk of any form of thrombosis, including the obese, and after severe pregnancy-related hypertension or the HELLP syndrome (haemolysis, elevated liver enzymes, low platelets) with persistent biochemical abnormalities: with alternative contraception for 7 days since the pill is therefore started beyond day 21.

■ The COC can be started immediately after injectables such as DMPA. But of more interest is the fact that the COC can also (and often very usefully) be given concurrently with DMPA: for example, on restarting after major or leg surgery that has been covered by DMPA (*see Q 6.17*) or to control bleeding problems (*see Q 8.47*). See *Q 8.52* for relevant advice if the prospective pill-taker is already overdue her most recent injection.

These and my other recommendations for starting the COC are summarized in *Table 5.4*. See *Q 7.55* for the POP.

CONTRACEPTION AFTER PREGNANCY

This important subject is discussed in much more detail in *Qs 11.18–11.32*, including, when there is amenorrhoea, how to avoid starting a new medical method (IUD, injectable or pill) when an implantation has (or might have) already occurred (*see Q 11.22*).

A point to mention here is that, after excluding pregnancy during amenorrhoea, the COC can often best be started on the next Sunday (plus additional precautions for 7 days); this avoids future bleeds at weekends (*see Q 5.52*).

5.51 What single question screens for accurate pill-taking?

Simply: 'What day of the week do you start each new pack?' If a pill-taker states the day with confidence, all is well. If she hums and haws or says 'It all depends', there's a problem!

5.52 Can I help my patients to avoid the withdrawal bleed (WTB) at weekends?

Yes, but only if you think to discuss the point! With most starting routines, depending on the weekday their first period happens to start and the length of their WTB, some three-sevenths of all pill-takers will bleed during part of one weekend in every four. This is completely unnecessary.

Starting the pill on the first Sunday of the next period is one option (*see Q 5.8*). This is popular in the US but must be combined with extra precautions until seven active tablets have been taken. Alternatively, at any time during follow-up, you can simply advise *shortening any one PFI so as to start the next pack on a Sunday or Monday*: thereby ensuring that future WTBs will occur only on weekdays.

MAJOR SYSTEMIC EFFECTS OF THE COC

5.53 Which studies have provided our present information about the wanted and unwanted effects of the COC?

 There have been many case–control and database studies (e.g. EURAS), but much of the most useful data has been generated by cohort studies. Wherever possible, statements made in this book are based on congruence

TABLE 5.4 Starting routines for combined oral contraceptives (as recommended by J Guillebaud – UKMEC recommendations differ slightly)

	Start when?	Extra precautions for 7 days?
1 Menstruating	Day 1	No* if starting with an active tablet
	Day 2	No[†]
	Day 3 or later	Yes[†]
	Any time in cycle ('Quick start')	Yes[†]
2 Postpartum		
(a) No lactation	Day 21 (low risk of thrombosis by then[‡], first ovulations reported day 28+)	No
(b) Lactation	Not normally recommended at all (POP/ injectable preferred)	
3 Post induced early abortion/miscarriage	Same day – or next day to avoid postoperative vomiting risk. Day 21 if was at/beyond 24 weeks' gestation	No
4 Post trophoblastic tumour	1 month after no hCG detected	As (1)
5 Post higher-dose COC	Instant switch[§] – or use condoms for 7 days after the PFI	No
6 Post lower- or same-dose COC	After usual 7-day break	No
7 Post POP	First day of period	No
8 Post POP with secondary amenorrhoea, not pregnant	Any day (Sunday? Has advantages, see Q 5.52)	No
9 Post DMPA (risk of pregnancy excluded, see Q 11.22)	Any day (see text, may overlap the methods)	No[¶]

TABLE 5.4—cont'd

	Start when?	Extra precautions for 7 days?
10 Other secondary amenorrhoea (risk of pregnancy excluded, see Q 11.22)	Any day (Sunday? – see Q 5.52)	Yes
11 First cycle after postcoital contraception (see Q 10.40)	First day/or no later than day 2	No
	Or: 'Quick start', i.e. immediately, as Q 10.41	Yes

*If planned 'Sunday start': extra precautions till 7 active tablets have been taken.
†Delay into day 2 can sometimes help, to be sure a period is normal. UKMEC and WHOSPR are less cautious and only after day 5 advise extra precautions for the 7 days that are believed to suffice to make any ovary quiescent (see Q 5.17). Starts beyond day 5 (i.e. not waiting for that elusive next period) are entirely acceptable if the prescriber is sure there has been no risk of conception up to the starting day.
‡Puerperal thrombosis risk lasts longer after severe pregnancy-related hypertension or the related HELLP syndrome, so delay COC use until the return of normal BP and biochemistry (see Q 5.50). But a history of HELLP in an earlier pregnancy is irrelevant (WHOMEC).
§This advice is because of anecdotes of rebound ovulation occurring at the time of transfer.
¶Unless was overdue most recent injection – if so, see Q 8.52.
Note: in presence of amenorrhoea, exclusion of there being either a blastocyst or sperm in the upper genital tract can be done by obtaining a negative sensitive pregnancy test after a minimum of 14 days of abstinence or 'very safe' contraception (see Q 11.22).

of the findings of all the studies, by different investigators in different populations. Three of the most important are:

- *The Royal College of General Practitioners' (RCGP) study*: in brief, 23 000 married pill-users were recruited from 1400 GP practices and matched (only for age) with a similar number of married control women not using the COC. The GPs informed the study coordinators of all subsequent medical effects, based on every surgery attendance or hospital referral for in- or outpatient care (including for pregnancy). Ex-users have been similarly followed up.
- *The Oxford/FPA study*: launched in the same year (1968), this study has similarly followed a total of over 17 000 clinic attenders since its start. In this study, users of different reversible methods of contraception act as controls for each other; 56% used oral contraceptives at the outset, compared with 25% who were diaphragm-users and 19% who were fitted with an IUD.
- *The Nurses' Health study*: In 1976, 121 700 female registered nurses in the US completed a mailed questionnaire including items relevant primarily to risk of cancer and circulatory disease. Follow-up questionnaires are sent every 2 years to update the risk factor data and to ascertain any major medical events.

The completeness of the follow-up in all the above studies is exemplary; for example, for fatal outcomes, ascertainment in the Nurses' study runs at about 98%.

5.54 What are the strengths and deficiencies of the main cohort studies?

They have the strengths of similar prospective epidemiological studies, particularly with regard to the completeness of data collection over the years, and the possibility of assessment of non-comparability between the groups compared, and of biases. However, they share obvious weaknesses:

- Random allocation was impossible, so pill-users are different from non-users in many important ways: in the Walnut Creek Study, for example, COC-users tended – as compared with non-users – to be on average taller, more physically active, more likely to smoke or drink in moderation (although not more likely to be heavy smokers or heavy drinkers), to sunbathe more frequently, to have initiated sex earlier and to have had more partners.
- All the studies tended to include fewer teenagers than are now normally found amongst a pill-using population, partly because the unmarried are so difficult to follow in long-term prospective studies.

- In the UK studies, a large number of initially recruited women were lost to follow-up just because they moved house. However, checks on the characteristics of a sample of the latter have not shown them to differ in such a way as to significantly bias the results.
- By the time the cohort studies report, they tend to be providing information about yesterday's contraceptives. Much of the data generated by the above studies relates to brands containing at least 50 µg of estrogen and the recently marketed progestogens are under-represented.

5.55 What are case–control studies and what can we learn about the COC from them?

Case–control studies are retrospective: cases are recruited with a condition of interest (e.g. VTE) and attempts are made to match the women with 'controls' (admitted to the same hospital or from the same community) who are free of the condition but otherwise as similar as possible. The basic idea is that if the frequency of pill use is greater in cases (relative risk more than 1), the pill might be causing the condition; if it is less (relative risk less than 1), the pill might be protective. Useful studies of this kind are quoted repeatedly in this book, many organized through WHO. Case–control studies never provide absolute rates (attributable cases per 100 000 of population) although these can be roughly calculated if the background prevalence of the condition is known. These studies have a number of problems we cannot discuss in detail here, but here are some:

- They are obligatory for very rare events like thrombosis and diseases that take many years of exposure for any causation to become apparent, such as arterial wall disease or cancer. But they are notorious for the problems of bias and confounding. Epidemiologists try very hard to correct for these but certain confounders (predisposing factors for which pill use or use of particular brands of pill might be a marker, leading to an association that is coincidental, not causative) might be unknown. *See Q 5.109* for a good example of this kind of problem..
- Epidemiology is always weak when it comes to assessing odds ratios (or relative risks) that are not much above or below unity (in the ranges 1–2 and 0.5–1). Yet for common conditions these could mean an important attributable risk or benefit.
- Because of the low prevalence of use, we are unlikely ever to have useful epidemiological data on the side-effects of the POP.
- It is more difficult to study beneficial than adverse relationships: 'nobody ever gets credit for fixing problems that never happened'. The death that does not take place as a result of protection against ovarian cancer is difficult to recognize, unlike the one from VTE that is linked

to COC use. However, adequate data are available for most of the benefits in *Q 5.57*.

5.56 Can we identify the 'best buy' among the different pills, for benefits versus risks?

In summary, no. We have to say that thus far all the methods of epidemiology, even when backed by 'biological plausibility', have proved too insensitive as research tools for this to be done with any specificity. Preoccupation with metabolic minutiae (common among rival drug firms in the 1980s and early 1990s) can also be misleading.

But there are good data to show that we should give formulations with the lowest acceptable dose of both the estrogen and progestogen. It is also clear that it is essential to have available a range of different products for prescribers and users to exercise effective choice – in relation both to the initial prescription and, subsequently, when minor side-effects occur.

ADVANTAGES AND BENEFICIAL EFFECTS

5.57 What are the beneficial effects of the COC?

These can be listed as follows:

CONTRACEPTIVE

1 Highly effective – and the regular withdrawal bleeds give regular reassurance of that fact.
2 Highly convenient, especially sexually (non-intercourse-related).
3 Reversible (*see Qs 5.62, 5.63*).

NON-CONTRACEPTIVE – MAINLY GYNAECOLOGICAL

4 A reduction in the rate of most disorders of the menstrual cycle:
   (a) less heavy bleeding, therefore
   (b) less anaemia
   (c) less dysmenorrhoea
   (d) regular bleeding, and timing can be controlled (*see Q 6.86*) with no bleeding at weekends (*see Qs 5.52, 6.87*) or arranged to occur only about four times a year through tricycling as an option (*see Q 5.32*) – or never (*see Q 5.34*)
   (e) fewer symptoms of premenstrual tension overall (*see Q 5.135*), especially if tricycling is tried, although some women do experience similar symptoms on the COC itself
   (f) no ovulation pain, which can be severe in some cycles.
5 Less pelvic inflammatory disease (PID) (*see Q 5.60*).
6 Fewer extrauterine pregnancies – because ovulation is inhibited, and possibly as a long-term result of (5).

7 Less benign breast disease (*see Q 5.97*).

8 Fewer functional ovarian cysts (*see Q 5.61*).

9 Less need for hospital treatment due to bleeding from or size of fibroids (*see Q 5.97*).

10 A beneficial effect on some cancers, notably carcinoma of the endometrium and epithelial cancers of the ovary (*see Qs 5.76, 5.77*) and almost certainly also a reduced risk of colorectal cancer (*see Q 5.75*).

MISCELLANEOUS

11 Fewer sebaceous disorders, especially acne (primarily with selected estrogen-dominant COCs) (*see Q 6.61*).

12 No acute toxicity if overdose is taken: only vomiting, and in prepubertal girls the likelihood of WTB a week or so later.

13 Protection from osteoporosis and control of climacteric symptoms in older women up to age 50 (as a valid alternative to natural estrogen replacement therapy, in risk-factor-free women needing contraception whose ovaries are beginning to function less well, *see Q 11.37*). The same can apply to younger women with premature ovarian failure or oligomenorrhoea (*see Qs 5.66–5.68*). But the COC has unsurprisingly been found not to improve bone density when the comparison is with normal cycling women – who of course receive estrogen from their own ovaries.

14 Beneficial social effects (e.g. *postponing childbirth until after tertiary education, as an option*). Other possible benefits have been identified in some studies but have yet to be fully confirmed:

15 Reduction in the rate of endometriosis (*see Q 6.52*).

16 Less trichomonal vaginitis (risk of toxic shock syndrome: *see Q 6.53*).

17 Maybe less risk of toxic shock syndrome (TSS: *see Q 6.54*).

18 Less thyroid disease (both overactive and underactive syndromes according to the RCGP study).

19 Maybe less rheumatoid arthritis (*see Q 6.60*).

20 Fewer duodenal ulcers. This apparent effect could well be a good example of confounding (*see Q 5.55*): anxious women prone to ulcers might also be more influenced by the media to avoid COCs.

5.58 What is thought to be the unifying mechanism of the benefits, especially the gynaecological benefits? How can this be useful in counselling prospective pill-takers?

The removal of the normal menstrual cycle and its replacement by a situation that more closely resembles the physiological state of pregnancy. Women who, due to frequent pregnancies and prolonged lactation, have few menstrual cycles during their reproductive lives (say 50 rather than the 450 plus that would now be typical in developed countries) are less likely 'naturally' to get all the symptoms and conditions listed at items (4), (7), (8), (9), (10), (15) and (19) in Q 5.57. The similarity of the protection that the COC gives against ovarian and endometrial cancers, for example, is probably because there is much less chromosomal activity in the endometrium and ovaries than in cycling women. Less chromosomal activity means less chance of harmful mutations during frequent epithelial cell divisions.

So, taking the pill is in some ways more 'normal' than using a barrier contraceptive and having numerous menstrual cycles, because the latter are in reality 'abnormal' and tend to promote gynaecological pathology, i.e. all the conditions at items (4), (7), (8), (9), (10) and (15) in Q 5.57. In a real sense, any woman who has been on the pill for 10 years has had iatrogenic amenorrhoea for 10 years, but of a benign, pregnancy-mimicking kind because estrogen and progestogen are still available to the relevant tissues.

Some women find this story reassuring, that in summary the pill can be truly said to tend to 'restore normality'. It reduces the dangers of too many menstrual cycles among those many who now do the 'unnatural' thing, by not having huge families (*see also* Q 5.135).

5.59 Does lowering doses to reduce the risks also reduce the benefits of gynaecological or non-gynaecological pathology, in comparison with the older high-dose formulations?

There has to be some real doubt about this. The protection against functional cysts (*see* Q 5.61) is definitely reduced by such pills, although there is certainly no proof that it no longer exists. The modern more estrogenic pills might well also be less protective against benign breast disease, fibroids and endometriosis, which are benefited by relatively more progestogen.

My own (unproven) concern is particularly about the triphasics (*see* Q 5.181), which imitate (albeit imperfectly) the normal cycle. This might not be such a good idea because eliminating the normal cycle seems, as we have just seen, to be relevant to the mechanism of the gynaecological benefits. But we can be sure of one good thing: any oral contraceptive that regularly blocks ovulation ought to retain the most valuable protective effect against ovarian cancer.

5.60 By how much does the COC protect against PID, and what is the mechanism?

The protective effect against symptomatic PID appears large, a 50% or more reduction in the risk of hospitalization for the disease. This is such a major cause of subfertility (*see* Q 9.48) that in many parts of the world it is probably a significant non-contraceptive benefit of the pill.

Although suggestions that the COC might facilitate transmission of HIV have been largely discounted (*see* Q 6.71), there is nothing to suggest protection against any of the sexually transmitted viruses (except there are data that all STIs are important in promoting the sexual transmission of HIV, hence the COC might reduce the risk of HIV infection indirectly through the reduced risk of PID).

MECHANISM

It seems likely that progestogens reduce not only the sperm penetrability of cervical mucus (*see Q 5.4*), but also its 'germ penetrability'. Indeed, the two might even be connected, in that spermatozoa can act as 'bio-vectors': there is some evidence that sexually transmitted organisms such as *Chlamydia* and the gonococcus actually 'hitch a lift', using the sperm as their means of transport to the upper genital tract!

Chlamydia carriage is actually more frequent in COC-takers than controls (not easy to interpret, as controls might be using more condoms). So infection and sexual transmission of organisms are probably not impeded at the level of the cervix/vagina: the beneficial effect of the progestogen is likely to be one of protection of the upper genital tract.

However, silent or less severe infection that can still occlude the tubes is not uncommon in pill-takers. There is some evidence that the COC attenuates the symptoms of *Chlamydia*, and this could be an adverse effect if it led to the condition being under-diagnosed and under-treated. Yet the overall effect of the COC on this cause of infertility is likely still to be positive, given the Farrow study (*see Q 5.62*).

Despite this, truly safer sex requires condom use as well ('Double Dutch').

5.61 By how much does the COC protect against functional ovarian cysts, and what is the mechanism?

 The reduction has been shown in practically all studies. In a study in Boston, pill-users were one-fourteenth as likely to develop such cysts as non-users. Although benign, such cysts often result in surgery.

Functional cysts are caused by abnormalities of ovulation. Most of the time, the COC abolishes all kinds of ovulation (both normal and abnormal). However, the POP increases the risk of cyst formation (*see Q 7.34 – and also Q 5.59* regarding the lowest-dose combined pills).

REVERSIBILITY OF THE COC

5.62 Are COCs fully reversible as just stated (*see Q 5.57*)? Do they impair future fertility?

The short answers to these questions are 'yes' to the first and 'no' to the second. In the Oxford/FPA study, for example, among previously fertile women who gave up contraception, by about 30 months over 90% of the ex-pill-users had delivered: a proportion that was indistinguishable from that for ex-users of the diaphragm and IUD. There was a definite delay of 2–3 months in the mean time taken to conceive, probably due in part to the advice pill-takers are often given (*see* Q 6.49).

More recently, a study by Farrow et al [*Human Reproduction* 2002;17:2754–2761] of 12 106 pregnant women showed that prolonged use (>5 years) of the COC before the 8497 planned conceptions was associated with a decreased risk of delay in conceiving – even for nulliparous women. Quite the opposite finding to what, since the very first day the COC was marketed, has been a prime concern. Indeed, I find in my visits to Africa that fear of infertility continues to put people off the pill unnecessarily (*see* Q 5.70).

It is also interesting that, when this study was done (it began in the early 1990s), so many (3545 or 29%) of the conceptions were admitted to be 'accidental'.

5.63 What, then, is 'post-pill amenorrhoea'?

This term should be abolished (*see* Q 5.64). It is commonly used to mean secondary amenorrhoea of more than 6 months' duration following discontinuation of the COC. Most authorities now believe that the association is casual rather than causal. Of 1862 inhabitants of Uppsala County, Sweden, 3.3% reported a history of amenorrhoea of longer than 3 months. Amenorrhoea of more than 6 months' duration occurred in 1.8% of the population, most frequently in women under the age of 24. So this is quite a common condition. If a woman is predisposed but instead takes the COC for many years, any episodes that would otherwise have been recognized will be masked by the regular withdrawal bleeds induced by her contraceptive. In such a woman, the pill could easily be unfairly blamed for her 'after pill' secondary amenorrhoea when it could only in fact be revealed 'after pill'.

Moreover, studies show that the probability is not associated with formulation, nor – in most studies – with duration of use. Professor Jacobs of University College London has shown that the distribution of diagnoses was the same in cases of secondary amenorrhoea after the pill as in non-post-pill cases; and in the two groups the types of treatment needed, the frequency with which they were employed and the excellent outcome in terms of cumulative conception rates were all the same. All this argues very strongly against a specific pill-induced syndrome causing secondary amenorrhoea.

5.64 What are the bad effects of continuing to use the term 'post-pill amenorrhoea' at all?

■ It leads to a tendency on the part of many doctors to defer investigation of patients with amenorrhoea that develops after the pill, thereby delaying the diagnosis and treatment of potentially serious conditions. Instead, as there is no specific syndrome, after 6 months without a period all cases of secondary amenorrhoea should be referred for investigation and appropriate treatment – whether they are 'post-pill' or 'post-condom'!

■ A second unfortunate result of accepting amenorrhoea after the pill as a real condition is that it deters doctors from prescribing oral contraceptives to women for whom they otherwise might be suitable. A past history of secondary amenorrhoea is a good example (*see Q 5.68*). In some conditions, as we shall see, the COC can be positively beneficial and it is still frequently being needlessly withheld.

■ Amenorrhoeic women often develop feelings of guilt that treatment with the pill has caused their amenorrhoea and has wrecked their chances of ever having a baby. In the first place, it is most unlikely that the pill had anything to do with their problem and, secondly, even if it did, modern therapy of amenorrhoea is so effective that cumulative pregnancy rates approaching 100% can be confidently expected.

5.65 How are such cases of secondary amenorrhoea managed?

It is beyond the scope of this book to go into details of the investigations for secondary amenorrhoea. See instead the evidence-based guideline by the Royal College of Obstetricians and Gynaecologists (RCOG) in association with NICE, entitled *Fertility: Assessment and Treatment for People with Fertility Problems* (2004).

It is important for all concerned to be clear that the assessment should include establishing whether the woman currently desires a pregnancy. It is crazy, but not unheard of, for high technology to be used to induce ovulation in a woman who promptly requests a termination when the resulting ovum is fertilized! (*see Q 11.17*)

5.66 What are the risks of prolonged amenorrhoea? How should women be treated subsequently if they do not want a pregnancy?

The management depends very much on the diagnosis and particularly on estrogen status, as well as whether the woman is actually ready yet for fertility enhancement.

Prolonged amenorrhoea and oligomenorrhoea (say, less than four periods a year) are not by any means always innocuous conditions. They should always be investigated, and management then depends on the diagnosis.

POLYCYSTIC OVARY SYNDROME (PCOS) VERSUS 'POLYCYSTIC OVARIES'

PCOS is not the same as the finding of polycystic ovaries on ultrasound scan: a very common finding in more than 20% of normal women, studied both on the pill and off it. So far as we know, it is only clinically of importance in the smaller number of cases where the ultrasound finding is linked with symptoms: irregular or absent menses with, usually, evidence of excessive androgen activity (acne or hirsutism). Those symptoms, with the scan findings, do then add up to the 'syndrome'. Such women, even if amenorrhoeic, have high levels of both estrogen and androgens, and with the latter goes a low level of sex hormone-binding globulin (SHBG). Their problem seems to be mediated through insulin-like growth factors, linked with carbohydrate and lipid metabolism (syndrome X), and putting on weight sets up a number of vicious metabolic circles – and risks, especially of arterial damage.

The most important therapeutic point therefore is to help a non-overweight PCOS woman to stay slim; if her BMI is already above 30, she will benefit greatly by losing weight through sensible dieting and taking more exercise. If hirsutism is a problem, she might require a consultant-led high-dose cyproterone acetate and estrogen regimen, followed by Dianette/Clairette 2000/35 (new generic marketed in UK since last edition) (see Q 6.65) or Yasmin and Yaz (see Qs 6.62–6.66) which, like the former contain an anti-androgenic progestogen (in this case drospirenone). Metformin or a related drug may be indicated if the above metabolic syndrome is diagnosed, and interestingly can lead inter alia to improvement in hirsutism and/or severe acne without hormone therapy.

If acne alone is the problem, perhaps with some irregular menstrual cycling, managing the PCOS in primary care is appropriate; there is usually no need to refer. Dianette (see Q 6.65) can be prescribed, usually followed (once the symptoms are controlled) by another oral contraceptive – mild acne is an indication, in my view, for one of the modern 20–35-μg estrogen varieties with desogestrel or gestodene. Yasmin or Yaz (Q6.64) are excellent for more severe cases, containing like Dianette an anti-androgenic progestogen and, unlike it, licensed for long-term use. This combined-pill treatment increases SHBG, so binding androgens, and also protects the endometrium from overstimulation.

Prolonged unopposed estrogen in PCOS, due to infrequent ovulation and corpus luteum formation, increases the risk of carcinoma of the endometrium: which is another advantage of COC use for these women (and others with simple obesity and oligo-/amenorrhoea).

Be very cautious, however, on VTE grounds, if the BMI is above 30; and all EE-containing products should normally be avoided above a BMI of 39.

SECONDARY AMENORRHOEA IN LOW-NORMAL OR UNDERWEIGHT WOMEN

This is often weight-related amenorrhoea and common in anorexia nervosa and in track athletes. The concern here is that they have no follicular estrogen, little extraglandular estrogen from peripheral conversion of androgen in fat depots and, moreover, have enhanced metabolism along the pathway that degrades estrogens to antiestrogens. All these mechanisms lead to low estrogen levels and a serious risk of osteoporosis. If the amenorrhoea has continued for more than 6 months, specialist referral including bone scanning for osteopenia is usually indicated. Note also that prolonged hypo-estrogenic amenorrhoea is now a contraindication (WHO 4) for DMPA (*see Q 8.25*).

These women are theoretically at risk of heart disease, like women with a premature menopause, if the hypo-estrogenic state were to continue for a very long time. They should certainly stop smoking, which also lowers plasma estrogen, and be encouraged to put on weight. They are usually opposed to being 'unnatural' by taking hormones, yet they might be better off healthwise on an estrogen-dominant and 'lipid-friendly' pill than using barrier contraception alone. Opposed natural HRT estrogens could be used if preferred – they would be as good for prevention of osteoporosis, but it is a myth that HRT would be any better than the COC for this indication. There would also be a conception risk once ovulation is restored.

HYPERPROLACTINAEMIA

This requires specialist treatment, e.g. with bromocriptine or another dopamine agonist drug. Hypo-estrogenism is not a problem in treated cases, with return of menstrual cycles and usually normal libido. The COC is usable simultaneously with a dopamine agonist but only under careful supervision (WHO 3). There is the risk of enlarging a macroadenoma, if present, potentially endangering eyesight, so the advice of the specialist in charge should always be sought.

AMENORRHOEA WITH NORMAL ESTROGENIZATION, NO PCOS (OVARIES SHOW NO OVULATION BUT WITH EVIDENCE OF FOLLICULAR ACTIVITY)

Here there is the contraceptive problem that at any time the woman might ovulate. A simple method of contraception (e.g. condom or perhaps a contraceptive sponge or spermicide) would be fine, until the first spontaneous period occurs. Because this suggests the return of ovulation, the woman would then be advised to consider transferring to a more effective method – not excluding the COC as an option.

5.67 In summary, what is the place of the COC for women with amenorrhoea?

It is positively beneficial to use the COC in a number of these cases. Its estrogen content definitely helps where the estrogen status is low, especially to prevent long-term problems such as heart disease and osteoporosis. And the progestogen content of the COC can also be of value in PCOS women with estrogen excess and no endogenous progesterone, to protect their uterus from carcinoma of the endometrium.

5.68 What advice should be given to a healthy woman who gives a past history of secondary amenorrhoea but is currently seeing normal periods?

All the evidence suggests that there is no reason to refuse the COC to such women, although they must understand that with or without the pill they might at some future time have difficulty in conceiving. Future fertility can never be proved in advance of becoming pregnant. Another important point is to investigate such a woman first if her current menses are in fact still erratic, for example, if she is experiencing less than four periods per year. An ultrasound scan might well show PCOS (*see Qs 5.66, 5.67*).

5.69 To preserve future fertility, should pill-users take regular breaks of say 6 months, every 2 or every 5 years?

The answer here is an unusually confident 'no'. This follows from *Q 5.62*: the pill is a reversible means of birth control, whose reversibility is not dependent on duration of use. Too often, breaks demonstrate very well to the woman that her fertility is unimpaired – by an unplanned pregnancy! *See also Qs 5.30, 5.31 and 6.73*, which add a health-related (rather than a fertility-related) perspective to this same issue of duration of use/taking breaks.

5.70 Contrary to the common myth about its reversibility, doesn't the COC in fact much reduce the likelihood of infertility?

Yes (see the Farrow paper quoted in *Q 5.62*). Many of the benefits of the pill (*see Q 5.57*) relate to conditions that can readily impair fertility and childbearing, specifically:

- less pelvic infection
- fewer ectopic pregnancies
- less endometriosis
- less growth of fibroids, a cause of miscarriage
- fewer functional ovarian cysts, a cause of unnecessary surgery with risk of adhesions
- less surgery altogether, for all the conditions listed here, a frequent cause of pelvic adhesions and consequent infertility
- fewer unwanted pregnancies: which can lead in various ways to secondary infertility (e.g. by infected abortions of all kinds, or by puerperal infection).

For the same reasons, there is no logic in pill-takers being specially earmarked for a regular annual bimanual examination (*see Q 6.3*)!

MAIN DISADVANTAGES AND PROBLEMS

5.71 What are the major established unwanted effects of COCs?

These are summarized here, before more detailed consideration. They fall under four main headings:

- Circulatory diseases (*see Qs 5.98–5.118*).
- Liver disease:
  - liver adenoma (*see Q 5.97*), or carcinoma (*see Q 5.96*)
  - cholestatic jaundice (*see Q 6.36*)
  - gallstones (*see Qs 6.37–6.38*).
- Adverse effects on some cancers (*see Qs 5.72–5.96*).
- Unwanted social effects.

The last are hotly debated. Discussion ranges over whether removal of the fear of pregnancy has in some societies tended to promote intercourse with multiple partners, with its consequences on marital and emotional stability, STIs and so on, or whether other simultaneous changes, such as the decline in religious belief, have been more important factors.

- There are, of course, numerous other possible but fortunately less 'major' unwanted side-effects.
- 'Minor' side-effects are never to be seen as 'unimportant' to the person concerned, though.
- Practically all that have been described will be considered in later sections of this chapter.

THE COC AND NEOPLASIA (BENIGN AND MALIGNANT)

5.72 Does the COC influence the rates of benign and malignant neoplasms?

It should not be surprising that artificial hormones can influence neoplasia but recent research has confirmed the expectation that the effect of hormones would not be all in one direction. Some benign neoplastic conditions are benefited by OC use (e.g. benign breast disease), some are promoted (e.g. liver adenomas). Similarly, two cancers are now clearly shown to be less frequent in pill-users (carcinoma of the ovary and endometrium); whereas the COC might possibly act as a co-carcinogen in the case of two other common cancers (cervix and breast). The literature is complex and the jury is still out.

5.73 Why has it taken so long to begin to show associations between the pill and neoplasia?

The main reason is summarized in the word 'latency'. There can be up to 30 years between first exposure to an agent and its manifestation in the incidence of tumours. Even the largest prospective studies tend to have too few numbers and take too long to give an answer. Hence, data have been obtained mainly from case–control studies, which are notoriously subject to bias. Other problems relate to the following:

- The specificity of any co-carcinogen to the species, to the tissue and to tumour histology.
- Time of life is relevant – in animal models, chemicals can have contrary actions, promoting or inhibiting tumours according to when, in the life of the individual, exposure takes place.
- Formulation: not only differing ratios of progestogen to estrogen, but also different progestogenic chemicals, are used around the world. It is particularly unfortunate that most studies cannot disentangle the effects of specific formulations (apart from generally showing that low-estrogen pills usually have a lesser effect).

5.74 What is the benefit/risk balance sheet for neoplasia and the pill, so far as is currently known?

The situation can best be explained to a patient in terms of 'swings and roundabouts' (*Fig. 5.6*). Some cancers are definitely less frequent in pill-users (e.g. endometrium and ovary, *see Qs 5.76 5.77*); others might be more frequent (but in none of those shown is a causative link proven beyond all doubt). For all remaining common malignancies (e.g. of the respiratory, gastrointestinal or renal tracts), there seems no association, or certainly no

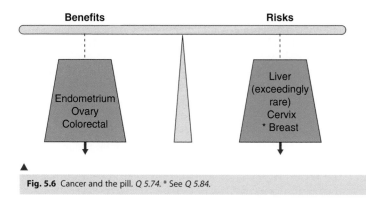

Benefits

Risks

Endometrium
Ovary
Colorectal

Liver
(exceedingly rare)
Cervix
* Breast

Fig. 5.6 Cancer and the pill. *Q 5.74.* * See Q 5.84.

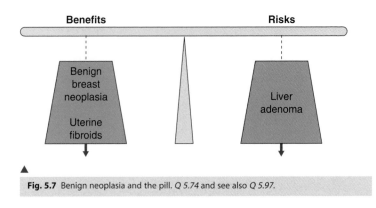

Fig. 5.7 Benign neoplasia and the pill. *Q 5.74* and see also *Q 5.97*.

adverse association, at all. A similar balance sheet can be struck for benign neoplasia (*Fig. 5.7*).

The bottom line in counselling is: Populations using the pill might develop different benign or malignant neoplasms from non-users, but computer models using the best currently accepted data and assumptions do not so far indicate that the overall risk of tumours is increased. (There is no proof of an overall reduction of risk either.) Now let us consider some of the details.

5.75 What is the influence of the COC on colorectal cancer?

Several studies, both cohort and case–control, now find that COC use reduces this risk. A large study [Fernandez E et al 1998 *Epidemiology* 9:295–300] found a 60% risk reduction among ever-users. This was confirmed in the 1 million woman-year RCGP database studied by Hannaford et al [*British Medical Journal* 2007;335:651–661]. So, although this protective effect was not shown in some other studies and the biological explanation for it is unclear, this benefit can now be moved into the 'highly probable' category.

5.76 What is the influence of the COC on carcinoma of the ovary?

Good news! Many studies have yielded results pointing in the same direction, namely that epithelial ovarian tumours are less frequent in COC-users. Overall, the risk is reduced by about half. There is increasing protection with increased duration of use, and in the Oxford/FPA study [Vessey M et al *British Journal of Cancer* 2006;95:385–389] the protective effect lasted for at least 20 years after pill-taking ceased. This is good news indeed, because ovarian cancer carries a high mortality.

5.77 What is the influence of COC use on carcinoma of the endometrium?

More good news, the risk of this cancer in ever-users is again reduced by about 50%. Numerous studies show increasing protection with increasing duration of use, and, again, according to Vessey (reference above), the effect persists for at least 20 years after stopping use.

The similarity of the beneficial effects of the COC on these two cancers is striking, but, given their epidemiology, not really surprising (*see* Q 5.58).

5.78 What is the influence of the COC on trophoblastic disease (hydatidiform mole)?

There is no evidence that the incidence of any form of this tumour of pregnancy is increased by past pill use.

However, workers at Charing Cross Hospital in London have shown that usage of the combined pill after this diagnosis, and before human chorionic gonadotrophin (hCG) has reached undetectable blood levels, doubles the likelihood that the patient will require chemotherapy for incipient choriocarcinoma. Other researchers, notably from America, have completely failed to show this association, but their chemotherapy policy is far more aggressive. See UKMEC.

The London team remains convinced of a causative link. They and UKMEC continue to recommend that combined hormonal methods are avoided (WHO 4, *see* Q 5.121), until the hCG levels are undetectable, in urine at first, then confirmed in the blood. Progestogen-only methods are all classified in the UK as WHO 3 until that time. Hormonal emergency contraception, however, is WHO 2 (*see* Q 10.28).

Thereafter, most importantly, this history is definitely WHO 1. IUDs and the LNG-IUS are WHO 4 while hCG levels are high but WHO 1 when hCG is no longer measurable. Fortunately, in the vast majority of cases the hCG levels do become undetectable within 2 months of evacuation of the mole.

The prohibition against hormonal methods, which is only precautionary (and not advised by WHO itself, or in the US at all), is therefore usually short-lived and not as long as until the next conception – which itself is usually advised after there have been at least 6 months with no hCG detectable.

5.79 What is the influence of the COC on carcinoma of the cervix?

Evidence exists of a modest increased risk of both squamous cell carcinoma and the much rarer adenocarcinoma of the cervix. Studies on cervical cancer are complicated by confounding with the sexual variables, i.e. by the problem of getting accurate information about different patterns of sexual activity, both for women and their partners. The prime carcinogen is clearly a sexually transmitted virus (specific high-risk types of the human papillomavirus [HPV] being the prime candidates). Cofactors are also important: cigarette smoking currently stands most accused in that role (at least doubling the risk in developed-country studies).

Yet most studies do show an association between incidence of, and now also in mortality from, this cancer, plus its premalignant forms (cervical intraepithelial neoplasia [CIN]), and use of the COC. But is the association causative or casual? The Oxford/FPA cohort study [latest report in *British Journal of Cancer* 2006;95:385–389] and the RCGP (Hannaford) study referenced at Q 5.75 both support causation by demonstrating a clear effect of duration of pill use among nearly 7000 parous women. In the FPA study the odds ratio was 2.9 after 4 years' usage, rising to 6.1 after 8 years and still maintained at 4.6 in ex-users after 8 years (though with wide confidence intervals). There were 59 cases of invasive cancer in women in the OC group, compared with only 6 cases in the never-users. The frequency of taking cervical smears for cytology was similar in both populations.

5.80 What is your overall assessment of the association with neoplasia of the cervix?

The COC does not increase the likelihood of acquiring HPV. But once a high-risk strain such as type 16 or 18 is present in the cervix, the data suggest that the COC is a cofactor, increasing the rate at which CIN progresses through the preinvasive stages to invasion. It is probably weaker in this respect than cigarette smoking.

Even if the two cofactors are combined, it is believed that routine 3-yearly screening by cervical cytology (especially now it will increasingly be liquid-based cytology) will suffice. Almost all preinvasive lesions should then be diagnosed in time to be treated pre-emptively, barring human errors (by patient or the screening service), which sadly do occur. Indeed, they explain nearly all the invasive cases in the UK studies reviewed in Q 5.79, since those cases would mostly pre-date the marked improvement in population coverage by the NHS Cervical Screening Programme that began in 1988.

Note that past treatment for CIN lesions is no more than WHO 2 for pill continuation (provided there is ongoing cytological surveillance, Q 5.81).

To sum up, COC-users should be reminded to ensure they have regular cytological and, as necessary, colposcopic surveillance. In the future, vaccination of young girls against high-risk types of HPV should dramatically reduce the incidence of this cancer and its premalignant stages.

5.81 Should women discontinue COC use once an abnormal cervical smear has been detected?

It is currently entirely acceptable to continue COC use during the monitoring of a mildly abnormal cervical smear, during definitive treatment of CIN and subsequently. These are weak, relative contraindications (WHO 2, *see Q 5.121*): although the recurrence risk for the problem would of course be minimized if the couple were prepared to use a barrier method instead or as well (*see Qs 3.26, 4.17*).

THE COC AND BREAST CANCER

5.82 What is the association between breast cancer and COC use?

The incidence of this disease is high and therefore it must inevitably be expected to develop in women whether they take COCs or not. As the recognized risk factors include early menarche and late age of first birth, use by young women was rightly bound to receive scientific scrutiny. However, if there is a real causative link with pill use, use by older women will obviously result in more attributable cases, because the incidence rises steeply with age above 35 years (*Fig. 5.8*).

The literature to date is copious, complex, confusing and contradictory! Research is complicated by the problems related to latency, changes in formulation, time of exposure and high-risk groups.

5.83 What is the main risk factor for breast cancer?

Age, because it affects everyone (unlike family history, or possession of the rare but certainly hazardous risk factor of carrying a *BRCA* gene). It seems

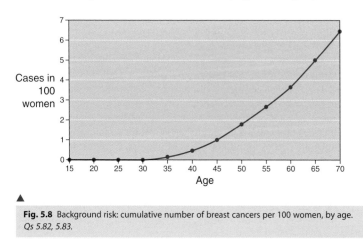

▲

Fig. 5.8 Background risk: cumulative number of breast cancers per 100 women, by age. *Qs 5.82, 5.83.*

that cumulative duration of exposure of breast tissue to ovarian hormones – or to substitutes thereof (notably those in the combined pill or HRT) – means a cumulative increased risk of cancer, starting in the mid-thirties, as shown in *Fig. 5.8.*

Is the risk from those substitutes the same as or greater than that from a woman's exposure (over the same duration) to the hormones from her own ovaries? For the usual combined HRT (estrogen plus progestogen), rather than estrogen alone, the answer for current users now appears to be 'greater' – but with no detectable added risk in ex-users after 5 years [see the Million Women Study, *The Lancet* 2003;362:419–427 for full details].

A study by Marchbanks et al in 2002 (*see Q 5.87*) was essentially negative for added breast cancer risk, in a population aged 35 to 64 at diagnosis, for any duration of previous use. Since all pill-takers are effectively 'menopausal' (i.e. their inactivated ovaries produce virtually no estrogen nor progesterone), this reassuringly means that replacement of ovarian hormones by EE plus progestogen for all those years had not affected their breasts more than functioning ovaries would have done – with respect to breast cancer risk later in life. However, as now to be discussed, earlier work still clearly suggests that the COC source of hormones slightly increases breast cancer risk compared with the ovarian source in two categories:

■ current users
■ recent ex-users.

5.84 So what was the model proposed in the 1996 paper by the Collaborative Group on Hormonal Factors in Breast Cancer (CGHFBC)?

The group reanalysed original data from 90% of all the available epidemiological data worldwide. This relates to over 53 000 women with breast cancer and over 100 000 controls from 54 studies in 25 countries. In its publication [Collaborative Group 1996 *The Lancet* 347:1713–1727], the group proposed a widely accepted model (*see Qs 5.88–5.91*) – of an increase in risk through pill usage of 24%, but with diminution in ex-users and complete disappearance of added risk by 10 years. The strongest risk factor was confirmed as age of the woman: this is believed to be linked, as just mentioned, to cumulative exposure of the breast to estrogen/progestogen hormones. They found that the most important predictor of added risk with the COC was recency of use.

This model showed disappearance of risk in ex-users, but recency of use of the COC was the most important factor: with the odds ratio unaffected by age of initiation or discontinuation, use before or after first full-term pregnancy, or duration of use. The main findings are summarized in *Table 5.5* and below.

TABLE 5.5 The increased risk of developing breast cancer while taking the pill and in the 10 years after stopping	
User status	**Increased risk**
Current user	24%
1–4 years after stopping	16%
5–9 years after stopping	7%
10 plus years an ex-user	No significant excess
(Collaborative Group on Hormonal Factors in Breast Cancer, 1996.)	

5.85 So what is the good news in the CGHFBC model of breast cancer and the COC?

COC-users can be reassured that:

■ Although the small increase in breast cancer risk for women on the pill noted in previous studies is confirmed, the odds ratio of 1.24 signifies an increase of 24% only while women are taking the COC and for a few years thereafter, diminishing to zero after 10 years.

■ Because of the rarity of breast cancer at young ages, the absolute attributable risk (in terms of cases of cancer) is acceptable, but may be less so whenever the background risk is higher (*see* Q 5.86).

■ Beyond 10 years after stopping there is no detectable increase in breast cancer risk for former pill-users.

■ The cancers diagnosed in women who use or have ever used COCs are clinically less advanced than those who have never used the pill; and are less likely to have spread beyond the breast.

This reanalysis shows that these risks are not associated with duration of use, the dose or type of hormone in the COC, and there is no synergism with other risk factors for breast cancer (e.g. family history – see below).

The risks for progestogen-only contraceptives (POPs and injectables) failed to reach statistical significance. However, this does not exclude a real effect, which in that case would be very similar for those methods to the model for the COC. *See* Qs 7.51 *and* 8.37 for the practical implications.

5.86 What is the not-so-good news?

Mainly, this affects use by those with pre-existing risk factors; and by older women, who are now permitted to use the COC to age 50 if they choose to do so, provided they are fully healthy non-smokers (*see* Q 6.76). If the background risk for the individual is greater, whether because of increased age or a family history, the applicable percentage increase in *Table 5.5*

TABLE 5.6 Cumulative risk of breast cancer by recency of use. Showing usage in different age groups, the cumulative number of breast cancer cases per 10 000 women in never-users of oral contraception and the cumulative number per 10 000 women who had used oral contraception for 5 years and who were followed-up for 10 years after stopping

Pill use for 5 years or any duration*	To age 20	To age 25	To age 30	To age 35	To age 40	To age 45
Breast cancers diagnosed by:	Age 30	Age 35	Age 40	Age 45	Age 50	Age 55
Never-users	4	16	44	100	160	230
Users who stopped 10 years earlier	4.5	17.5	49	110	180	260
Excess number of cases of breast cancer per 10 000 women	0.5	1.5	5	10	20	30

*Because the CGHFBC researchers state that for a given age at last use the excess risk is little affected by a woman's prior duration of oral contraceptive use.

necessarily means more attributable cases (than in women without any breast cancer risk factor).

As *Fig. 5.8* shows, irrespective of the use of hormonal contraception the cumulative risk of breast cancer in young women is very small, being 1 in 500 in women up to age 35. But the cumulative risk increases with age thereafter, to 1 in 100 at age 45 and 1 in 12 by age 75. The increase in COC-attributable cases as age of last use increases has been calculated, and is shown in *Table 5.6*. Most importantly, for a given age at last use, the excess risk is little affected by a woman's prior duration of oral contraceptive use. Everything seems to depend on recency of use (i.e. current or within 10 years) at the given age.

5.87 In 2002, and again in 2006, what was the good news about breast cancer and the pill?

■ A large, well-conducted study by the US Centers for Disease Control (CDC) [Marchbanks PA et al 2002 *New England Journal of Medicine* 346:2025–2032] of 4575 women aged 35–64 with breast cancer, and matched controls, reported no increased COC-related risk – odds ratio of 1 or less. This applied across the board and for all the following: current users, past users, long-term users, users with a family history, and users starting COCs at young age. The latter was particularly comforting, negating the so-called 'time-bomb' for ex-users in this older age group with a high incidence for breast cancer – even for those exposed before a first full-term pregnancy. This study is very reassuring, given that COC exposure in the population was >70%, although it is not the last word by any means.

■ The RCGP and Oxford/FPA cohort studies described at *Q 5.53* above also showed no increased risk of breast cancer among takers or ex-takers of COCs and even an apparent slight protective effect some 20 years after cessation [Vessey M et al 2006 *British Journal of Cancer* 95:385–389].

5.88 Why do we not now simply go with anyone's first impression from the CDC study that it is no worse for the breast if sex hormones come from the COC instead of the ovaries?

The CGHFBC study (*see Q 5.84*) does have the virtues of size, plus the data coming from numerous different centres. Moreover, technically:

■ The upper confidence interval of the overall odds ratio was 1.3. This places the 24% increase shown in the 1996 pooled analysis within the bounds, i.e. that analysis might still be corresponding to reality.

■ Crucially, most of the cancers in the CDC study would have been diagnosed more than 10 years after stopping the COC and hence would be non-pill-caused ones on the CGHFBC model anyway (*see Q 5.85* and last line of *Table 5.5*).

■ The CDC study unfortunately tells us nothing about those few women (often with genetic predispositions) who are diagnosed with cancer under age 35 (this important group was not recruited).

■ The CDC study also has very little data about women who carry on taking the COC until the menopause. Very few of the latter were in the studied population, although such long-term use has been permitted as a choice in more recent years.

So the CGHFBC model should certainly continue to be applied to the last two important groups (*see Qs 5.92, 5.93*).

5.89 Can the adverse CGHFBC findings be explained by surveillance bias?

If reality is as the CDC study suggests – that there is truly no increase in risk when the breasts are exposed to the pill's hormones as opposed to those produced by the ovary, at least for cancer diagnosis at age 35–64 and when exposure to the COC has been mainly before age 35 – what explains the earlier findings?

The Collaborative Group conceded from the outset that their findings, of less advanced cases being identified in current or recent takers of the pill but more of them being found at each given age, could actually be explained wholly or in part by surveillance bias. This would imply that pill-takers, both during and after the years of use of the method, were relatively more 'breast aware' than non-takers, and so would have more excision biopsies.

But as already stated, the CDC study amplifies the reassurances of the earlier analysis rather than refuting it: because most of the cancers studied would have been diagnosed more than 10 years after stopping the COC and hence on the CGHFBC model would be background-risk cancers, not connected with the pill, anyway (see *Table 5.5*).

5.90 So what are the clinical implications for routine pill-counselling?

The Faculty of Sexual and Reproductive Healthcare in the UK states that pill-users should be informed of/counselled about the uncertainties with regard to breast cancer and the COC, but reiterates the advice given by the CSM that there need be no fundamental change in prescribing practice.

One effect of the essentially negative CDC study of 2002 is to remove pressure to raise this issue proactively at the first visit with young pill-users. However, any questions they have should be answered with complete transparency and, even if they are not asked, at an appropriate time the topic should always be addressed. Women should be encouraged to practise breast awareness and report any unusual changes promptly.

In summary, women using COCs can be reassured that:

■ There might be little or no added breast cancer risk for women through using the pill. If it exists, the highest likely estimate is 24% and then it applies only while women are taking the COC and for a few years thereafter; it reduces to zero after 10 years.
■ Beyond 10 years after stopping there is no detectable increase in breast cancer risk for former pill-users.
■ No excess COC-related mortality from this has been shown [Beral V et al 1999 *British Medical Journal* 318:96–100].
■ The cancers diagnosed in women who use or have ever used COCs are clinically less advanced than in those who have never used the pill and are less likely to have spread beyond the breast.
■ The risks, even if existing, are not associated with duration of use or the dose or type of hormone in the COC and there is no synergism with other risk factors for breast cancer (e.g. family history).
■ Women who do have a strong family history (breast cancer under age 40 in a sister or mother) do indeed have a pre-existing problem: but the percentage extra risk is the same for them as for girlfriends without the family history. They might certainly use the COC (WHO 2) if they so wish. But they should be advised to request reassessment whenever new data are obtained, and every 5 years.

■ The balancing protective effects of COCs against malignancy of the ovary and endometrium and now probably large bowel are always worth mentioning.

The known contraceptive and non-contraceptive benefits of COCs might seem so great to many (but not to all) as to compensate for the likely very small excess risk of breast cancer.

5.91 How do you explain the worst-case scenario to a pill-taker if the CGHFBC model continues to be the one we fundamentally accept?

I use the fourth column of *Table 5.6*, divide the numbers by 10, and ask her to visualize two concert halls, each like that shown in *Fig. 5.9 and each* holding 1000 women. Imagine that the first hall is filled with 1000 pill-takers, all now aged 45 – but all having used the COC for varying durations of time, then stopping when they reached age 35 (a common situation). The (cumulative) number of cases of breast cancer would be 11 in concert hall 1. However, in hall 2, which is filled with never-takers of the pill, also all currently aged 45, there would be 10 cases. Therefore there is only one extra pill-attributable case per 1000 in hall 1.

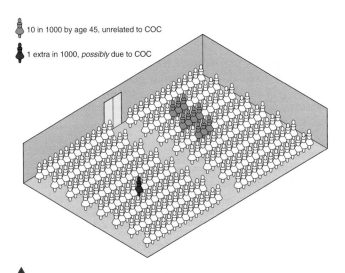

10 in 1000 by age 45, unrelated to COC

1 extra in 1000, *possibly* due to COC

▲

Fig. 5.9 Cumulative incidence of breast cancer during and after use of COC until age 35. *Q 5.91* (from Guillebaud 2007 *Contraception today*, 6th edn, p. 25. London, Informa Healthcare. With permission. Based on data from the Collaborative Group on Hormonal Factors in Breast Cancer 1996). See also *Table 5.6*.

Moreover, if the pill truly acts only as a cofactor, then it is very possible that this woman had had her disease initiated independently of the COC and without it would still have developed the disease – only at a later age.

Importantly, the remaining 989 women in hall 1 will, from this time on, have only the same risk of breast cancer as the women in hall 2, i.e. no ongoing added risk because it is over 10 years since their last pill. This is a very reassuring point for many.

Finally, the cancers diagnosed among the pill-takers in hall 1, already and in future, will tend to be less advanced than those in hall 2.

5.92 What about pill use by an older woman?

As *Table 5.6* shows, without any change in relative risk there is an increased attributable risk with age. For example (changing the denominator of the table to 1000), there are 3 extra cases per 1000 for ex-users now aged 55 who stopped the COC 10 years before, rather than the 1 extra case shown in *Fig. 5.9*. This must be explained and might be acceptable to many with the balancing from the established protection against cancer of the ovary and endometrium.

But, to my mind, these data, along with the age-related increase of all the circulatory diseases – even in risk-factor-free women – should lead more older women to choose from other more long-acting options (especially IUDs and the IUS).

5.93 What about COC use in high-risk groups for breast cancer, specifically (A) those with a family history of a young (under 40) first-degree relative with breast cancer or with a predisposing *BRCA* gene? And (B) women with benign breast disease (BBD)?

■ A sister or mother developing breast cancer this young means an approximate twofold greater background risk than the generality of women. Rather as just discussed for older women, the 24% increment in risk is not believed to be greater, but when applied to a bigger background rate means more attributable cases. Therefore, though UKMEC classifies it as WHO 1, this history in my view is a relative contraindication (WHO 2, *see Qs 5.121, 5.138*).

■ The *BRCA* genes, though rare, greatly increase the background risk of eventually getting breast cancer and are therefore classified WHO 3, meaning another method is definitely preferred.

■ BBD in all forms is classified by UKMEC as WHO 1. However, if a breast biopsy has been done and showed epithelial atypia, this in my view is at least WHO 3, and warrants obtaining the advice of the patient's oncologist/histologist.

■ Pending diagnosis, an undiagnosed breast mass is similarly WHO 3 for the COC.

Different women will react differently to the same information, given, as it should always be, in a balanced way. Some will ask for a different method, where no possible increase in breast cancer risk has been suggested – over and above that she has to live with. If, however, the woman chooses the COC, as she is entitled to do in all WHO 2 and sometimes in WHO 3 circumstances, given its balancing benefits on ovarian, endometrial and colorectal cancer, it should be a low-estrogen formulation with reassessment every 5 years or so.

5.94 What is the prognosis if a woman develops breast cancer while on the COC? Should women with this history ever use hormonal methods in future?

The prognosis is actually better than for a woman not on the COC at the time of diagnosis (see above). Nevertheless, most authorities advise that the pill should be discontinued and women with a history of this cancer should avoid COCs thereafter (WHO 4). In my view the COC should always be in the WHO 4 category, but I agree with UKMEC that all the progestogen-only methods are acceptable (WHO 3) with caution during remission: defined by WHO as after 5 years. This would be following discussion with the oncologist and with continued surveillance.

5.95 Has the last word been spoken on this issue?

No way! Research continues. The above (*Qs 5.82–5.94*) seems the best that we can make of available data at present.

5.96 What is the influence of the COC on other cancers?

PRIMARY HEPATOCELLULAR CARCINOMA

Case reports and case–control studies have suggested that COC use might promote this rare cancer. The annual attributable risk is estimated as less than 4 per million users. It might very well be much less: given that liver cancer is usually fatal within 1 year of diagnosis, yet there has been no increase in deaths in the US or Sweden, where the COC has been widely used since the 1960s. Instead, there has been a gradual increase in incidence and mortality in Japan, where the COC is seldom used.

Moreover, the pill association is not established in hepatitis-B-infected livers – fortunately, as that is the main risk factor for this cancer.

Once again, smoking rears its ugly head: increasing the relative risk of this cancer by a factor of four, even without the COC. A past history of liver tumours (benign as well as malignant) absolutely contraindicates (WHO 4) the COC thereafter. *See also Q 6.66* regarding cyproterone acetate.

MALIGNANT MELANOMA OF THE SKIN

An increased risk among COC-users, particularly of the superficial spreading type of this cancer, was suggested by early work. More recent studies show no link. It is becoming increasingly probable that the association was not causal – related to the pill itself – but rather due to the confounding variable (in those days) of exposure to ultraviolet light. In other words, pill-takers were more likely to sunbathe!

Women in long-term remission after melanoma – and *also* after apparent cure following fertility-conserving treatment for gynaecological cancers – can use COCs – provided their oncologist agrees.

No association has been shown with malignancy involving any other organ or tissue.

5.97 What is the influence of the COC on benign neoplasms?

See *Fig. 5.7*, page 160.

■ *Benign breast disease (BBD)*: a definite protective effect has been shown, which increases with duration of use and is probably attributable to the progestogen component of the pill. The protection in some studies seems to be restricted to the most common but less serious forms of the disease without epithelial atypia, the latter being considered the premalignant variety (*see Q 5.93*). This might explain the paradox that COCs protect against BBD developing in the first place but have no demonstrable protective effect against breast cancer.

■ *Hepatocellular adenoma*: though benign in histology, this tumour may present with a life-endangering haemoperitoneum and treatment is by major liver surgery (*see Q 6.40*). It occurs more frequently in COC-users than in other women, but the background prevalence is so low that the incidence among users of old-type COCs was found to be very small (around 1/100 000 users per year). The risk appears greatest in older women using relatively high-dose pills for a long period of time, and indeed has not been quantified for modern low-dose varieties. *See also Q 5.96 above.*

■ *Focal nodular hyperplasia (FNH) of the liver*: this has also been linked, and can regress with COC withdrawal (*see Q 5.136* for prescribing implications).

■ *Other benign tumours showing no association*: these include benign trophoblastic disease (but *see Q 5.78*) and prolactinoma of the pituitary gland. For some years it was widely held that COC use increased the risk of the latter, but good case–control studies have provided strong evidence against the association (*see also Q 5.138*).

■ *Fibroids*: while older high-estrogen OCs were believed to cause fibroids to increase in size, current more progestogen-dominant brands have been shown to reduce the risk of hospital referral for fibroids. However, this benefit has not been confirmed for the most recently marketed COCs.

THE COC AND CIRCULATORY DISEASES

5.98 Which circulatory diseases have been shown to be more common in COC-users?

To expand from Q 5.71:

- *Systemic hypertension*: this is not so much a disease in its own right, as it predisposes to and does its damage through the arterial circulatory diseases below. Detection of this is crucial, in determining eligibility for the COC and for ongoing safety in use of the method.
- *Venous disease*:
  - deep venous thrombosis
  - pulmonary embolism
  - rarely, thrombosis in important single veins, e.g. mesenteric, hepatic or retinal.
- *Arterial diseases*:
  - myocardial infarction
  - thrombotic strokes
  - haemorrhagic strokes
  - other arterial events affecting solitary but vital vessels, such as mesenteric or retinal arteries.

5.99 Can any of these risks be explained by known metabolic changes induced by the artificial hormones of the COC? In particular, what is the influence of the estrogen content?

- Over the years, biochemistry has been of only very limited help. Very many studies have been done but the true meaning of many of the findings has been difficult to interpret – particularly those thought to relate to arterial disease (*see Q 5.100* and *Table 5.7*).
- Alterations in clotting factor levels induced by estrogen might be thrombogenic. More important changes include reduced levels of antithrombin III and protein S but there are also increased levels of fibrinogen and several of the vitamin K-dependent coagulation factors. These changes help to explain the increased risk of venous thrombosis, particularly if the woman already has a congenital or acquired predisposition such as factor V Leiden and antiphospholipid antibodies (*see Qs 5.113, 5.115*).
- However, it is likely that if there is already significant arterial wall disease, estrogen might also promote superimposed arterial thrombosis. There is evidence of a compensatory increased fibrinolytic activity, also

TABLE 5.7 Some metabolic effects of combined oral contraceptives

	Blood level	Remarks
Liver		
Liver functioning	Altered in all	These many changes cause no
(a) generally	users	apparent long-term damage to the
(b) specifically		liver itself. The liver is involved,
Albumin	↓	however, in the production of most
Transaminases	↑	of the changes in blood levels of
Amino acids	Altered	substances shown elsewhere in this
Homocysteine	↑	table, including the important
		changes in carbohydrate and lipid
		metabolism, and coagulation
		factors
Blood glucose after	↑	These change, barely detectable
carbohydrate ingestion		with the latest pills, can partly
Blood lipids	Altered, mostly ↑	explain the increased risk of arterial
HDL-C – in low estrogen/	↓	disease with earlier preparations
progestogen-dominant		
COCs		
Clotting factors		
(a) generally	Mostly ↑	Both the pill and smoking affect
(b) specifically		these interrelated systems
Antithrombin III,	↓	Fibrinolysis is enhanced by COC in
Protein S		the blood, but reduced in the vessel
(anticlotting		walls
factors)		Protein S is lowered less by EE-
Fibrinolysis	↑	containing pills combined with LNG
Tendency for platelet	↑	than with DSG (see *Q 5.112*)
aggregation		
Hormones		
Insulin	↑	These hormone changes are related
Growth hormone	↑	to those affecting blood sugar and
Adrenal steroids	↑	blood lipids (above)
Thyroid hormones	↑	
Prolactin	↑	
LH	↓	These effects are integral to
FSH	↓	contraceptive actions. However, the
Endogenous estrogen	↓	first three tend to rise in some
Endogenous	↓	women during the pill-free week.
progesterone		Hence, any effective lengthening of
		the pill-free time can lead to an LH
		surge and ovulation

TABLE 5.7—cont'd

	Blood level	Remarks
Minerals and vitamins		
Iron	↑	This is a good effect for women prone to iron deficiency
Copper	↑	Effects unknown, but not believed to cause any health risk for most pill-users. Pyridoxine is discussed in *Q 6.23*
Zinc	↓	
Vitamins A, K	↑	
Riboflavin, folic acid	↓	
Vitamin B$_6$ (pyridoxine)	↓	
Vitamin B$_{12}$ (cyanocobalamin)	↓	
Vitamin C (ascorbic acid)	↓	
Binding globulins (including SHBG)	↑	These globulins carry hormones and minerals in the blood. Because their levels increase in parallel with the latter, the effective blood levels of the hormones or minerals are usually not much altered
Blood viscosity	↑	
Body water	↑	This retention of fluid explains some of the weight gain blamed on the pill
Factors affecting blood pressure	Altered	Drospirenone in Yasmin & Yaz might lower COC-associated ↑ aldosterone secretion and sodium retention (see *Qs 5.101, 6.9, 6.64*)
Renin substrate	↑	Changes do not correlate as well as expected with the rare incidence of frank pill-related hypertension
Renin activity	↑	
Angiotensin II	↑	
Immunity/allergy		
Number of leucocytes	↑	See *Qs 6.70–6.72*
Immunoglobulins	Altered	
Function of lymphocytes	Altered	

Notes:
1. In the table ↑ means the level usually goes up, ↓ down.
2. 'Altered' means that the changes are known to be more complex, with both increases and decreases occurring within the system.
3. The changes are generally (a) within the normal range, (b) similar to those of normal pregnancy.
4. These effects are obviously highly relevant to the interpretation of many laboratory tests. See *Q 6.80.*

an estrogen effect. This might in part explain the rarity of overt disease, especially arterial disease, in non-smoking pill-users.

■ Hepatic secretion of many different proteins is stimulated by estrogens. These proteins are involved in: the transport of hormones, vitamins and minerals, the control of BP and immunological processes. When estrogen is given, the stimulatory effect can sometimes be suppressed by concomitant administration of a progestogen. But the interactions are complex: there might also be synergism or independence of the effects (see *Table 5.7*), and there are differences between progestogens.

■ Finally, synthetic estrogens have been shown to raise arterial BP both in short-term challenge experiments and in longer-term studies.

> The protective increase in fibrinolysis is impaired by heavy smoking.

5.100 What is the influence of the progestogen content on metabolism and risk?

■ The risk of VTE, which still seems to be primarily caused by estrogen, might be modified by progestogens in some way as yet to be fully explained (*see Qs 5.108–5.112*).

■ Provided estrogen is also given, increasing the dose of progestogen leads to an increased rate of diagnosis of clinical hypertension. (However, when given without estrogen, as in the POP or DMPA, progestogens have not been shown to have an important adverse effect on BP.)

■ When estrogen was kept constant, the incidence of arterial diseases – both as a group and individually – was correlated with the progestogen dose in some early epidemiological studies. This has only been shown for levonorgestrel (LNG)–norethisterone (NET) group progestogens, often unhelpfully referred to as the 'second generation'.

■ Many studies, including an RCT at the Margaret Pyke Centre, have shown that if a constant dose of estrogen is given, then the estrogen-induced HDL-C increase is reversed by LNG- and NET-containing pills, whereas it is permitted by desogestrel or gestodene if present (*see Q 5.110*).

■ When arterial risk factors are present, however, it remains a tenable hypothesis that these apparently 'lipid-friendly' products might reduce arterial disease risk, relative to other products (*see Q 5.116*).

5.101 Given the importance of blood pressure in arterial disease, what effects does the COC have?

In the majority of COC-users there is a slight, measurable increase in both systolic and diastolic BP within the normotensive range. Early large studies showed a 1.5–3 times higher relative risk of clinical hypertension. Modern varieties with reduced biological impact of the estrogen and progestogen (both are relevant because there is synergism once estrogen is being taken) have reduced but not eliminated this risk.

However, the new progestogen drospirenone in combination with EE as Yasmin led in one pre-marketing clinical study to a very small but significant fall in mean BP. Whether using this or Yaz (*Q6.64*) translates into greater safety of those formulations for arterial disease, especially when there are risk factors, warrants further clinical studies.

Predisposing factors include:

- strong family history
- a tendency to water retention and obesity
- the metabolic syndrome (*see Q 5.66*).

Past pregnancy-associated hypertension (toxaemia) does *not* predispose to hypertension during OC use, in controlled studies. But the RCGP study showed that past toxaemia history (which might be a 'marker' for essential hypertension, not diagnosed before the pregnancy) does predispose to myocardial infarction, especially in smokers (*see Q 5.138*).

Hypertension is of course an important risk factor for the arterial diseases to be considered in detail below, especially heart disease and both types of stroke.

5.102 As of 2008, what do we really know about how the COC affects the various cardiovascular diseases?

On 3–7 November 1997, WHO convened in Geneva a Scientific Group Meeting on Cardiovascular Disease and Steroid Hormone Contraception. The background papers prepared for the meeting have been published in the journal *Contraception* (March 1998, vol. 57). The final report of the Scientific Group Meeting was published in 1998 by WHO (Technical Report Series, No. 877). A most useful summary was published by the WHO in 1998 in their periodical *Progress in Human Reproduction Research* (which also contains all the most important references). WHO's main findings have stood the test of time since then.

Venous thromboembolism (VTE)
The Scientific Group concluded that:

■ Current users of COCs have a low absolute risk of VTE, which is nonetheless 3–6 times that in non-users. The risk is probably highest in the first year of use and declines thereafter, but persists until discontinuation.

■ After use of COCs is discontinued, the risk of VTE drops rapidly to that in non-users.

■ Among users of COC preparations containing less than 50 μg of ethinylestradiol, the risk of VTE is not related to the dose of estrogen. [JG: Rather, this expected link has as yet neither been shown, nor disproved.]

■ COCs containing desogestrel or gestodene probably carry a small risk of VTE beyond that attributable to COCs containing levonorgestrel [JG: which appears to reduce the risk – but see EURAS study Q 5.119 below].

■ There are insufficient data to draw conclusions with regard to COCs containing norgestimate.

■ The absolute risks of VTE attributable to use of oral contraceptives rise with increasing age, obesity, recent surgery, and congenital or acquired thrombophilia.

■ Raised blood pressure, which is an important risk factor for arterial disease, does not appear to elevate the risk of venous thromboembolic disease. [JG: WHO made this point also about cigarette smoking: but newer data now suggest there is a true causative link with smoking.]

■ There are insufficient data to conclude whether there is a relation between VTE and the use of progestogen-only contraceptives. [JG: Yet in practice WHO and UKMEC classify a past history of VTE as no more than WHO 2 (see Q 5.121) for all the progestogen-only contraceptives. I agree, since there is no established causative link (Vasilakis C et al 1999 *The Lancet* 354:1610–1611)].

■ The relative risks of venous thromboembolic disease observed in users of COCs in developed countries appear to be applicable to developing countries.

Acute myocardial infarction (AMI)
Data are available which show that increasing age, cigarette smoking, diabetes, hypertension and raised total blood cholesterol are important risk factors for AMI in young women. The Scientific Group concluded that:

■ The incidence of fatal and non-fatal AMI is very low in women of reproductive age. Women who do not smoke, who have their blood pressure checked and who do not have hypertension or diabetes were, in the WHO and a number of other studies, including the EURAS study (see Q 5.119), at no increased risk of AMI if they used COCs, when compared with never-users of the same age. However, a small risk even in non-smokers was shown in two meta-analyses quoted by the Faculty of Sexual and Reproductive Healthcare in: http://www.fsrh.org/admin/uploads/FirstPrescCombOralContJan06.pdf.

■ There is no increase in the risk of AMI with increasing duration of use of COCs.

■ There is no increase in the relative risk of AMI in past users of COCs. **[JG: This is not the pattern to be expected if the COC alone, in the absence of arterial risk factors, were atherogenic.]**

■ Women with hypertension have an increased absolute risk of AMI. The relative risk of AMI in current users of COCs with hypertension is at least three times that in current users without hypertension.

■ The increased absolute risk of AMI in women who smoke is greatly elevated by use of COCs, especially in heavy smokers. The relative risk of AMI in heavy smokers who use COCs might be as high as 10 times that in non-smokers who do not use COCs. **[JG: See *Table 5.8*.]**

■ Although the incidence of AMI increases exponentially with age, the relative risk of AMI in current users of COCs does not change with increasing age.

■ There are insufficient data to assess whether the risk of AMI in users of low-dose COCs is modified by the type of progestogen. [*But see Q 5.116.*]

■ The above conclusions appear to apply equally to women in developed and developing countries.

Ischaemic stroke

The Scientific Group concluded that:

■ The incidence of fatal and non-fatal ischaemic stroke is very low in women of reproductive age, but increases with increasing age.

■ In women who do *not* smoke, who have their blood pressure checked, and who do not have hypertension, the risk of ischaemic stroke is nevertheless increased about 1.5-fold in current users of low-dose COCs compared with non-users.

■ There is no further increase in the risk of ischaemic stroke with increasing duration of use of COCs.

■ Women who have stopped taking COCs are at no greater risk of ischaemic stroke than women who have never used oral contraceptives.

■ Women with hypertension have an increased absolute risk of ischaemic stroke. The relative risk of ischaemic stroke in current users of COCs with hypertension appears to be at least three times that in current users without hypertension.

TABLE 5.8 Estimated number of cardiovascular events (per million woman-years) at different ages among non-users and users of combined oral contraceptives in developed countries by smoking habits

Cardiovascular event	Age (years)		
	20–24	30–34	40–44
Non-smokers – Non-users			
Acute myocardial infarction	0.13	1.69	21.28
Ischaemic stroke	6.03	9.84	16.05
Haemorrhagic stroke	12.73	24.28	46.30
Venous thromboembolism	32.23	45.75	59.28
Total	51.12	81.56	142.9
Non-smokers – Users*			
Acute myocardial infarction	0.20	2.55	31.92
Ischaemic stroke	9.04	14.75	24.07
Haemorrhagic stroke	12.73	24.28	92.60
Venous thromboembolism	96.68	137.30	177.80
Total	118.70	178.90	326.40
Smokers – Non-users			
Acute myocardial infarction	1.08	13.58	170.20
Ischaemic stroke	12.06	19.67	32.09
Haemorrhagic stroke	25.46	48.55	138.90
Venous thromboembolism	32.23	45.75	59.28
Total	70.83	127.60	400.50
Smokers – Users*			
Acute myocardial infarction	1.62	20.36	255.30
Ischaemic stroke	18.09	29.51	48.14
Haemorrhagic stroke	38.19	72.83	231.50
Venous thromboembolism	96.68	137.30	177.80
Total	154.60	260.00	712.70

*Blood pressure was checked in users.
Source: Farley TMM, Collins J, Schlesselman JJ. Hormonal contraception and risk of cardiovascular disease: an international perspective. *Contraception* 1998;57:211–230.

- The absolute risk of ischaemic stroke in women who smoke is about 1.5–2 times that in non-smokers; this risk is multiplied by a factor of 2–3 if such women are also current users of COCs.
- The risk of ischaemic stroke in users of COCs containing high doses of estrogen is higher than that in users of COCs containing low doses of estrogen.

■ These conclusions appear to apply equally in developed and developing countries.

[JG: NB This WHO report does not mention migraine with focal aura (though this does feature in WHOMEC UKMEC, *see Qs 5.153–5.161).* **It is believed that universally better prescribing in relation to this predisposing factor ought further to reduce the risk of this catastrophic complication.]**

Haemorrhagic stroke
The Scientific Group concluded that:

■ The incidence of fatal and non-fatal haemorrhagic stroke is very low in women of reproductive age.
■ In women aged less than 35 years who do not smoke and who do not have hypertension, the relative risk of haemorrhagic stroke associated with use of COCs is not increased.
■ The incidence of haemorrhagic stroke increases with age, and current use of COCs appears to magnify this effect of ageing.
■ There is no increase in the risk of haemorrhagic stroke with increasing duration of use of oral contraceptives.
■ Women who have previously used oral contraceptives are at no greater risk of haemorrhagic stroke than women who have never used them.
■ Women with hypertension have an increased absolute risk of haemorrhagic stroke. The relative risk of haemorrhagic stroke in current users of COCs with hypertension might be 10 times that in current users without hypertension.
■ The risk of haemorrhagic stroke in women who smoke is up to twice that in non-smokers; in women who are current users of COCs and who smoke, the relative risk is about 3.
■ There is no evidence that either the estrogen or the progestogen constituent of COCs is related to the risk of haemorrhagic stroke.
■ These conclusions appear to apply equally in developed and developing countries.

Possible biological mechanisms for cardiovascular effects
COCs affect lipoprotein and carbohydrate metabolism, haemostasis, and mechanisms regulating blood pressure. An influence on the functioning of the endothelium of blood vessels and arterial tone also seems likely. The Scientific Group concluded that:

■ The biological mechanisms underlying cardiovascular disease involve a complex interplay between lipoprotein metabolism, humoral regulators such as insulin, coagulation and fibrinolysis, the renin–angiotensin–

aldosterone system, and the functioning of the endothelium of blood vessels.

■ COCs do not increase the risk of developing diabetes mellitus. They have little effect on fasting plasma concentrations of glucose and insulin but cause modest elevations in the plasma levels of glucose and insulin after an oral glucose challenge and might increase insulin resistance.

■ The changes in metabolism of lipoproteins in plasma induced by use of COCs have been extensively studied. Low-dose COCs increase fasting plasma levels of triglycerides but have only minor effects on low-density lipoprotein–cholesterol (LDL-C) or total cholesterol. The effect on HDL-C depends on the balance of estrogen and progestogen. The clinical significance of such changes is uncertain in the context of current low-dose formulations.

■ COCs alter the plasma concentrations of many components (including their activation markers) of both the coagulation and fibrinolytic systems. These changes are less marked with COCs containing low doses of ethinylestradiol and even less so with progestogen-only contraceptives. Hereditary conditions such as antithrombin III defect and factor V Leiden mutation predispose women to VTE. These disorders might underlie a large proportion of idiopathic venous thromboembolic events, perhaps one-third of those seen in Caucasian women. This effect is increased in women using COCs.

■ The prevalence of hereditary conditions such as antithrombin III defect and factor V Leiden mutation is about 5% in Caucasian women but is lower in other populations. The positive predictive value of screening for these disorders is very low. [JG: *See Qs 5.113 and 5.114.*]

■ Even low-dose COCs cause modest elevations in blood pressure that might increase the risk of arterial disease. In healthy young women with a low background risk of arterial disease, small increases in blood pressure attributable to use of COC are likely to have minimal effects on the absolute risk of arterial disease.

Making informed choices about COCs
It is clear that mortality rates from each of the above cardiovascular diseases are extremely low among women of reproductive age, and that the added risk of using steroid contraceptives is also very low. Within the context of the everyday risks of modern life, steroid contraceptives are safe. Factors that need to be taken into account when determining a woman's risk of cardiovascular disease while using COCs include:

■ the age-specific incidence of each cardiovascular condition
■ the strength of the association between use of COCs and each cardiovascular outcome

- the woman's age and presence of other risk factors for cardiovascular disease, such as smoking and a history of hypertension
- whether there are important differences in risk between particular formulations of COC, and, if so, the choice of formulation.

The number of cardiovascular events attributable to the use of COCs is very small, especially among users of all ages who do not smoke and among younger users who smoke. [**JG: This is shown very clearly in *Table 5.8*, which comes from the same WHO publication, especially as the numbers shown are per million women per year.**] The number of associated deaths is even smaller and, again, is highly dependent on whether the user is a smoker. Any small increase in risk of cardiovascular disease must be considered against the very high contraceptive efficacy of COCs and the rapid reversibility of this effect after they are stopped. The use of less reliable alternative methods of contraception (or the avoidance of any contraception) exposes women to an increased risk of pregnancy, a condition that is associated with a higher incidence of venous thromboembolic disease than that associated with the use of any of the currently available low-dose COCs. In addition, COCs are associated with many non-contraceptive benefits, including a reduced risk of endometrial and ovarian cancer.

The Study Group concluded with respect to total cardiovascular disease risk, that:

- Among users of COCs who do not have risk factors for cardiovascular disease, the annual risk of death attributable to use of oral contraceptives is approximately 2 deaths per million users at 20–24 years of age, 2–5 per million users at 30–34 years of age and approximately 20–25 per million users at 40–44 years of age. [**JG: In *Fig. 5.11* I use a summary risk of 10 per million for the total all-age and all-cause mortality risk of the COC. This seems about right even if the EURAS findings (Q 5.119) are confirmed.**
- The risk of mortality from all cardiovascular disease attributable to use of oral contraception is much greater (up to 10-fold) among women aged 40–44 years than among women aged 20–24 years. [**JG: A very relevant point this, now we have several new highly effective long-acting choices for the older woman, despite the convenience for her of the COC (*see Q 11.38*).**]
- *At any given age a woman who smokes but who does not use oral contraceptives is at greater risk of death from arterial disease than a user of oral contraceptives who does not smoke . . .*
- Venous thromboembolic disease is the most common cardiovascular event among users of oral contraceptives. However, it contributes very little (sic – *but see Q. 5.119)* to any increase in the number of deaths,

since the associated mortality (maximum 2%) is relatively low compared with that associated with arterial diseases. Long-term disability from non-fatal venous thromboembolic disease is also low.

5.103 What is the difference between relative risk and absolute or attributable risk?

This is a most important distinction, which is not often understood by either patients or journalists. Twice almost nothing out of a million is still almost nothing! Many pill-takers can relate to the analogy that being given a second lottery ticket does not make you hugely more likely to win, even though doubling your chances:

A small relative risk might easily cause more attributable cases than a large one, if the background prevalence is high – and vice versa.

In *Table 5.9* the first set of figures (A) actually apply to the frequency of hepatocellular adenoma in controls as compared with COC-users taking older 50-μg-plus pills. The second set (B) come from *Table 5.8* (*see Q 5.102*), which itself is from the 1998 report of the WHO's special Scientific Group. They apply to smokers aged 40–44, who would have an increase in relative risk of AMI of only 1.5 if they additionally took the modern low-dose pills at that age; but the attributable number of extra cases (absolute risk) is 85 per million. Contrast only 19 extra cases of hepatoma in the first set of figures (A), despite a 20-fold greater relative risk.

Neither statistic is good news (both are dangerous conditions). But the difference in the excess number of cases caused explains why it was reasonable to accept, for the old-type 50-μg-plus pills, a 20-fold increase in the risk of benign liver tumours. However, a mere 50% increase in AMI through more modern pills is widely considered unacceptable for smokers above age 40.

5.104 Patients are naturally anxious about the known adverse effects of the combined pill on cancer and circulatory disease. Assuming they otherwise wish to use the method, how can this anxiety be reduced?

See Q 5.102, the section on 'making informed choices', and *Figs 5.10* and *5.11*. The media do the general public a disservice by tending to exaggerate

TABLE 5.9 Attributable risk			
Background prevalence	Relative risk	No. of cases	No. of cases attributable
(A) 1 in 10^6	×20	20	19
(B) 170 in 10^6	×1.5	255	85

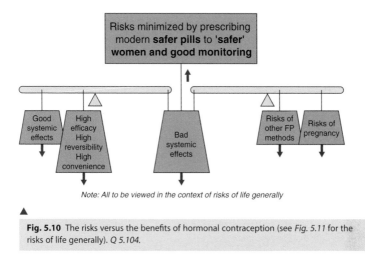

Fig. 5.10 The risks versus the benefits of hormonal contraception (see *Fig. 5.11* for the risks of life generally). *Q 5.104.*

the bad systemic effects and by not pointing out the counterbalancing non-contraceptive benefits, aside from the advantages of efficacy, reversibility and convenience. Another form of counterbalancing is shown on the right-hand side of *Fig. 5.10*, namely the comparison with the risks of pregnancy (so effectively avoided by the COC) and the avoidance of the risk and inconvenience of the alternative methods.

- Potential users can be reminded that there are many other risks in life. However intelligent and educated, most of us are amazingly 'risk-illiterate'. Many risks are far greater than pill-taking, yet cause minimal concern: for example, having babies or travelling by car (*Figs 5.11, 5.12*). Life is pretty risky: believe it or not, each year one has a 1:1000 chance of having to visit a Casualty Department through a home injury from a bottle or a can. At least three deaths have been reported at the Brompton Hospital through allergy to hamsters.
- For those who are not very numerate, risks are best expressed by, for example: 'The risk of dying through pill-taking is less than one-hundredth of the risk of death through smoking 20 cigarettes a day'.
- Others find it helpful to look at *Fig. 5.12*, which shows the time taken to achieve a one-in-a-million risk of dying: e.g. by 1 h of car-driving. On that basis, since the highest likely estimate of all-cause pill mortality risk (based on high-dose products) comes to about 10 per million (*see Q 5.102*), if a new pill-taker drives for 10 fewer hours than normal in the whole of the coming year, it will be as though she is 'not on the pill at all!' – in terms of risk.

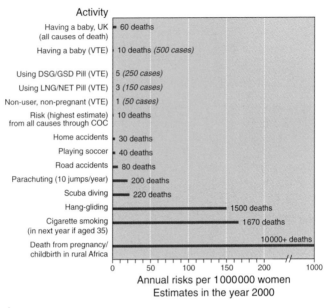

Fig. 5.11 The risks of various activities (annual number of deaths per 1 000 000 exposed). *Q 5.104.* With regard to cancer, in this figure, excess cancer mortality is assumed to be zero (see *Q 5.74* and *Fig. 5.6*) (sources: Dinman 1980 *Journal of the American Medical Association* 244:1226–1228; Mills et al 1996 *British Medical Journal* 312:121; Anonymous 1991 *British Medical Journal* 302:743; Strom 1994 *Pharmacoepidemiology*, 2nd edn, pp. 57–65. Chichester, John Wiley; Guillebaud 1998 *Contraception today*, 3rd edn, p. 20. London, Martin Dunitz). COC, combined oral contraceptive; DSG, desogestrel; GSD, gestodene; LNG, levonorgestrel; NET, norethisterone; VTE, venous thromboembolism. *Note:* The EURAS study 2007 gives much higher VTE rates across the board, for reasons not yet fully explained: see *Q 5.119.*

■ Finally, prospective pill-takers can be reminded that the tiny risks of the COC can be further reduced: by careful prescribing of lower-dose preparations, with good subsequent monitoring (*see Qs 5.120, 5.138, 6.1*).

5.105 What effect does smoking have on the mortality of arterial disease in pill-users?

Given the relevance of smoking as a serious risk people take for granted, it is salutary to note that the 1983 report of the RCGP showed (and later data are congruent) that the pill-user who also smoked not only was more likely to suffer a heart attack but also was much more likely to die as a consequence – a higher case-fatality rate was noted in smokers.

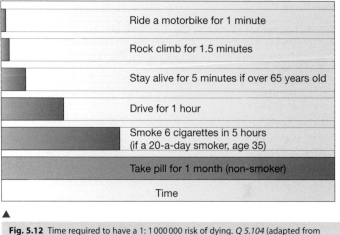

▲

Fig. 5.12 Time required to have a 1: 1 000 000 risk of dying. *Q 5.104* (adapted from Minerva, *British Medical Journal*, 1988; from Guillebaud 2007 *Contraception today*, 6th edn, p. 25. London, Informa Healthcare. With permission).

5.106 How can a busy doctor ever convey enough information about COCs to enable worried women to make a fully informed decision?

So much is now known about the method that this is becoming ever more difficult to do. The advice of the Medical Defence Societies is:

A doctor has the duty to give such warnings and carry out such checks as are considered by his/her peers to be necessary having regard to the relevant circumstances of the case. There is no obligation to explain every risk but there is the need to be forthright in explaining risks.

In other words, you should be frank about what is known and honest about what is not yet known; communicate the main pros and cons of the method as in *Qs 5.57 and 5.71–5.104*; explain the practicalities, rules for missed pills, minor side-effects – most especially BTB; and allow time for questions. Full records should be kept. A pretty tall order!

For most busy practitioners who wish to maintain high standards, 'allow time' means more accurately:

■ 'make time', plus
■ delegate.

In the real world, how do women present? In the middle of a busy surgery, as like as not needing postcoital contraception first (*see Chapter 10*, a whole chapter to take account of there!), and then to start the COC before their follow-up visit.

> A useful tip: make it the Practice's norm that all new starters on the pill (or any 'medical' method) have a second 10–15-min appointment later in the same week, often with the Practice Nurse, to answer any questions – which often arise later, after they have read the fpa leaflet (see below).

5.107 What else is important as an adjunct to good counselling?

The written word! In my view, counselling should always be supplemented by a leaflet and I think the best is still the fpa's leaflet on the combined pill. At the time of writing (July 2008), I have concerns about their Flow Diagram for missed pills, but the wording of the rest of the current leaflet is excellent. Among other things, this has a medico-legally important bulleted list of those side-effects that should lead the woman to seek urgent medical advice (*see Q 6.13*).

But new pill-takers must *always* also receive the PIL (licensed patient information leaflet) that relates to the specific product.

Finally, much medical time can be saved if those women who desire the impossible, a 2-h consultation about oral contraception, are referred to my comprehensive paperback entitled *The Pill* (see Further Reading)!

THE 1995 CONTROVERSY ABOUT VENOUS THROMBOEMBOLISM (VTE) – WHERE ARE WE NOW?

5.108 Now that the dust has settled, what is your take on that letter from the UK Committee on Safety of Medicines (CSM) on 18 October 1995 regarding VTE?

There is still a range of expert views about the four publications on COCs and VTE published in December 1995 and January 1996, mentioned above in the long WHO extract. They were carefully performed and reasonably congruent with each other. They reported a doubling of the odds ratio for users of desogestrel/gestodene-containing products (DSG/GSD-containing or so-called 'third generation' progestogens) in comparison with the 'second generation' levonorgestrel- or norethisterone-containing ones (here called 'LNG/NET pills').

[The 'generation' terminology is ambiguous and best avoided. I now much prefer to refer to the *relative estrogen dominance of each formulation* (*see Q 5.111*).]

5.109 Yet has not the accuracy of this finding been queried?

Indeed: many authorities continue to believe that the whole of the apparent association can be explained not by cause-and-effect but by:

■ Prescriber bias (prescribers being selectively more likely, prior to October 1995, to use DSG/GSD products for first-timers and women thought to be at risk of VTE).

■ The 'attrition of susceptibles' or 'healthy-user effect' (LNG/NET pills being more commonly used by longer-term users and parous women who would be less likely as a population to suffer a VTE, because those who had had this disease would no longer be using the method).

■ Diagnostic bias resulting from prescriber bias, in that women put on DSG/GSD pills because of a perceived higher risk might then also be more likely to be referred for accurate investigations, leading to this easily overlooked diagnosis being made more often than among users of LNG/NET pills.

Evidence for these alternative explanations for the finding comes from:

■ In 1996, Lewis and co-workers on the Transnational study showed a significant trend of increasing risk of VTE for the progestogens in COCs, related solely to the recency of their introduction to the market.

■ There is also the very odd WHO finding that Mercilon with 20 µg of EE, the artificial estrogen well recognized as creating prothrombotic coagulation changes, was significantly associated with more cases of VTE than Marvelon with 30 µg.

Neither of the above is biologically plausible, yet they might be readily linked to prescriber bias and the healthy-user effect.

But for honest seekers after the truth (you – the reader – and I!) the question remains whether there could yet be some real difference between DSG and GSD versus LNG or NET combined products in allowing EE to cause VTE events despite the non-causative explanations – although clearly these must apply in part.

5.110 In your opinion, where does that leave us as prescribers?

At the time of writing (July 2007), personally, I am sure the apparent doubling is a worst-case scenario, because of the exaggerating effects of the above biases and confounders. But even allowing for these, I am prepared to accept some difference of VTE risk when comparing the DSG/GSD pills with the LNG and NET ones (*see Q 5.111*), which is so small as to be almost negligible. See Q 5.119 (EURAS study), below.

5.111 Is it biologically plausible that the same 30-µg dose of EE would have different effects when combined with the two different types of progestogens?

There is a degree of biological plausibility, yes, because we have known for years that NET (somewhat) and LNG (more so) behave in some respects as antiestrogenic progestogens:

■ A dose of 30 µg EE raises SHBG, raises HDL-C and tends to improve acne.

■ In an RCT at the Margaret Pyke Centre we found that if LNG 150 µg is combined with the same 30-µg dose of EE, as in Microgynon/Ovranette, then SHBG goes up less than with EE alone and HDL-C is actually lowered (i.e. the EE effect is reversed). See *Fig. 5.13*. Moreover, clinically, acne may be worsened. Therefore, LNG (and, in high enough dose, NET) is clearly capable of opposing the estrogenicity of EE in its biochemical effects (e.g. SHBG) and in some of its somatic effects (e.g. acne).

■ However, combined with DSG 150 µg, as in Marvelon, or with GSD 75 µg, as in Femodene/Katya 30/75 (new generic marketed in UK since last edition), the same dose of EE raises SHBG more, raises HDL-C and tends to improve acne – all very like EE would do on its own. See *Fig. 5.13*.

Thus, on those three criteria (among others), DSG/GSD pills allow EE to have more of its estrogenic effects than LNG ones do. As prothrombotic coagulation changes are also primarily estrogen-related, a similar difference in VTE potential has always been possible.

What about the POPs (in *Chapter 7*) and thrombosis, specifically Cerazette, which is the only one that has a 'third generation' progestogen, i.e. desogestrel?

Following from the data in *Fig. 5.13* above, that LNG and NET oppose a number of estrogen-mediated effects – and the extra evidence in *Q 5.112* that this opposition effect extends specifically to procoagulant clotting changes affecting protein S etc. – there is no cause for concern with the desogestrel-containing Cerazette. This is because:

■ The product itself is estrogen-free, devoid of any EE in it to cause worries about thrombosis.

■ The progestogen it contains is one of the 'neutral' ones, not one that influences the effects of estrogen. It leaves all estrogens – including the body's own estradiol – alone, to have their usual effects, including on clotting factors.

Therefore there is at present no evidence against the view that desogestrel in Cerazette is neutral in the matter of thrombosis. It won't reduce the risk of VTE below normal for that woman – but neither should it increase it. *See Qs 7.40 and 7.41.*

Fig. 5.13 Prospective randomized controlled trials of four pills: desogestrel (DSG) + ethinylestradiol (EE) 30; gestodene (GSD) + EE30; norethisterone acetate (NETA) + EE30; levonorgestrel (LNG) + EE30. **A.** Increment in sex hormone-binding globulin (SHBG). **B.** Change in high-density lipoprotein (HDL) cholesterol. (Margaret Pyke Centre Study.) Q 5.111 (from Guillebaud 2007 *Contraception today*, 6th edn, p. 22. London, Informa Healthcare. With permission).

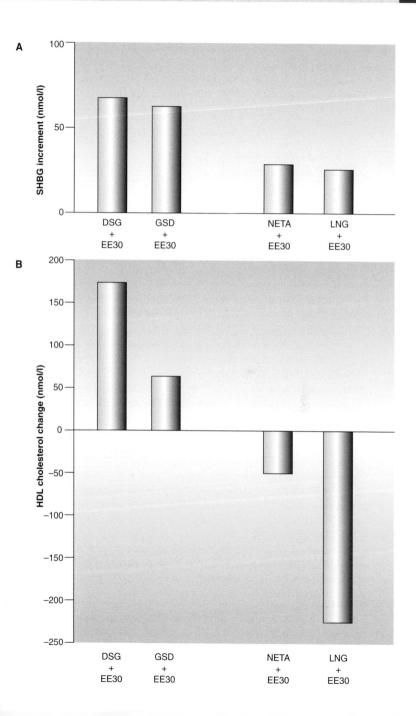

5.112 But surely no one has been able to show a consistent difference in the effects of the two types of progestogen upon the coagulation factors that are altered by estrogen?

On the contrary, such differences are now emerging in relation to so-called acquired activated protein C resistance (the work of Rosing and others in the Netherlands) and to the lowering of protein S, which are both estrogenic effects. In a further study on volunteers, we showed [Mackie IJ et al 2001 *British Journal of Haematology* 113:898–904] that protein S was reduced more in users of DSG than in those taking LNG formulations ($P < 0.0001$). Protein S decreased significantly when switching from LNG to DSG pills, mirrored by a similar and significant *increase* with switching from DSG to LNG formulations. Yet both products (Marvelon and Microgynon) contain the same 30-μg dose of the protein-S-lowering estrogen EE.

This fits well with my hypothesis that LNG 'opposes the estrogenicity' of EE in the COC. For actual thrombosis to occur, we suggested a further triggering factor was a likely prerequisite.

5.113 What are the main hereditary predispositions to VTE? And what action should be taken if one is suspected?

Women with possible hereditary thrombophilia, or who give a clear family history of idiopathic thrombosis in a parent or sibling under 45 (see *Table 5.10*, p. 200), should ideally not be prescribed any COC until thrombophilia has been excluded. The most prevalent abnormality is factor V Leiden (the genetic cause of activated protein C resistance). If this, and rarer problems like deficiencies of protein C, protein S and antithrombin III and the G20210 mutation in the prothrombin gene are known to exist, they absolutely contraindicate all EE-containing pills. This is so albeit, actually, the attributable risk from having any of them is not great (*see Q 5.114*).

On the other hand, even if they are not found the woman cannot be totally reassured. The haemostatic system is immensely complicated. Almost half of truly idiopathic cases of VTE are not explainable by modern coagulation testing since by no means all the predisposing abnormalities of the haemostatic system have yet been characterized. Therefore, in *Table 5.10* (p. 200) the COC is still WHO 2 if a woman with a positive family history has negative test results. She might indeed use the pill method, but should be specifically advised about the early symptoms of thromboembolism. Moreover, like all with a single relative contraindication for VTE, she should normally receive an LNG/NET pill.

5.114 If resources are available, why do we not simply screen everyone who asks to go on the pill for a predisposing factor to VTE?

Because it is neither cost-effective nor good practice to screen for the hereditary thrombophilias in cases without well-defined family history criteria (i.e. thrombophilia in the family or idiopathic thrombosis in a parent or sibling under 45). Given that each year there are only three extra cases of VTE among 1000 pill-takers with the most common thrombophilia, factor V Leiden, compared with pill-users without this predisposition, 997 of 1000 never actually get a thrombosis. They prove, in a real sense, to be 'false positives'; and then there are other predispositions that are not yet measurable (leading to many 'false negatives'). Given the cost of comprehensive testing, it would cost £100 000s to save one life by untargeted screening. More harm than good would result.

5.115 What are the acquired thrombophilias, and when should they be looked for/screened for?

Antiphospholipid antibodies (such as the unhelpfully named lupus anticoagulant) can appear in various connective tissue disorders, especially systemic lupus erythematosus (SLE). They should be looked for whenever such a disorder is suspected. However, screening for these in *healthy* women is not cost-effective because, once again, of the number of false positives (women with a detectable abnormality who never get a thrombosis, even during years of pill-taking) and false negatives (women who suffer an idiopathic thrombotic event with or without the COC yet have no congenital or acquired abnormality which modern technology can detect).

Antiphospholipid antibodies increase the risk of both VTE and arterial disease and therefore if present they absolutely contraindicate the COC – but are not an issue for any of the progestogen-only methods (*see Q 7.41*).

5.116 Which progestogens might be best for the least arterial wall disease risk (chiefly AMI and strokes)?

There still remains the possibility of a relative benefit to the arterial walls and hence arterial disease from what appear to be the 'good' effects of DSG/GSD-containing and other more estrogen-dominant COC brands: they do not lower HDL-C as some of the higher-dose LNG and NET brands do.

Some epidemiological data on AMI are now available, but not enough to be conclusive. Both the Transnational study and the Tanis study [Tanis BC et al 2002 *New England Journal of Medicine* 345:1787–1793] have shown – among smokers – that users of low-dose formulations containing LNG had a statistically significant increased risk of AMI, but no such increase if they used DSG/GSD products. The 1999 MICA study was not confirmatory of this, but a later report from the same group's data did show a lower *mortality* from myocardial infarction if the smokers who became AMI patients had been using GSD or DSG formulations. More studies are needed to confirm these findings.

5.117 How would you put the VTE risks in perspective?

See *Table 5.8* (p. 180) and *Figs 5.11 and 5.12* (pp. 186 and 187). The new studies confirm that all low-dose COCs carry an extremely low risk for healthy women. The UK Department of Health (DoH) issued a helpful statement in April 1999, which has not been revoked, as follows:

An increased risk of venous thromboembolic disease (VTE) associated with the use of oral contraceptives is well established but is smaller than that associated with pregnancy; which has been estimated at 60 cases per 100 000 pregnancies. Some epidemiological studies have reported a greater risk of VTE for women using combined oral contraceptives containing desogestrel or gestodene (the so-called third generation pills) than for women using pills containing levonorgestrel (LNG) – the so-called second generation pills **[JG: sic, actually this category also includes norethisterone (NET) pills]**. The spontaneous incidence of VTE in healthy non-pregnant women (not taking any oral contraceptive) is about 5 cases per 100 000 women per year. The incidence in users of second generation pills is about 15 per 100 000 women per year of use. The incidence in users of third generation pills is about 25 cases per 100 000 women per year of use: this excess incidence has not been satisfactorily explained by bias or confounding. The level of all of these risks of VTE increases with age and is likely to be increased in women with other known risk factors for VTE such as obesity.

Women must be fully informed of these very small risks. . . . Provided they are, the type of pill is for the woman together with her doctor or other family planning professionals jointly to decide in the light of her individual medical history [JG: my emphasis].

Note in the above DoH quotation that even though the DoH accepts a real difference between the two 'generations' of COCs – and this is still hotly disputed by some – the estimated annual 'spontaneous' VTE risk per 100 000 users for DSG/GSD pills is assessed at only 25 cases versus 15 for LNG/NET pills.

■ Multiplying by 10, therefore, the difference – being the annual attributable number of cases through using DSG/GSD brands rather than one of the less estrogen-dominant ones – is small, 100 VTE cases per million.

■ Using these estimates and taking the upper estimate of about 2% *mortality* for VTE, there is only a 2 per million difference in annual VTE mortality between DSG/GSD products and LNG/NET products.

■ Now, it has been estimated that there is a one-in-a-million risk in each hour of travel by car (see *Fig. 5.12*, p. 187). Even if the whole of the above difference is accepted as real, therefore, it is small enough, in comparison with other risks (see *Fig. 5.11*) that are taken in everyday life, for a well-informed woman to take if she so chooses.

> ■ If, for example, she wishes to use or to switch to a DSG/GSD brand on the grounds of 'quality of life', to control so-called minor side-effects such as acne, headaches, depression, weight gain or breast symptoms: if her previous COC was Microgynon she can be told that if she simply avoids 2 h of driving in the whole of the next year, in risk terms it remains as if she never left off taking the Microgynon.

5.118 Is intolerance of the LNG/NET pill brands through non-life-endangering but nevertheless 'annoying' side-effects acceptable as sufficient grounds for a woman to use a DSG/GSD brand?

Yes, this is clear in the above DoH quote; indeed, it was accepted from the outset, in the original letter circulated by the CSM – provided the woman understood and accepted the tiny excess risk of VTE. In my experience as a counsellor of pill-takers, the difference in risk compared with an LNG/NET brand as described in the above Box is often seen as unimportant to the point of irrelevance, compared with the risks of life generally (once those are better understood). *See also Q 5.119.*

5.119 How different are the estimates of VTE incidence from the EURAS (European Active Surveillance Study) report of 2007, compared with those used in the above discussion?

A paper in *Contraception* [2007;75:344–354] reports on EURAS, a massive post-marketing surveillance cohort study of 58 674 COC-users with only 2.4% loss to follow-up, mainly recruiting in Germany – and a parallel study of 48 961 women of reproductive age in a representative sample of the German population – who were questioned about their use of OCs, pregnancy and the occurrence of VTE during the last 12 months.

■ The authors conclude that, for reasons not yet fully explained, VTE risks both off and on the COC appear to be much higher than those used hitherto by the DoH (*see Q 5.117*) and by the European regulatory authorities.

■ If the data in their parallel study are adjusted for the age profile of the EURAS population, the incidence for non-pregnant non-users is 440 VTE events per million woman-years (95% confidence interval, 2.4–7.3).

■ Users of COCs in EURAS all had a similar elevated VTE risk of approximately 900 per million woman-years overall: with no difference shown between the different formulations. This implies the VTE risk for OC-users is roughly twice as high as for non-pregnant non-users.

■ In relative terms, this difference is smaller than previously assumed. However, as previously explained, the absolute attributable risk is higher: a COC-attributable increase of over 400 cases per million users with a 2% mortality would mean 8 extra deaths per million woman-years just from VTE.

■ However, reassuringly, no increase was seen in EURAS in the risks of arterial disease for any formulation, compared to non-users of the COC.

■ Since arterial disease has a much higher mortality risk than VTE, if EURAS is right then one can remain fairly comfortable with the approximate 10 per million (10 h of driving) estimate for annual mortality risk overall for COC-taking, as used in *Q 5.104*. It would simply mean there were more venous but fewer arterial deaths than we had previously assumed, within the same total.

■ BMI was a crucial risk factor, causing a threefold increase in VTE incidence for women with a BMI over 30 compared with those with a normal BMI of 20–24. *See Q 5.122.*

The authors discuss these rates of VTE at some length, both in the above paper and in a Review [*Contraception* 2007;75:328–336]. Why are the absolute risks so much higher both for controls and for women using the COC than for those on which most discussions have been based ever since 1995, as used in *Fig. 5.11* and *Q 5.117*?

■ On the one hand, the cohort design, careful ascertainment and high follow-up rates suggest validity of the new estimates.

■ On the other hand, some other studies may have found lower rates, appropriately, because they were more focused on 'idiopathic' VTE rather than *all* VTE – which includes predisposing factors such as leg fracture or surgery.

The truth remains elusive here and the interested reader should read the above papers in *Contraception*.

SELECTION OF USERS AND FORMULATIONS: CHOOSING THE 'SAFER WOMEN' AND THE 'SAFER PILLS'

5.120 What is your recommended framework for good pill management?

We want safer pills for what I call the 'safer women', maximum safety as well as efficacy. We need a framework for choice of users as well as choice of pills:

1 Who should never take the pill? (i.e. what are the absolute contraindications, WHO 4?)

2 Who should usually or often not take the pill? Maybe – but then with special advice and monitoring (the relative contraindications now classified by WHO as either WHO 3 or 2, as described in *Q 5.121*). All these contraindications are described in detail later (*see Qs 5.136–5.140*).

3 Which is the appropriate pill?

4 Which second choice of pill? This means taking account of:
   (a) biological variation in the pharmacokinetics of contraceptive steroids (*see Qs 5.162, 5.163*)
   (b) endometrial bleeding as a possible biological measure of their blood levels (*see Qs 5.164–5.170*)
   (c) what is known about their side-effect profile (*see Qs 6.21, 6.22*).

5 What is necessary for monitoring during follow-up? Including:
   (a) the implications of the PFI (*see Qs 5.16–5.33*)
   (b) BP (*see Qs 6.5–6.8*)
   (c) headaches, especially migraines (*see Qs 5.153–5.161*)
   (d) management of important new risk factors or diseases (*see Qs 6.1–6.18, 6.23–6.72*)
   (e) management of minor side-effects (*see Qs 6.19– 6.22*).

The answers to the next questions regarding prescribing are based now primarily on UKMEC, see below, along with my leading article [*British Medical Journal* 1995;311:1111–1112], the statement from the Clinical and Scientific Committee of the Faculty of Sexual and Reproductive Healthcare, UK [*British Medical Journal* 1996;312:121] and the above DoH statement in *Q 5.117*. See also *Q 5.102* and the article on evidence-guided prescribing of COCs by Hannaford and Webb [*Contraception* 1996;54:125–129]. In my view, none of the later literature substantially challenges this pragmatic scheme.

5.121 What is the WHO system for classifying contraindications?

This system, which I was able to help to devise at a small WHO working group in Atlanta early in 1994, is described in a WHO document, *Medical Eligibility Criteria for Contraceptive Use* (2004), along with its UK adaptation known as UKMEC. See www.who.int/reproductive-health.htm for the former and http://www.fsrh.org/admin/uploads/298_UKMEC_200506.pdf for the latter. See also *Appendix B* (p. 555ff.).

Essentially there are four categories, as shown in the Box on page 198. Numbers 1 and 4 are unchanged when compared to what we are used to (i.e. when the method is always or never usable). The useful new feature of the classification is separation into two categories of relative contraindication.

WHO classification of contraindications [with amplifications by J. Guillebaud]

WHO 1
A condition for which there is no restriction for the use of the contraceptive method, indeed the condition might even be an indication for it.
  'A' is for ALWAYS USABLE [**e.g. COC with history of candidiasis; uncomplicated varicose veins**]

WHO 2
A condition where the advantages of the method generally outweigh the theoretical or proven risks.
  'B' is for BROADLY USABLE [**e.g. COC in smoker age 20; history of pregnancy-related hypertension**]

WHO 3
A condition where the theoretical or proven risks usually outweigh the advantages, so the prospective user should be advised that another method would be preferable. But – respecting her autonomy – if she accepts the risks and relevant alternatives are contraindicated or rejected, given the risks of pregnancy as an alternative, the method can be used with caution/additional care and monitoring.
  'C' is for CAUTION/COUNSELLING, if used [**e.g. COC in diabetes without known tissue damage; long-term treatment with enzyme-inducer drugs**]

WHO 4
A condition that represents an unacceptable health risk.
  'D' is for DO NOT USE, at all [**e.g. COC with personal history of thrombosis; migraine with aura**]

Notes:

1 Although the A–B–C–D scheme is a helpful aide-mémoire to what each category signifies, I will stick with the WHO's 1–2–3–4 classification in this book to avoid any confusion. So, wherever WHO 3 is mentioned, 'Caution, extra counselling' is intended.

2 Clinical judgment is required in consultation with the contraceptive user, especially:
  (a) in all category 3 conditions – since another method would usually be an even better choice?
  (b) if more than one condition applies. As a working rule, two category 2 conditions moves the situation to category 3; and if any category 3 condition applies, the addition of either a 2 or a 3 condition normally amounts to category 4 (DO NOT USE).

3 This scheme is extremely valuable and is used extensively in the rest of this book. However, it is important for the reader to appreciate that the WHO's and UKMEC's own classification may differ for some conditions, either from

UK practice, or my personal considered judgment of what would be optimal for clients in the UK. Moreover, numerous conditions have not as yet been considered at all by WHO or the UKMEC. It should not therefore be assumed that my judgment that a condition is (say) WHO 3 for the POP is necessarily the same as WHO's view. To learn if WHO and therefore UKMEC do have a view, and to note where I sometimes differ, see *Appendix B*.

4 One of the main purposes of this scheme is to 'loosen up' with respect to contraindications, destroying pill myths that WHO 3 or 4 applies when whatever it is might actually be an *indication* for the method (WHO 1) – the best example being a woman's concern about conserving her future fertility (Q 5.70)! The intention is to remove 'medical barriers' to contraceptive use, i.e. wrong or misclassified contraindications, which end by depriving people of what would be the best method for them and so may well result in avoidable pregnancies. The system can be applied to *any* medical method, not just the COC.

5.122 What should happen at the first visit?

■ Prescribers should first take a comprehensive personal and family history to exclude the established absolute and relative contraindications to the use of COCs. A personal history of definite VTE remains an absolute contraindication to any COC containing EE combined with any progestogen. For others, *see Q 5.136.*

■ The risk factors for VTE and arterial wall disease must be assessed, separately and carefully. *Tables 5.10* and *5.11* and their footnotes are crucial in this process. Note that in either table, any one risk is WHO 2 or 3 (second or third column of each table) unless it is severe enough on its own to warrant the category WHO 4.

■ Multiple risk factors: as a working rule, two category 2 conditions moves the situation to category WHO 3; and if any category 3 condition applies, the addition of either a 2 or a 3 condition normally amounts to category 4.

■ The *blood pressure* should be properly measured, to obtain a good baseline reading. Beware if it is already above 160/95 (WHO 4) or even above 140/90 on repeated measurements, which is WHO 3 (*Table 5.11*) for COCs. That classification always means another method would be preferable – and obligatory (WHO 4) if another risk factor also applies.

■ The woman's *body mass and height* should be available at this visit so her BMI may be derived and used for decisions based on *Tables 5.10* and *5.11*. High BMI is very important because of its major effect on VTE risk in the EURAS study (*see Q 5.119*) and it is relevant to arterial risk also. Routine weighing at follow-up visits has rightly been discontinued for

TABLE 5.10 Risk factors for venous thromboembolism (VTE)

Risk factor	Absolute contraindication	Relative contraindication		Remarks
	WHO 4	WHO 3	WHO 2	
Personal or family history (FH) of thrombophilias, or of venous thrombosis in sibling or parent	Past VTE event; or identified clotting abnormality in this person, whether hereditary or acquired FH of a defined thrombophilia or *idiopathic* thrombotic event in parent or sibling <45 and thrombophilia screen not (yet) available	FH of thrombosis in parent or sibling <45 with recognized precipitating factor (e.g. major surgery, postpartum) and thrombophilia screen not available	FH of thrombotic event in parent or sibling <45 with or without a recognized precipitating factor and *normal* thrombophilia screen FH in parent or sibling ≥45 or FH in second-degree relative [classified WHO 2 but tests not indicated]	*Idiopathic* VTE in a parent or sibling <45 is an indication for a thrombophilia screen if available. The decision to undertake screening in other situations (including where there was a recognized precipitating factor) will be unusual because very cost-ineffective – might be done on clinical grounds, in discussion with the woman Even a normal thrombophilia screen cannot be entirely reassuring, as some predispositions are unknown
Overweight – high body mass index (BMI)	BMI ≥40	BMI 30–39	BMI 25–29	For most UK prescribers BMI >35 is *de facto* WHO 4
Immobility	Bed-bound, with or without major surgery; or leg fractured and immobilized	Wheelchair life, debilitating illness	Reduced mobility for other reason	Minor surgery such as laparoscopic sterilization is WHO 1

TABLE 5.10—cont'd

Risk factor	Absolute contraindication	Relative contraindication		Remarks
	WHO 4	WHO 3	WHO 2	
Varicose veins (VVs)	Current superficial vein thrombosis in the upper thigh Current sclerotherapy or similar by laser for VVs (or imminent VV surgery)		History of superficial vein thrombosis (SVT) in the lower limbs, no deep vein thrombosis	SVT does not result in pulmonary embolism, although this past history means some caution (WHO 2) in case it might be a marker of future VTE risk Uncomplicated VVs are irrelevant to VTE risk (WHO 1)
Cigarette smoking		≥15 cigarettes per day	<15 cigarettes per day	On balance the literature now suggests a VTE risk from smoking, though less than the arterial disease risk it causes
Age			>35, if relates to VTE risk alone	Arteries are more relevant to risk than veins

Notes:

1 A single risk factor in the relative contraindication columns indicates use of an LNG/NET pill, if any COC used (as in the BNF).

2 Beware of synergism: more than one factor in either of relative contraindication columns. As a working rule, two WHO 2 conditions makes WHO 3; and if WHO 3 applies (e.g. BMI 30–39) addition of either a WHO 3 or WHO 2 (e.g. reduced mobility) condition normally means WHO 4 (do not use).

3 Acquired (non-hereditary) predispositions include positive results for antiphospholipid antibodies – definitely WHO 4 since they also increase the risk of arterial events (*Table 5.11*).

4 There are also important acute VTE risk factors, which need to be considered in individual cases: notably, major and all leg surgery, long-haul flights and dehydration through any cause.

5 There are minor differences in the above table from UKMEC, notably the author's more cautious categorization of BMIs above 25.

TABLE 5.11 Risk factors for arterial disease

Risk factor	Absolute contraindication	Relative contraindication		Remarks
	WHO 4	WHO 3	WHO 2	
Family history (FH) of atherogenic lipid disorder or of arterial CVS event in sibling or parent	Identified familial hyperlipidaemia in this person, persisting despite treatment	FH of known familial lipid disorder or *idiopathic* arterial event in parent or sibling <45 and client's lipid screening result: ■ not available, or ■ confirmed and responding to treatment	Client has the less problematic common hyperlipidaemia and responding well to treatment FH of arterial event with risk factor (e.g. smoking), in parent or sibling <45, and lipid screen not available	FH of premature (<45) arterial CVS disease without other risk factors, or a known atherogenic lipid disorder in a parent or sibling, indicate fasting lipid screen, if available (Check with laboratory re clinical implication of abnormal results) Despite any FH, normal lipid screen in client *is* reassuring, means WHO 1 (in contrast to thrombophilia screening)
Cigarette smoking	≥40 cigarettes/day	15–39 cigarettes/day	<15 cigarettes/day	Cut-offs here are somewhat arbitrary
Diabetes mellitus (DM)	Severe, longstanding or DM complications (e.g. retinopathy, renal damage, arterial disease)	Not severe/labile and no complications, young patient with short duration of DM		DM is always at least WHO 3 (safer options available)
Hypertension (consistently elevated BP, with properly taken measurements)	Systolic BP ≥160 mmHg Diastolic BP ≥95 mmHg	Systolic BP 140–159 mmHg Diastolic BP 90–94 mmHg On treatment for essential hypertension, with good control	BP regularly at upper limit of normal (i.e. near to 140/90) Past history of pre-eclampsia (WHO 3 if also a smoker)	BP levels for categories are consistent with UKMEC but different from WHOMEC (see Q 6.6)

TABLE 5.11—cont'd

Risk factor	Absolute contraindication	Relative contraindication		Remarks
	WHO 4	WHO 3	WHO 2	
Overweight, high body mass index (BMI)	BMI ≥40	BMI 30–39	BMI 25–29	High BMI increases arterial as well as venous thromboembolic risk
Migraine	Migraine with aura Migraine without aura if attacks last >72 h + no overuse of medication	Migraine without aura plus a strong added arterial risk factor	Migraine without aura	Relates to *thrombotic* stroke risk Triptan treatment does not affect the category
Age >35	Age >35 if a continuing smoker Age >51 for all others, even if risk-factor-free	Age 35–51 if ex-smoker	Age 35–51 if free of all risk factors (yet even safer options are available)	In all persistent smokers, age >35 best classified as WHO 4 In ex-smokers, WHO 3 is because arterial wall damage may persist; but UKMEC permits WHO 2 after 1 year of *not* smoking

Notes:

1 Beware of synergism: more than one factor in either of relative contraindication columns. As a working rule, two WHO 2 conditions makes WHO 3; and if WHO 3 applies (e.g. smoking ≥15 per day) addition of either a WHO 3 or WHO 2 (e.g. age >35) condition normally means WHO 4 (as in table).

2 In continuing smokers, COC is generally stopped at age 35, in the UK. But, given the rapid risk reduction shown in studies of complete smoking cessation, according to UKMEC ex-smokers are classified WHO 3 only until 1 year, dropping to WHO 2 thereafter. In my view, WHO 3 is the best category for truly ex-smokers, regardless of time since cessation at age 35.

3 WHO numbers also relate to use for contraception: use of COCs for medical indications such as PCOS often entails a different risk/benefit analysis, i.e. the extra therapeutic benefits might outweigh expected extra risks.

4 There are minor differences in the above table from UKMEC, notably the author's more cautious categorization with respect to smoking and DM.

many years, but weight measurement might be indicated later by there being a marked change.

5.123 Which pill for ordinary first-time users of COCs?

■ All marketed pills can now be considered 'first line'. See the section in bold of the DoH statement (*see Q 5.117*). Given the tiny, not yet finally established difference in VTE mortality between the two 'generations', the woman's own choice of a DSG or GSD product or other estrogen-dominant product (see below) must be respected – and the discussion fully documented:

The informed user should be the chooser.

■ Young first-time users: despite what has just been said, the usual first choice should be a low-dose LNG/NET pill, containing no more than 35 µg EE and no more than 150 µg LNG or 1000 µg NET. Reasons: first-timers include an unknown subgroup who are VTE-predisposed; also, VTE is a more relevant consideration than arterial disease at this age; plus the pills are cheaper. The 'default pill' for pill starters in the UK is Microgynon 30.

■ Single risk factor for venous thrombosis *or* for arterial disease, including age above 35: *see Qs 5.124 and 5.125*.

5.124 Which pill for a woman with a single risk factor for venous thrombosis (e.g. BMI anything above 25)?

An LNG or NET product would be preferred, if the COC is used at all. BMI 30–39 is a WHO 3 situation (*Table 5.10*)

The choice of type of COC is more difficult if she has a BMI above 30 but also has PCOS (*see Q 5.66*), because estrogen dominance is important in this condition to raise SHBG and control acne. In such cases, the fact that the COC chosen (such as Marvelon) might increase VTE risk more than an LNG-containing brand can often be justified by the medical indication, i.e. the extra therapeutic benefits – beyond just contraception – would be held to justify the anticipated but very small extra risks.

Beware also that VTE risk rises with increasing age.

5.125 Which pill for a woman with a single definite arterial risk factor (from *Table 5.11*) or who is healthy and risk-factor-free but above age 35?

Many studies, including the RCGP study, the Oxford/FPA study, the American Nurses study, WHO (1998), MICA (1999) and EURAS (*Q 5.119*), were unable to detect any increased risk of AMI in non-smokers, whether they were current or past pill-takers. This means the arterial event risk of using all the modern low-estrogen brands must be very small, though probably not absent (*see Q 5.102*), for women free of arterial risk factors. But it is high when they are present (the RCGP's relative risk estimate was 20.8 for pill-takers who smoked), the risk increases with age (see *Table 5.8*, p. 180) and the case-fatality rate for AMI is also much higher (*see Q 5.105*). Fortunately, it is always of benefit to stop smoking, so that in genuine ex-smokers COCs are acceptable for use above 35 – see Footnote 2 to *Table 5.11* and *Q 6.77*.

There are suggestive data (*see Q 5.116*) that DSG/GSD pills might have relative advantages for arterial wall disease in higher-risk women. Therefore, switching to a low-estrogen (20 μg) DSG (Mercilon-20) or GSD (Femodette/Sunya 20/75 [new generic marketed in UK since last edition]) pill may be mooted:

■ with smokers (and others with a single arterial risk factor) as they get older (normally no later than age 35 though, because of multiplication of risk factors; see Box in Q 5.121, p. 198)
■ for the few completely risk-factor-free women who choose (despite the availability of the LARCs, which are usually a better choice) to continue to take the COC from 35 to 51 years of age.

Loestrin 20 is another option and is slightly less estrogenic.

5.126 Which pill for a woman who finds she does not tolerate an LNG/NET COC because of persistent BTB or androgenic/other 'minor' side-effects – or who just wants a change?

As already stated, the differential risk between pill types is very small. If a woman does not tolerate an LNG or NET COC because of persistent BTB or 'minor' side-effects such as acne, headaches, depression, weight gain or breast symptoms, or if she wants a change for personal reasons, use of a DSG or GSD product is medico-legally very secure. Once again, the informed user should be the chooser.

5.127 Presumably the verbal consent of women not using the pill brands recommended by the CSM must be well recorded?

Yes: if DSG/GSD pills are chosen (whether for this arterial risk factor indication or just because the woman prefers one of them on quality-of-life grounds), given the fact that they were singled out by the CSM in 1995 and that advice has not been revoked, there should, for medico-legal security, always be a full contemporaneous record:

■ of the risk factor history
■ that the woman accepts a possibly increased risk of VTE (conveyed in a non-scary way, e.g. as equalling 2 h of driving in a whole year, *see Q 5.117*).

This counselling should additionally be backed by a user-friendly leaflet, such as the COC leaflet produced by the UK fpa (along with the PIL).

5.128 What about norgestimate, the progestogen in Cilest? And the antiandrogenic progestogens?

There remains considerable uncertainty here, through lack of epidemiological data. Intriguingly, one of the main metabolites of norgestimate is biologically active (levo)norgestrel (22% by weight, equivalent to about 55 μg of the 250 μg in each tablet). As we saw above, this is a relatively antiestrogenic progestogen, so one might expect some counteraction of the estrogenicity, and maybe therefore the VTE thrombogenicity, of the 35 μg of EE that Cilest contains.

We need more data. In practice, we can continue to use Cilest without the specific medico-legal anxieties raised by the CSM letter of 18 October 1995. Cilest seems to be working out as a useful choice for many women, more estrogen-dominant than, say, Microgynon 30 but not markedly so.

The same considerations with regard to VTE apply to Evra, the new contraceptive skin patch (*see Q 6.81*).

Another progestogenic substance used in UK combination pills is cyproterone acetate, which is an antiandrogen used in the formulation Dianette and considered later (*see Q 6.65*). It is marketed primarily for the treatment of moderately severe acne and hirsutism. Recent work confirms that it is clearly an estrogen-dominant product, with a statistically increased risk of VTE compared to LNG-containing products. *See also Qs 6.61 and 6.62* with regard to the other antiandrogenic progestogen drospirenone, and its use in Yasmin – which (unlike Dianette) is marketed as a long-term COC.

MORE ABOUT THE AVAILABLE PILL FORMULATIONS

5.129 Which are now considered the 'safer pills'?

It is much easier to say what they are not! The doses in the first brands marketed in the 1960s, on which indeed much of the early epidemiology was based, were clearly too high. On the market then was a brand that gave more of the same estrogen in a day than is now given in a week; and virtually the same daily dose of a progestogen as now covers a complete cycle (see *Table 5.12*)!

In short, safer pills seem generally to be 'smaller pills'. Both the constituent hormones are capable of unwanted metabolic effects and their epidemiological consequences. After saying that, the question is still, after all these years, impossible to answer more specifically. And it will depend on whether one is considering arterial or venous disease.

TABLE 5.12 Reduction in doses since combined pills were first introduced			
	Dose of sex steroid per tablet in 1962	Minimum of same as used in 2008	Compared with 1962 same dose in 2008 from
Ethinylestradiol (EE)	150 µg in Enovid-10	20 µg in Femodette/ Sunya 20/75, Mercilon-20, Loestrin 20	One week of tablets
Norethisterone (NET)	10 000 µg in Ortho-Novum-10	500 µg in Ovysmen/ Brevinor	One month of tablets

Note: 15-µg EE pills are now marketed in continental Europe.

Above all, we must retain a range of formulations so as to have flexibility in prescribing when 'minor' side-effects occur (*see Qs 6.19–6.22*).

A policy based on preferring 'smaller' pills should reduce the risk of major side-effects. Clinical experience with the lowest doses also shows that, with one exception, minor side-effects are less frequent and less severe.

What is the exception? The obvious one is cycle control: but that can be handled, as part of the follow-up prescribing scheme to be described (*see Qs 5.162–5.179*).

5.130 What are the fundamental problems in applying a 'safer pills' policy?

■ Almost no RCTs, and too few cohort studies comparing formulations, have large enough numbers and relevant epidemiological end-points. And now that the VTE story that led to the 'pill scare' of October 1995 is largely accepted, it is clear that we all had our hands burnt by relying on (the more easily obtainable) metabolic surrogate markers like HDL-C.

■ Then there is individual variation. A medium-dose pill for one woman could be in its biological effect a low-dose pill for another, or a high-dose pill for a third.

It is thus a false expectation that any single pill will suit all women. We return to this point below (see *Fig. 5.14* [p. 231] and *Qs 5.162–5.179*).

5.131 What are the pill brands available, and how can they be classified?

The practitioner is faced with a variety of formulations (*Table 5.13*). All contain the same estrogen, EE (or, in the case of Norinyl-1, a prodrug for it called mestranol, *see Q 5.38*).

TABLE 5.13 Formulations of currently marketed combined oral contraceptives

Pill type	Preparation	Estrogen (µg)	Progestogen (µg)	
Monophasic				
Ethinylestradiol/ norethisterone type	Loestrin 20	20	1000	Norethisterone acetate*
	Loestrin 30	30	1500	Norethisterone acetate*
	Brevinor	35	500	Norethisterone
	Ovysmen	35	500	Norethisterone
	Norimin	35	1000	Norethisterone
Ethinylestradiol/ levonorgestrel	Microgynon 30 (also ED)	30	150	
	Ovranette	30	150	
Ethinylestradiol/ desogestrel	Mercilon	20	150	
	Marvelon	30	150	
Ethinylestradiol/ gestodene	Femodette/Sunya 20/75	20	75	
	Femodene (also ED)/Katya 30/75	30	75	
	Minulet	30	75	
Ethinylestradiol/ norgestimate	Cilest	35	250	
Ethinylestradiol/ drospirenone	Yasmin	30	3000	
	Yaz	20	3000	(24 active tablets then 4 placebos)
Mestranol/ norethisterone[†]	Norinyl-1	50	1000	
Bi/triphasic				
Ethinylestradiol/ norethisterone	BiNovum	35	500	833[‡] (7 tabs)
		35	1000	(14 tabs)
	Synphase	35	500	(7 tabs)
		35	1000	714 (9 tabs)
		35	500	(5 tabs)
	TriNovum	35	500	(7 tabs)
		35	750	750 (7 tabs)
		35	1000	(7 tabs)
Ethinylestradiol/ levonorgestrel	Logynon (also ED)	30	50	(6 tabs)
		40 — 32[‡]	75	92[‡] (5 tabs)
		30	125	(10 tabs)
	Trinordiol	30	50	(6 tabs)
		40 — 32	75	92 (5 tabs)
		30	125	(10 tabs)

TABLE 5.13—cont'd

Pill type	Preparation	Estrogen (µg)		Progestogen (µg)		
Ethinylestradiol/ gestodene	Tri-Minulet	30 ⎫ 40 ⎬ 32 30 ⎭		50 ⎫ 70 ⎬ 79[‡] 100 ⎭		(6 tabs) (5 tabs) (10 tabs)
	Triadene	30 ⎫ 40 ⎬ 32 30 ⎭		50 ⎫ 70 ⎬ 79 100 ⎭		(6 tabs) (5 tabs) (10 tabs)
Also: Ethinylestradiol/ cyproterone acetate (marketed primarily as acne therapy, not as a standard COC; see Qs 6.22, 6.23)	Dianette/Clairette 2000/35	35		2000		

*Converted to norethisterone as the active metabolite.
[†]Has to be converted to ethinylestradiol, approx. 35 µg, as active estrogen, so Norinyl-1 approximates to Norimin (see Q 5.38).
[‡]Equivalent daily doses for comparison with monophasic brands.

In previous editions of this book these were grouped in a figure, in ladders according to the particular progestogen they contain, each lower rung representing a lower hormone content than those above. The philosophy behind this display was that the lower down a ladder one is, the less likely is injury if one falls off! The POPs were seen as the least likely to cause side-effects – and depicted on ground level.

That 'ladder' approach will no longer be used here as it has become less and less useful with the arrival of new data (*see Qs 5.132, 5.108–5.112*).

5.132 In *Table 5.13*, how do the pills using different progestogens differ from each other?

Because norethisterone acetate is converted in vivo (with more than 90% efficiency) to norethisterone, all formulations using it are part of the norethisterone group.

As discussed, levonorgestrel and, to a lesser extent, norethisterone appear to reduce the effective estrogenicity of a given dose of EE, with a probable beneficial effect on prothrombotic blood changes and thrombosis risk. All other progestogens that are used in COCs make, in general, more estrogen-dominant pills, although obviously a change in the estrogen dominance can also be produced by changing the dose of EE itself. In the UK the lowest dose available is 20 μg, but elsewhere 15-μg doses are now also available.

5.133 Why is D-norgestrel called levonorgestrel? Please explain.

Norgestrel is a racemic mixture of a D-isomer and L-isomer. The former is given the prefix 'D' because it shares the same spacial orientation as other molecules that, by the conventions of stereochemistry, are all called the D-forms. However, when in solution it deviates light in the opposite direction (i.e. to the left) and is therefore known as levonorgestrel.

The opposite applies to L-norgestrel, which rotates light to the right. It is also biologically inactive but it has to be metabolized. Hence, where there is a choice, it is preferable to use the nearest equivalent brand that uses pure levonorgestrel.

INDICATIONS AND CONTRAINDICATIONS FOR THE COC METHOD, IN MORE DEPTH

5.134 For whom is the COC method particularly indicated?

The woman who is not ready/willing for a LARC and decides that maximum protection from pregnancy and independence from intercourse are the most important features in her own view. But she can also use it for its non-contraceptive benefits without currently needing contraception (*see* Q 5.135).

It is particularly valuable for the healthy young sexually active non-smoking woman who is sufficiently motivated to be a reliable pill-taker. If and when she is at risk of STIs she should be advised to use condoms as well.

5.135 For what (primarily gynaecological) disorders and diseases is the combined pill prescribed?

Because the extra requirement for treatment increases the benefit side of the benefit–risk equation, it might sometimes be acceptable to prescribe higher-dose pills or to give the COC to women with one or more relative contraindications. A specialist's advice should be sought where appropriate. The COC can be invaluable therapy to:

- Relieve *spasmodic dysmenorrhoea*.
- Treat *other menstrual cycle disorders*: in cases of prolonged bleeding with no demonstrable pathology, but also for true secondary amenorrhoea once characterized. Indeed, the reason for any cycle irregularity or secondary amenorrhoea should always be determined first, but then the pill might well be the most appropriate treatment, especially for

hypo-estrogenic states (*see Qs 5.66–5.68*). Tricycling (*see Q 5.32*) or 365/365 pill-taking (*see Q 5.34*) are options to consider.

■ Relieve premenstrual syndrome (PMS). This is not always successful, indeed some women develop similar symptoms when taking the COC. It is certainly the case that any treatment that ablates the normal menstrual cycle benefits PMS. Using a monophasic COC for that purpose but replacing with a 10–13-week pill cycle through tricycling (as described in Q 5.32), or perhaps continuous pill-taking (*see Q 5.34*), minimizes the likelihood that the COC-replacement itself reproduces the symptoms. Some data suggest that Yasmin and Yaz (*Qs 6.62–6.64*) are better for PMS than other COCs. These also might be expected to give even better results if taken by one of the continuous regimens: but we need more comparative data.

■ Control *menorrhagia*. A relatively progestogen-dominant pill should be chosen. If in addition fibroids are present and surgery is not indicated, their size should be monitored by ultrasound.

■ Control *endometriosis* as maintenance therapy after first-line treatment. Use a progestogen-dominant brand like Microgynon 30, and a continuous 365/365 or tricycle regimen (*see Qs 5.32, 5.34, 6.52*).

■ Control *functional ovarian cysts* (*see Q 5.61*) and *ovulation pain* if severe.

■ Relieve estrogen deficiency:
  – in marathon athletes or anorexics with *amenorrhoea* (*see Q 5.66*)
  – to control gynaecological/menstrual cyclical symptoms in selected healthy non-smoking perimenopausal women under age 51 and still requiring contraception, although becoming estrogen ± progesterone deficient: i.e. as a contraceptive form of HRT.

■ Control *acne* and other manifestations – including an increased risk of endometrial cancer due to unopposed estrogen – of the *polycystic ovarian syndrome (PCOS)* – see Q 5.66. Estrogen-dominant pill brands are also useful for acne treatment without evidence of PCOS.

■ As prophylaxis against *ovarian cancer*, for women at high risk (*see Q 5.58*).

Nowadays, other means to control many of the gynaecological conditions above – notably the LNG-IUS (*see Q 9.143ff*) and Cerazette (*see Q 7.11*) – might be chosen instead.

Triphasic pills are usually not appropriate for these indications because the intention is often to abolish the normal cycle, and they might too closely simulate it.

5.136 What are the absolute contraindications to (all formulations of) COCs, i.e. WHO 4 in the WHO classification of Q 5.121?

Any compilation of contraindications reflects the judgment of the compiler, as much as the available science at the relevant date. The answers to this and the following questions are as assessed by me in 2007! They are largely but not completely congruent with WHO's and UKMEC's classification (see *Appendix B*); but many of these conditions have yet to be assessed by WHO.

Many important diseases mentioned below are considered in more detail elsewhere – please see the Index. Conditions in this first list are WHO 4 for the COC.

More detailed discussion and numerous references relevant to *Qs 5.136–5.161* here (and to the whole of Chapter 5) may be found by visiting the following excellent sources:

1 First Prescription of the Combined Oral Contraceptive. FFPRHC (now FSRH) Guidance of the Faculty of Family Planning. July 2006, updated Jan 2007. http://www.fsrh.org/admin/uploads/FirstPrescCombOralContJan06.pdf

2A The searchable database of the Faculty, which by 2007 had answered 1900 questions from members. Visit http://www.fsrh.org/ then click Clinical Enquiries.

2B An invaluable book *Family Planning Masterclass* edited by G Penney, S Brechin and A Glasier is available which is based on the same database, published by the FFPRHC (now FSRH) in 2006.

Both sources under (2) above consider *all* methods of contraception, not just the COC.

ABSOLUTE CONTRAINDICATIONS TO COCs (AND OTHER EE-CONTAINING METHODS SUCH AS THE CONTRACEPTIVE SKIN PATCH), i.e. WHO 4 IN THE WHO CLASSIFICATION:

1. **Past or present circulatory disease**
   - Any past proven arterial or venous thrombosis
   - Ischaemic heart disease or angina or coronary arteritis (Kawasaki disease – past history is usually WHO 2 with complete recovery, but may be WHO 4 if there is persistent cardiac or coronary vessel damage following the acute phase)
   - Severe or combined risk factors for venous or arterial disease (see *Tables 5.10* and *5.11*) can be WHO 4 – e.g. BMI 40 or above is sufficient on its own for the WHO 4 category

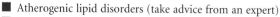

- Atherogenic lipid disorders (take advice from an expert)
- Known prothrombotic states:
  - abnormality of coagulation/fibrinolysis, meaning any of above congenital or acquired thrombophilia states
  - Klippel–Trenaunay–Weber syndrome, which greatly increases VTE risk, though the specific thrombophilia has not been identified [Penney et al, Family Planning Masterclass 2006, p. 445]
  - from at least 2 (preferably 4) weeks before until 2 weeks after mobilization following elective major or leg surgery (do not demand that the COC be stopped for minor surgery such as laparoscopy)
  - during leg immobilization (e.g. after fracture) or varicose vein injection sclerotherapy or intraluminal laser treatment – or equivalent
  - when going to high altitudes if there are added risk factors (otherwise WHO 3 – see below)
- Migraine with aura
- Definite aura *without* a headache following
- Transient ischaemic attacks
- Past cerebral haemorrhage
- Pulmonary hypertension, any cause
- Structural (uncorrected) heart disease such as valvular heart disease or shunts/septal defects is only WHO 4 if there is an added arterial or venous thromboembolic risk (persisting, if there has been surgery). Always discuss with the cardiologist – could be WHO 3, especially if the patient is always on warfarin. See *Table 5.14*. In other structural heart conditions, if there is little or no direct or indirect risk of thromboembolism (this being the crucial point to check with the cardiologist), the COC is usable (WHO 3 or 2)

2. **Liver**
- Active liver cell disease (whenever liver function tests are currently abnormal, including infiltrations, severe chronic hepatitis B and C, and cirrhosis)
- Past Pill-related cholestatic jaundice; if this was in pregnancy, it can be WHO 3 (contrast WHOMEC and UKMEC, who say WHO 3 not 4 for the former – and WHO 2 for the latter)
- Dubin–Johnson and Rotor syndromes (Gilbert's disease is WHO 2)
- Following viral hepatitis or other liver cell damage: but COCs may be resumed once liver function tests have become normal and a dose of ≤2 units of alcohol consumption is tolerated
- Liver adenoma, carcinoma

TABLE 5.14 Eligibility for COC use in some varieties of heart disease

Absolute contraindication	Relative contraindication	
WHO 4	**WHO 3 (must lack features in first column)**	**WHO 2**
Atrial fibrillation or flutter, sustained or paroxysmal, as high risk of emboli – unless well controlled on warfarin (WHO 3)	Heart disease or past thrombosis well controlled on warfarin with very careful supervision of INR, which may alter with hormones. [Three exceptions – 'even on warfarin' in first column – plus in all cases the situation reverts to WHO 4 if warfarin stopped]	Dysrhythmias other than atrial fibrillation or flutter
Pulmonary hypertension or pulmonary vascular disease		Valve lesions not yet surgically corrected but uncomplicated, including mitral valve prolapse and bicuspid aortic valve; lacking any of the WHO 3 or 4 features of first & second columns
Pulmonary arteriovenous malformation	Bi-leaflet mechanical valve in mitral or aortic position on warfarin	
Poor left ventricular function (LV ejection fraction <30%)		Any prosthetic or tissue heart valves lacking any WHO 3 or 4 features
Dilated cardiomyopathy or previous cardiomyopathy with residual LV dysfunction	All known inter-atrial communications (ASD, PFO) – as always risk of paradoxical embolism, e.g. with Valsalva manoeuvre	Fully surgically corrected congenital heart disease lacking any of the WHO 3 or 4 features
Dilated left atrium (>4 cm)	Repaired coarctation with aneurysm and/or hypertension	Non-reversible trivial left-to-right shunt, e.g. small VSD; trivial patent ductus arteriosus
Cyanotic heart disease, even taking warfarin	Marfan's syndrome with aortic dilatation, unoperated	Repaired coarctation without aneurysm or hypertension

TABLE 5.14—cont'd

Absolute contraindication	Relative contraindication	
WHO 4	WHO 3 (must lack features in first column)	WHO 2
The (post-surgery) Fontan heart, even taking warfarin		Uncomplicated Marfan's syndrome
		Uncomplicated pulmonary stenosis
Björk–Shiley or Starr–Edwards valves, even taking warfarin		Hypertrophic obstructive cardiomyopathy (HOCM))
Any past venous or arterial thromboembolic event with the heart disease – not on warfarin (see second column)		Past pregnancy-related or other cardiomyopathy, fully recovered and with now normal heart on echocardiography

Notes:

1 **There is a paucity of published information, a very small evidence-base, about contraception in women with heart disease. Hence this table (which in any event cannot deal with all possible cases) is based on best evidence and opinions available at the time of writing (2007) as here interpreted by the author, with due thanks to the committee mentioned in Q 5.141. This may change as new evidence is obtained.**

2 The prime consideration in decisions about using the COC is *whether or not the condition itself increases the risk of venous or arterial thromboembolic events.*

3 If a patient can be classified in more than one WHO category, the more cautious category should be applied.

4 The risk of pregnancy should always be balanced against the thrombotic risk of taking the combined oral contraceptive. Thus, a high risk in pregnancy due to the heart condition may make COC risks justifiable if alternative effective methods are unacceptable, on the usual WHO 3 basis.

5 Most patients will require discussion with the cardiologist, and periodic reassessment of the suitability or otherwise of the COC in their individual circumstances – because cardiac status is not static.

ASD, atrial septal defect; INR, international normalized ratio; LV, left ventricle; PFO, patent foramen ovale; VSD, ventricular septal defect.

- Acute hepatic porphyrias; other porphyrias are usually WHO 3, but a non-steroid hormone method is usually preferable

3. **History of serious condition affected by sex steroids or related to previous COC use**
    - SLE – also a VTE risk mediated by possible antiphospholipid antibodies
    - COC-induced hypertension
    - Pancreatitis due to hypertriglyceridaemia
    - Pemphigoid gestationis
    - Chorea
    - Stevens–Johnson syndrome (erythema multiforme), if COC-associated
    - Trophoblastic disease – but only until hCG levels are undetectable
    - Haemolytic uraemic syndrome (HUS) and thrombotic thrombocytopenic purpura (TTP); a recent history of either of these poorly understood but related thrombotic syndromes is WHO 4 for the COC if there is continuing disease activity, especially nephropathy. *See also Q 5.137* below

4. **Pregnancy**
5. **Undiagnosed genital tract bleeding**
6. **Estrogen-dependent neoplasms**
    - Breast cancer
    - Past breast biopsy showing premalignant epithelial atypia
7. **Miscellaneous**
    - Allergy to any Pill constituent
    - Past benign intracranial hypertension
    - Amaurosis fugax: this transient complete loss of vision usually signifies transient retinal ischaemia, so obviously contraindicates the COC (WHO 4)
    - Specific to Yasmin: because of the unique spironolactone-like effects of the contained progestogen drospirenone, this particular brand should be avoided – should a COC be appropriate – in anyone at risk of high potassium levels (including severe renal insufficiency, hepatic dysfunction and treatment with potassium-sparing diuretics)
    - Sturge–Weber syndrome (thrombotic stroke risk)
    - Postpartum for 6 weeks if breastfeeding (according to UKMEC)
8. **Woman's anxiety about COC safety unrelieved by counselling**

This is not necessarily a complete list of relevant diseases or dis-eases – *see* Q 5.139 for how to assess any new condition affecting your patient.

Note that several of the above (e.g. existing or possible pregnancy, undiagnosed genital tract bleeding, estrogen-dependent neoplasms) are *not necessarily permanent* contraindications.

5.137 Relative contraindications – how are they assessed and how applied?

Here we have the impact not just of my judgment as compiler, but yours as prescriber! The art of medicine is nowhere better shown than in assessing how strong each of the contraindications at Q 5.138 is for the individual being counselled and then:

- balancing the risk of each against the benefits to each pill-taker
- allowing for synergism between risk factors and the general teaching that two or more relative contraindications equal one absolute contraindication – see also Box in Q 5.121, note 2(b)
- all in the light of everything relevant, like her probable fertility and her other contraceptive choices
- and all, most emphatically, being discussed openly with the woman, so that she makes the final decision.

5.138 What are the relative contraindications to the COC?

- Risk factors for circulatory disease are all relative contraindications, mostly WHO 3, sometimes WHO 2: provided normally that only one is present, and not to so marked a degree that it alone would absolutely contraindicate this method. See *Tables 5.10* and *5.11* (pp. 200 and 202). This category of increased circulatory risk includes:
  - postpartum in the first 3 weeks (WHO 3), due to VTE risk – but very low fertility at that time anyway
  - past toxaemia of pregnancy (pregnancy-related hypertension), which increases the risk of AMI in smokers, therefore WHO 3 for them (shown in the RCGP and MICA studies)
  - the HELLP syndrome, which is WHO 3 postpartum as long as the tests are still abnormal, but WHO 2 thereafter (*see Q 5.140*)
  - essential hypertension provided it is well controlled by treatment (WHO 3); also
  - warfarin treatment, which is usually WHO 3 (*see Q 5.141*), and
  - travelling to high altitude (*see Q 5.142*)
  - an isolated past history of an attack of HUS which was preceded by diarrhoea – as occurs with *E. coli* 0157 infection – with complete recovery would allow use of COC (WHO 2).
- Long-term partial immobilization (e.g. in a wheelchair). This is WHO 3 (*Table 5.10*). Complete flaccid paralysis of the lower limbs is viewed by some as WHO 4, especially if the BMI is >30.

■ Sex-steroid-dependent cancers in remission. Seek the specialist's advice. Any history of breast cancer is generally seen as an absolute contraindication (WHO 4) to the COC (see Q 5.136), though UKMEC follows WHO in permitting the COC (WHO 3) after 5 years' remission. Better options can usually be found, e.g. IUD, LNG-IUS or a progestogen-only method.

■ Oligo- and/or amenorrhoea should be investigated but the pill might subsequently be prescribed – WHO 2 – or even positively indicated (WHO 1; see Qs 5.62–5.67).

■ Gallstones causing symptoms or being treated medically are WHO 3, but WHO 2 if asymptomatic or have been treated by cholecystectomy.

■ Hyperprolactinaemia: this is now considered a relative contraindication (WHO 3) for patients under specialist supervision, as long as the woman is on dopamine agonist therapy (see Q 5.66).

■ Very severe depression, if likely to be exacerbated by COCs (WHO 3). But unwanted pregnancies can be very depressing!

■ Chronic systemic diseases. These are discussed further below (see Qs 5.139–5.148). In general they are weak relative contraindications, category WHO 2, mainly signifying extra counselling and above-average monitoring. Examples in the stronger WHO 3 category are: Crohn's disease with major small-bowel involvement (see Q 5.147), diabetes (see Q 5.149), chronic renal disease, and mild (not steroid-treated, in remission) SLE, although the presence of antiphospholipid antibody absolutely contraindicates the COC (see Qs 5.137, 5.148).

In all these, the reason in common for special caution is that the condition might lead in various ways to an increased risk of circulatory disease. If that risk became established, as in a diabetic with evidence of arteriopathy, it would be an absolute contraindication WHO 4 (see Q 5.138). In the case of SLE and Crohn's there is also the risk of sex hormones causing deterioration of the condition. Splenectomy, for whatever reason performed (e.g. in the treatment of sickle-cell disease), is only a relative contraindication (WHO 2). However, the platelets should be monitored, initially at least annually, and a count rising to above 500×10^9 per litre would absolutely contraindicate the estrogen of the COC (WHO 4).

■ Diseases requiring long-term treatment with enzyme-inducing drugs, which might reduce the efficacy of the pill (see Qs 5.36, 5.38): provided the recommended regimen is followed, this is WHO 3. But DMPA (see Q 8.11) or an IUD, or the LNG-IUS (see Q 9.147) are preferable options.

■ Other relative contraindications include:
   (a) if a young (<40 years) first-degree relative has had breast cancer (WHO 2) or the woman herself has benign breast disease (WHO 2 – but UKMEC says either of these is WHO 1)

(b) if a breast biopsy shows atypia: WHO 3 (*see Q 5.93*). Being a known carrier of one of the *BRCA* genes is also WHO 3

(c) during the monitoring of abnormal cervical smears (WHO 2)

(d) during and after definitive treatment for CIN (WHO 2).

Women in groups (a) and (b), if they do take the COC, need recounselling after about 4–5 years' use.

5.139 On what criteria can one decide whether the COC can be used for patients with intercurrent disease?

First, there are some conditions that are positively benefited (*see Qs 5.57, 5.135*) or at least not affected. There are persistent medical myths (*see Q 6.78*), and it is unfortunate that women continue to be unnecessarily deprived of the COC for the wrong reasons, like thrush, uncomplicated varicose veins, past amenorrhoea, current hypo-estrogenic amenorrhoea (e.g. weight-related) or fibroids.

It is impossible to list every known disease or state that might have a bearing on pill prescribing, but here are some useful criteria:

In general, discover first what the disease does in relation to known risks or effects of the COC. Does it cause changes that summate with adverse effects of the COC? Does it:

1 Increase the risk of arterial or venous thrombosis, anywhere? This includes consideration of restricted mobility even if the disease is otherwise unrelated to thrombosis risk.

2 Predispose to arterial wall disease or severe hypertension?

3 Adversely affect liver function?

4 Show a tendency to an important degree of sex hormone dependency, either generally (usually then a relative contraindication), or in that individual in the past (absolute contraindication).

5 Require treatment with an enzyme-inducing drug?

If (5) is true, the pill can still be an option, but special conditions apply (*see Q 5.38*) and there are better choices.

If (1) to (4) apply, there is the real problem of deciding whether the COC should be absolutely or (as at *Q 5.138*) relatively contraindicated (meaning not WHO 4 but WHO 3). Obviously the category will be WHO 4 if she has an added risk factor from *Table 5.10* or *5.11* such as smoking or obesity.

Note that in some chronic diseases the added risk obtaining in pregnancy can fully justify some increased risk due to the COC, at least in young and hence more fertile women, primarily because it is so effective. Its other benefits might also be highly relevant in some conditions. This is not so, however, for the list at *Q 5.136* (WHO 4, absolute contraindications).

If none of the above criteria apply, then the condition could normally be added to the following list in Q 5.140

5.140 Can you list those medical conditions in which the COC is broadly usable since there is no convincing evidence that deterioration might be caused or of any summation with effects of the pill?

According to current information, the following diseases all come into this 'Broadly usable' category (WHO 2):

Aids/HIV (*see* Q 6.71, although the category would change to WHO 3 if an enzyme-inducing antiretroviral drug were to be prescribed; and there are usually better contraceptive choices for these women; always along with condoms); asthma; Gilbert's disease; treated Hodgkin's disease (if fertility preserved); hereditary lymphoedema; past HELLP syndrome once the pregnancy-related changes (haemolysis, elevated liver enzymes, low platelets) have returned to normal; multiple sclerosis; myasthenia gravis; primary Raynaud's disease (*unless* the phenomenon proves to be symptomatic of a contraindicating condition such as SLE); renal dialysis; retinitis pigmentosa; rheumatoid arthritis (beware immobility); sarcoidosis; spherocytosis; thalassaemia major; thyrotoxicosis and Wolff–Parkinson–White syndrome (WHO 4 if atrial fibrillation associated). Also most cancers under treatment, if hormone dependency or an increase in the risk of thrombosis are not suspected.

Despite the condition featuring above (COC probably usable), in individual cases the prescriber should first review the checklist in Q 5.139 and might need to consult with the hospital specialist(s) supervising treatment for the main disorder: to obtain their support to use the COC and also to guard against unforeseen drug interactions, etc. Such women need extra supervision within primary care as well (shared care).

There are of course many other illnesses in the textbooks, too numerous to mention here: the solution to prescribing queries is to evaluate each condition as described in Q 5.139 above.

5.141 Can the COC be taken by some women with structural heart disease?

Yes, indeed. It is a myth that all such should be in category WHO 4. Every year a number of women – particularly after successful surgery, so-called 'grown-up congenital heart' or GUCH cases – conceive unwanted pregnancies using less effective methods because the COC was unnecessarily denied to them [see Leonard H et al 1996 *Heart* 76:60–62]. Yet those with more severe disease may be at high risk in pregnancy. For example, maternal mortality is >50% for women with pulmonary vascular disease. These women should never use the COC (and need alternative highly effective protection). Yet most woman with hypertrophic obstructive cardiomyopathy (HOCM), for example, though requiring intensive obstetric care, would have no particular added risk through using a COC (WHO 2, see *Table 5.14*).

The criteria of *Q 5.139* (chiefly whether there would be any added risk of arterial or venous thromboembolism) were discussed for a range of cardiac conditions by an *ad hoc* committee (of which I was a member), based at the Hammersmith Hospital in London during 2002–2003. *Table 5.14* lists these, categorized as WHO 4, 3 or 2, as the committee classified them. Note the disclaimer (and other footnotes).

Note also that the committee decided that certain cardiac patients – even those who have had an arterial or venous thrombotic event – who are taking warfarin might be allowed the COC on a WHO 3 basis. This, as usual, means that another method such as Cerazette, Implanon or an intrauterine method would actually be preferable. But if these are unacceptable, the COC is usable with careful supervision of the blood INR; the risk of thrombosis should be minimal, though warfarin dose adjustments may need to be made to allow for any effect of the COC hormones to increase the INR, by impeding the metabolism of the warfarin (*see Q 5.46*). Whenever anticoagulation ceases, of course, WHO 4 applies. Much more useful information may be found in *Table 5.14*.

5.142 Is the combined pill best avoided at very high altitudes?

Sometimes, yes. This is certainly something to discuss with the woman concerned. The issue is not whether the COC causes altitude illness – not suggested by the evidence – but if it might increase risks associated with that illness. Acute mountain sickness can kill, through hypoxia leading to acute pulmonary oedema and cerebral oedema, and blood clots in the small arteries are a feature post-mortem. In milder attacks well short of that, which can occur if unacclimatized people ascend rapidly to above about 2500 m (>8000 feet), there is an increasing risk of venous or arterial thromboembolism, including strokes. Although fibrinolysis is increased at altitude and during exercise, other circumstances in climbing are thrombogenic: dehydration through fluid loss or inadequate intake, trauma, immobility in tents when the weather closes in. Risk factors for developing altitude illness of all degrees of severity include the rate of ascent, the altitude at which the traveller will sleep and individual susceptibility [Barry PW, Pollard AJ 2003 *British Medical Journal* 326:915–919].

Acetazolamide (Diamox), which has been shown to improve climbing performance and prevent acute mountain sickness, acts as a mild diuretic and, as a consequence of mild dehydration, might exacerbate the thrombotic risk. Moreover, in high-altitude pulmonary oedema (were it to occur) there is patchy pulmonary hypertension.

In summary, considering the principle of summation discussed at *Q 5.139*, going to altitudes well above 2500 m has to be seen as in the category WHO 3 – in my view. If there were added risk factors from *Table 5.10* or *5.11* (pp. 200–203), WHO 4 would apply – after all, with more than one such risk factor the woman should not use the EE-containing pill even at sea level!

But for healthy Himalayan trekkers following the guidelines in the above *BMJ* article – summarized as 'climb high and sleep low' – the COC would be WHO 2. All should be informed of the possible minimal increase in risk of venous/arterial thrombosis.

From the practical point of view, at high altitude, the COC is very useful to control menstrual bleeding, especially if tricycled. Yet BTB is a common problem for some women at altitude.

Autonomy is an important principle here: rock-climbing is orders of magnitude more dangerous (see *Fig. 5.12*) than any risks modifiable by choice of contraceptive! The woman must have freedom to take an added risk, but prescribers have autonomy too if they think the risk of COC unacceptable (i.e. WHO 4, rather than 3, for that individual after consideration of *all* the relevant risk factors).

5.143 Is there a continuing problem for those who live long term at high altitude?

In residents, after acclimatization there is a physiological polycythaemia that normally increases blood viscosity; but this alone would be only a weak relative contraindication (WHO 2) to EE in the combined pill.

5.144 What about long-haul aeroplane flights and thrombosis risk?

As the sole risk factor this is WHO 2 – the COC is broadly usable and need not, indeed should not, be stopped (the risks of pregnancy would be far greater!). However, although all commercial flights are pressurized to the equivalent of about 2000 m, there are now numerous case reports of pulmonary embolism and some deaths (with or without the pill). As at high altitude, some extracellular to interstitial fluid shift is common; mild ankle oedema results but more important is the likelihood of intravascular volume depletion and haemoconcentration. Other important factors are the maintained sedentary position — which is equally a risk of course during long car or coach journeys – coupled with a diuresis due to alcohol and caffeine, all perhaps superimposed on dehydration due to prolonged sunbathing on a Far Eastern beach just before boarding!

Evaluation of risk factors, especially for VTE (see *Table 5.10*, p. 200), is again essential. If the woman has a high BMI, she should forget glamour and wear support hose. She also might consider stopping HRT just to cover the intercontinental flight. But normally as far as the pill itself is concerned, to quote my book *The Pill*:

There is no necessity to come off the pill – many flight attendants use it all the time. But follow their example and take some exercise during the flight: such as a brief walk around the plane every hour or so.

NB: *See also Q 6.92* concerning the important matter of how to maintain COC and POP efficacy when flying west through numerous time zones.

5.145 Can the combined pill be prescribed to patients with sickle-cell disorders?

'Yes' is the answer for those with sickle-cell trait; the situation with regard to homozygous sickle-cell disease (SS and SC genes) is more uncertain. There is an increased risk of thromboembolic disease, especially strokes, in such women and pregnancy can precipitate a crisis. The COC imitates pregnancy and the estrogen of the pill might in theory lead to superimposed thrombosis during the arterial stasis of a crisis. Therefore, until recently, most manufacturers and many authorities have included the frank sickling diseases among absolute contraindications to the COC. However, studies in the West Indies and West Africa have shown that the COC ought now to be considered only a relative contraindication (WHO 2, especially when balanced against the great risks of pregnancy in sicklers). Injectables, especially DMPA, are usually an even better choice (*see Q 8.15*).

5.146 Can a woman who has made a complete recovery from a subarachnoid haemorrhage, and had her intracranial lesion treated, use the combined pill?

UKMEC says WHO 4 for all stroke events. In my view, in this instance, the COC is relatively contraindicated (WHO 3) assuming a close subsequent watch for hypertension, but the POP or an injectable would be preferable. This is because almost all women on the combined pill have a detectable slight increase in systolic and diastolic BP, and one can never be certain that such a woman would not have some other weakness of a cerebral artery or angiomatous malformation.

5.147 Why are the inflammatory bowel diseases (Crohn's or ulcerative colitis (UC)) relative contraindications?

■ Both occur more commonly in COC-takers in some studies. Crohn's (but not UC) is also strongly linked with smoking. However, 300 pill-takers with stable disease had no more flare-ups over time than non-takers [Cosnes J et al 1999 *Gut* 45:218–222]. Hence, the COC may be used (WHO 2, except as below).

■ In exacerbations of either illness there is a high risk of thrombosis, especially VTE. Therefore, the COC should be used only in cases not prone to severe hospitalized exacerbations, and if such occur the pill should be stopped at once and would be absolutely contraindicated so long as the disease remained severe (WHO 4).

■ Malabsorption: as contraceptive steroids are so well absorbed, mainly in the jejunum (which is unaffected), malabsorption of the COC is usually not a problem. However, if there is major small-bowel involvement by Crohn's, absorption could be affected (WHO 3) and a non-oral method would be preferable (*see also Q 6.41*).

5.148 Can the COC be used by women with systemic lupus erythematosus (SLE)?

Increasingly, this is being seen as an absolute contraindication (WHO 4) except in the mildest, very stable, fully investigated cases not on steroids, with close supervision (WHO 3 – but a progestogen-only method would be preferable). This is because:

■ There are now numerous case reports and some comparative studies describing the onset or flaring-up of symptomatic SLE when estrogen was given, either in the COC or even, interestingly, as HRT postmenopausally. SLE can deteriorate seriously with renal involvement for the first time during use of COCs, but not with progestogen-only therapy.

■ There has been a recurring theme of recovery or improvement once the artificial estrogen was discontinued.

■ Cases can develop the lupus anticoagulant/antiphospholipid antibody, and once detected, the COC is definitely contraindicated for fear of thrombosis.

Obviously each patient has to be taken on her own merits. But as progestogen-only pills and injections have been tried in SLE women with no significant increase in episodes of active disease, these are usually preferred to the COC.

5.149 Can the combined pill be used by patients with established diabetes mellitus (DM)?

Arterial disease is a major hazard for diabetics; hence, ideally, they should avoid estrogen with its prothrombotic risks. Condoms and/or the POP, especially Cerazette (*see Q 7.44*), or Implanon or an IUD/IUS are all to be preferred.

In practice, however, some young diabetics are permitted use of an ultra-low-estrogen combined pill (WHO 3) using a 'lipid-friendly' progestogen. Mercilon or Femodette/Sunya 20/75 with only 20 µg estrogen would be good choices. Necessary criteria are:

- Young, ideally under age 25, and preferably having had DM for a short time.
- Free of any signs of complications of the disease, affecting arteries, nerves, kidneys or retina (these 'opathies' *always* make DM a WHO 4 condition).
- Free of the other risk factors in *Table 5.11* (p. 202). It is vital that such a patient is not also a smoker, hypertensive or with a BMI above 25.
- Perceived to need maximum protection against pregnancy and there really is no satisfactory alternative. In short: WHO 3 at best, otherwise WHO 4.

Diabetics occasionally then need to increase their total dose of insulin, which is not in itself a problem. They should be on the COC for the shortest possible time, encouraged to have their family as young as their circumstances allow, and then be transferred to another long-term method – ideally IUD/IUS or possibly sterilization.

5.150 Can potential or latent diabetics take the COC?

Yes. Caution used to be advised because the early pills did impair glucose tolerance and create hyperinsulinism. However, the RCGP study and others have shown absolutely no increase in the incidence of late-onset-type DM among current or former pill-users. Moreover, the more recent lowest-dose COCs do not even raise plasma insulins significantly. None of the following need therefore be considered as contraindications: a strong family history of DM (maturity-onset); gestational diabetes; birth of a baby weighing more than 4.5 kg (10 lb).

Such women are just supervised a little more closely than usual and need particular advice to avoid obesity.

5.151 If a young woman suffers a thrombosis in an arm vein after an intravenous injection, does this mean a predisposition to thrombosis? Should she avoid the COC (WHO 4) in future?

The answer is 'no'. The episode would be due to a chemical thrombophlebitis. This is not associated with any tendency to venous thrombosis elsewhere in the body.

5.152 In what way does the possession of blood group O influence prescribing policy?

Women with blood group O have been shown to have a lower risk of thrombosis than those with other blood groups. The protective effect probably applies to arterial as well as venous disease. Knowledge of her blood group might therefore be helpful in a positive way, when prescribing to a woman who is otherwise not an ideal pill-user. For example, one might be happier to prescribe the COC to a 34-year-old smoker if she were known to be blood group O rather than A.

MIGRAINE HEADACHES, WITH AND WITHOUT AURA

5.153 What is a working definition of migraine and why is it so important in pill prescribing?

Please see the three superb migraine Reviews by Dr E. Anne MacGregor [*Journal of Family Planning and Reproductive Health Care* 2007, vol. 33, pp. 36–47, 83–93 and especially 159–169, specifically dealing with combined hormonal contraceptives].

Migraines are:

- unpleasant headaches lasting 4–72 h that
- 'stop the person doing things' for at least one day, are
- usually one-sided and often pulsating,
- accompanied during the headache phase by
  - nausea/vomiting and/or
  - photophobia/phonophobia
- always associated with a refractory phase of some days thereafter – so 'daily' headaches cannot be migraine.

Migraine with aura differs only and crucially by what happens before the headache actually starts (see below).

 The importance of migraine is that studies showed early on that there is an increased risk of ischaemic stroke in COC-users. There is good evidence that this risk – and probably also the risk of myocardial infarction – is further increased in *migraine with aura*, especially if the women have other arterial risk factors like smoking. It is therefore crucial to identify the women *with* aura: the 1-year prevalence of this being 5%. But given that the 1-year prevalence of migraine *without* aura is about 11% of women, identifying them is important too: in order not to exclude them unnecessarily from a useful contraceptive, thereby adding in the risks of pregnancy.

5.154 What are the clinically significant symptoms of migraine with aura (formerly classical or focal migraine)?

The timing is crucial: they should begin before the headache itself, evolving over several minutes and typically lasting around 20—30 min. There might be a gap of up to 1 h from resolution of aura before the headache begins or headache might start as aura resolves. Visual symptoms occur in 99% of true auras:

■ A bright rather than dark loss of part or whole of the field of vision, on one side in both eyes (homonymous hemianopia). Note that the complete loss of vision (amaurosis) in one eye is very different from aura. It would require (even more) urgent action, as it might be due to retinal artery or vein thrombosis: stopping the COC forthwith plus urgent referral to an ophthalmologist.

■ Teichopsia/fortification spectra are often described, typically a bright scintillating zig-zag line gradually enlarging from a bright centre on one side, to form a convex C-shape surrounding the area of lost vision (bright scotoma).

The above are the main symptoms, visual in nature. The other sensory symptoms occur in only about one-third of auras, are usefully confirmatory but rarely occur without visual aura:

■ Unilateral sensory disturbance, typically in the form of pins and needles (paraesthesia) spreading up one arm or affecting one side of the face or the tongue; the leg is rarely affected.

■ Disturbance of speech (usually nominal dysphasia).

■ Motor disturbance (e.g. loss of motor function of a limb) is very unusual and more likely to indicate an organic lesion (*see Q 5.156*), not migraine with aura.

Note the absence in the above list of photophobia or symmetrical blurring or *generalized* 'flashing lights' or any other symptoms that occur during the headache itself. Relevant symptoms are generally asymmetrical, meaning that they are 'focal'.

Premonitory symptoms: Aura symptoms must not be confused with these, which occur in some women 1–2 days before any migraine, i.e. with or without aura. They include sensitivity to light or sound, food cravings, fatigue, poor concentration, yawning and pallor.

5.155 How should one take the history of migraine with aura?

Q 5.154 above may well seem rather a nightmare for history-takers! Anne MacGregor has devised some tips to make things much simpler:

■ Diary cards are invaluable: downloadable from www.migraineclinic.org.uk.

■ Ask the woman to describe a typical attack.

■ Then enquire, 'Do you have any visual disturbances:
   – starting before the headache
   – lasting up to 1 h
   – resolving before or with onset of the headache?'

■ Listen to what she says and match it up with the symptoms in Q 5.154, but *at the same time watch her carefully*. A most useful sign that it is likely to be true aura is, if, when asked to describe what she sees, the patient draws a zig-zag line in the air with a finger to one or other side of her own head.

In summary, aura has three main features:

- Characteristic **timing**: onset *before* (headache) + duration up to 1 h + resolution before or with onset of headache.
- Symptoms **visual** (99%).
- Description usually **visible** (using a hand).

Note that aura can sometimes occur without any headache following. If the aura description is clear and unequivocal, it has the same significance as it would have if a headache followed (*see* Q 5.157).

5.156 What important symptoms or features are not typical of migraine with aura, and how should they be managed?

These are:

- *sudden onset* or much longer duration, for *more than 1 h*, of the same symptoms as in Q 5.154
- a *black scotoma*, or amaurosis fugax (loss of vision in one eye)
- *motor loss*, or sensory loss affecting the whole of one side of the body or the lower limb only.

These suggest possible cerebral or retinal thromboembolism or a true transient ischaemic attack (TIA) – and of course do mean that the COC should immediately be stopped. But, as with loss of consciousness or epilepsy, they also (unlike a straightforward history of migraine with focal aura) signify *urgent referral to a neurologist*.

It is reported also that it is possible in scuba divers to confuse with migraine the symptoms of compression sickness (which of course requires urgent transfer to a decompression chamber).

5.157 So what are the absolute contraindications to commencing or continuing the COC (i.e. WHO category 4)?

- *Migraine with aura* or true *aura without headache*. The *artificial estrogen* EE of the COC (or patch or ring) is what needs to be avoided (or stopped, at once and forever) to minimize the additional risk of a thrombotic stroke.
- *Other migraines (even without aura) that are exceptionally severe in a COC taker* and last more than 72 h despite optimal medication.
- *All migraines treated with ergot derivative* (rare nowadays), due to their vasoconstrictor actions.
- *Migraine without aura* **plus** multiple risk factors for arterial disease, or a relevant interacting disease (e.g. connective tissue diseases already linked

with stroke risk), and, according to UKMEC, above age 35 the COC should be discontinued in *all* migraine sufferers (WHO 4).

5.158 What action should be taken apart from stopping the COC?

Above all, organize with the woman an acceptable effective alternative contraceptive method! It is not a 'pill or nothing' situation.

In all the above circumstances, any of the progestogen-only, estrogen-free hormonal methods can be offered – immediately: warn the woman that similar headaches might continue but now without the potential added risk from prothrombotic effects of the EE. Particularly useful choices are DMPA, Cerazette, Implanon and the LNG-IUS (*see Q 9.143*), which are all WHO 2 – disregard UKMEC, which classifies them as WHO 3 for continuation – or a modern banded copper IUD.

5.159 So when is migraine a 'strong' relative contraindication to the combined pill (WHO category 3)?

The COC (or EE-containing patch or ring) is usable with caution and close supervision:

- In troublesome migraine without aura where there is also an important risk factor for ischaemic stroke present. A good example is heavy smoking, which itself is a significant risk factor for ischaemic stroke.
- A clear past history of typical migraine *with aura* ≥5 years earlier or only during pregnancy, with no recurrence, may be regarded as WHO 3. COCs may be given a trial, with counselling and regular supervision, along with a specific warning that the onset of definite aura (carefully explained) means that the user should:
  - stop the pill immediately
  - use alternative contraception
  - seek medical advice as soon as possible.

5.160 When would migraine be only a WHO 2 risk, and how would you counsel such women?

In my opinion, the COC is 'broadly usable' (WHO 2) in all the following cases:

- *Migraine without aura*, and also without any arterial risk factor from *Table 5.11* and still under the age of 35: it is indeed disputed whether migraine without any aura is truly a risk factor for thrombotic stroke.
- *Use of a triptan drug* (they have been shown not to increase stroke risk in women not otherwise at risk).
- *The occurrence of a woman's first-ever attack of migraine without aura while on the COC*. It is a reasonable precaution to stop the pill if she is

seen during the attack. But as soon as there has been full evaluation of the symptoms – provided there were no features of aura or marked risk factors – the COC can be later restarted (WHO 2), with the usual counselling/caveats about future aura.

> The counselling of all such women (WHO category 3 and 2) must include specific instruction to the woman regarding those changes in the character or severity of her headache symptoms which means she should stop the method and take urgent medical advice. These symptoms are listed in *Q 5.154.*

5.161 Which COC brands or regimens are best for headaches and migraines without aura ('common' migraines)?

There are insufficient data regarding which brands, or even about 'second' versus 'third' generation pills, but *monophasic pills are generally preferred* to triphasic pills (fully described in *Qs 5.181–5.186*). The latter are not good for women with a tendency to any variety of headaches because the extra fluctuations of the hormone levels might act as a trigger. In addition, since in many such women their headaches tend to occur in the PFI, it can be enormously helpful to prescribe one of the continuous regimens (*see Qs 5.32, 5.34*), but again with a monophasic pill.

INDIVIDUAL VARIATION IN BLOOD LEVELS OF SEX STEROIDS: THE IMPLICATIONS FOR TREATMENT OF THE SYMPTOM OF BREAKTHROUGH BLEEDING (BTB)

5.162 As women vary, if the first pill brand does not suit, what guidelines are there to help to individualize the second or subsequent pill prescription?

Some women do react unpredictably and several brands might have to be tried before a suitable one is found. Some are never suited. This is hardly surprising. Individual variation in motivation and tolerance of minor side-effects is well recognized, and the management is fully discussed later. But, as we shall see, there is also marked individual variation in *blood levels* of the exogenous hormones and in responses at the end-organs, especially the endometrium.

5.163 What are the implications of individual variation in absorption and metabolism for the blood levels of the exogenous steroids in the average pill-user?

■ Blood levels, whether of EE or of all the progestogens that have been studied, vary at least 10-fold between women who are apparently

Titration of COC dose

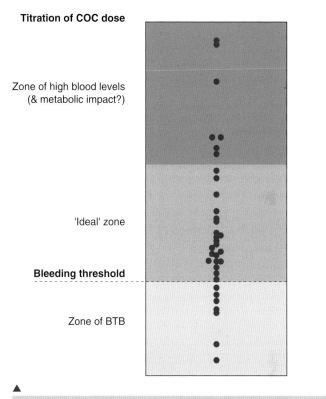

Zone of high blood levels
(& metabolic impact?)

'Ideal' zone

Bleeding threshold

Zone of BTB

▲

Fig. 5.14 Schematic representation of the approximately 10-fold variability in peak blood levels (though only 3-fold in AUC) of both contraceptive steroids: and the rationale of suggested titration against the bleeding threshold. *Q 5.163ff.*

similar, taking the same formulations and sampled exactly 12 h after their last tablet was swallowed (*Fig. 5.14*). The pharmacokinetic AUC varies less, but still about threefold. This is due to individual variation in:

– absorption
– metabolism, in the gut wall and in the liver (*see Qs 5.35, 5.36*)
– degree of binding to transport proteins, especially SHBG, in the blood plasma, which themselves are variably altered by different pills
– the efficiency with which normal EE is reformed and reabsorbed by the activity of the large-bowel flora (*see Q 5.36*).

■ In addition to variable blood levels between women, there is a superimposed variation in target organ sensitivity. This is very difficult to assess and complicates matters further (*see Q 5.177*).

■ Then there is a further 5- to 10-fold fluctuation in any woman, between the peaks after absorption and the troughs when the next daily tablet is taken. This saw-tooth pattern is shown in *Figs 5.2* and *8.1* (*see Q 8.5*). *Fig. 8.1* also conveys one of the presumed advantages of slow-release systems of administration, namely relatively constant daily blood levels.

5.164 What is the relevance to pill prescribing of this great variation in blood levels and AUC between different women taking the same formulation, as in *Fig. 5.14*?

First, as already discussed fully above (*see Q 5.40*), there is pretty good evidence from research on enzyme-inducers that women whose blood levels are low tend to suffer problems with BTB.

5.165 What about those women with relatively high circulating blood levels of artificial steroids? What evidence is there that side-effects can be correlated?

It is a very tenable hypothesis that metabolic changes and both major and minor side-effects of the COC are more common and more marked in those women whose blood levels are exceptionally high. In support, pill-takers in a US study who developed clinical hypertension were statistically more likely to have high blood levels of EE than control takers of similar pills without any rise in BP.

5.166 Is it feasible to measure the levels of either the estrogen or progestogen in body fluids?

This is not yet practical as a clinic procedure, although a simple testing kit for levels in the saliva or urine would be useful.

5.167 Without blood level measurements, how might one attempt to 'tailor' the pill to the individual woman?

I believe that one can, to a degree, but not by the approach that used to be recommended, namely attempting to base the choice on assessed features of that woman's normal menstrual cycle. This was, in my view, always illogical when one recalls that all COCs remove the normal cycle and replace it with an artificial one. That being so, it is surely preferable to make the replacement cycle as good as it can be for all. The aim is that it should, after adjustments during follow-up (*see Qs 6.21–6.22* along with *Tables 6.1* and *6.2*), eventually be 'better' than each woman's normal cycle, rather than a slavish imitation of it.

I therefore promote the 'tailoring' approach that follows, designed to discover with the woman's cooperation the 'smallest' pill that gives her adequate control of her cycle.

5.168 In *Fig. 5.14*, what does absence of BTB mean?

On the hypothesis of Q *5.165*, it could mean two different things. Absence of BTB means either that the woman has ideal blood levels of the artificial hormones or that they are higher than necessary for the desired effect of contraception – with plausibly a greater risk than necessary of causing unwanted effects.

5.169 How then might we avoid giving the woman who tends to the higher blood levels (or larger AUC) a stronger pill than she really needs?

By attempting during follow-up to give each woman the 'smallest' (lowest dose) pill her uterus will allow, without bleeding. *See Q 5.176*. I say 'attempting', as for most of the combinations the manufacturers have not helped by providing a range of doses (two sub-50-μg doses at the most).

5.170 What if BTB does occur? Does she need a higher dose or different formulation?

 Maybe! A higher-dose pill – or a phasic or gestodene variety (*see Qs 5.180, 5.181*) – might be appropriate. Or an alternative route for the hormones (contraceptive patch or ring, *see Qs 6.81–6.84*) to bypass the gut and ensure steady absorption. But, first and foremost, important alternative causes of the bleeding must first be excluded (**The 'D' Checklist**, see *Table 5.15*). I am aware of a 37-year-old woman who was seen by a number of different doctors and nurses during 1991, complaining of BTB. They kept trying different brands without success until someone passed a speculum and, tragically, found an inoperable carcinoma of the cervix. She had had a reportedly negative cervical smear 1 year previously but this was no excuse for the failure to examine (not at the first visit perhaps, especially if she had been only 25: but definitely when there was no response to treatment).

Moreover, 'missed pills' should not be one's first thought when COC-users present with spotting or BTB: among pill-takers positive for *Chlamydia*, about 13% in a 1993 US study by Krettek had spotting as a symptom, compared with only 5% of uninfected pill-takers.

Note carefully all the other possibilities in *Table 5.15*; also Q *5.32* regarding BTB in later packets during tricycling.

Cigarettes, under Drugs, are also now clearly linked – Oxford/FPA study and that by Rosenberg et al [*American Journal of Obstetrics and Gynecology* 1996;174:628–632] – to BTB, both in the pill cycle and in the normal cycle. This is thought to be the effect of increased catabolism of estrogen through constituents of tobacco smoke.

TABLE 5.15 Checklist in cases of possible 'breakthrough bleeding' (BTB) in pill-takers

---

A note of caution: First eliminate other possible causes . . . She is a woman, not just a pill-taker!

The following checklist is modified from the classic book by Esther Sapire (*Contraception in Health and Disease*. New York: McGraw-Hill, 1990):

Disease – Consider examining the cervix. It is not unknown for bleeding from an invasive cancer to be wrongly attributed to BTB on the pill. *Chlamydia* often causes a bloodstained discharge due to endometritis. Or a polyp might be present

Disorder of pregnancy causing bleeding (e.g. because of recent abortion, trophoblastic tumour)

Default – missed pill(s). Remember that the BTB may start 2 or 3 days later and be very persistent thereafter

Drugs – especially enzyme-inducers (see *Qs 5.36, 5.40*) – cigarettes are also relevant Drugs (see *Q 5.171*)

Diarrhoea with VOMITING – diarrhoea alone has to be exceptionally severe to impair absorption significantly (see *Q 5.26*)

Disturbance of absorption – likewise, to be relevant has to be very marked, e.g. after massive gut resection

[Diet] – gut flora involved in recycling ethinylestradiol might be reduced in vegetarians. An entirely theoretical factor, no obvious increase in BTB risk in vegetarians has ever been reported

Duration of use too short – BTB that the woman can tolerate might resolve if she can persevere for 3 months with any new formulation (see *Q 5.174*). See also *Q 5.33* regarding management of BTB during tricyling (possible need to take a bleeding-triggered break in continuous tablet-taking)

Finally, after the above have been excluded:

Dose – if she is taking a monophasic, try a phasic pill (see *Qs 5.174, 5.181– 5.184*)
   – increase the progestogen or estrogen component (see *Qs 5.174, 5.175*) if possible
   – try a different progestogen
   – try a different route to ensure absorption (e.g. contraceptive patch or ring, see *Qs 6.81–6.84*)

5.171 What other 'Ds' can be added to those in *Table 5.15*?

Since the last edition, during my lectures around the world, a number of other 'Ds' have been suggested from the floor, with varying degrees of seriousness.

More causes of BTB:

■ D for Doctor-caused (poor instruction/advice).

- ■ D for Dud pills: iatrogenic causes (which have really happened) include wrong prescriptions for POPs and HRT products instead of the COC. Overdue Date (time-expired product) or other cause of Damaged product are other possibilities!
- ■ D for Diathesis/Dyscrasia: a coincidental bleeding disease could first manifest itself this way.
- ■ D for Drink: alcohol and other non-therapeutic substances, i.e. drugs, chiefly because their abuse is a likely cause of default (liver enzyme induction by alcohol is not thought to be important).

INITIAL CHOICE OF PREPARATION, AND EARLY FOLLOW-UP

We are now in a position to consider how best to put the above facts and principles into practice. The objective is that each woman receives the least long-term metabolic impact that her uterus will allow, i.e. the lowest dose of contraceptive steroids that is just above her own bleeding threshold.

5.172 What is the normal choice for the first pill prescription?

As previously stated, there is no proven 'best buy'. In general, one does not choose the more complicated triphasics (*see Qs 5.181–5.186*) or 20-μg pills when future compliance is suspect. Pills known to have a relatively high rate of BTB are also best kept for trial later, when a new user is better able to cope (but all users must be advised about BTB in case it should occur, because forewarned is forearmed; *see Q 6.97*).

Microgynon 30 in its ED ('Every Day') version is my own first choice for a healthy first timer for the reasons described at *Q 5.6ff.*

5.173 Which women might need consideration of a stronger formulation (50–60 μg) from the outset?

Those women who are known to have reduced bioavailability of the COC:

- ■ Women on long-term enzyme-inducing drugs (*see Qs 5.36–5.38, 6.27*).
- ■ Rarely, women with established malabsorption problems (e.g. massive small-bowel resection).

However, for women who have had a *previous contraceptive failure* with the COC, yet claiming perfect compliance or having missed no more than one tablet, it is preferable to provide a standard formulation, often the same (monophasic) as they previously had, only now tricycling the packets plus a shortened PFI after every third or fourth pack (*see Q 5.28*) – and there is also the option at *Q 5.34*.

5.174 What pill should follow if BTB is unacceptable after 2–3 months' trial and there is no other explanation?

Provided that the other causes in the list in *Table 5.15* have all been carefully excluded, if BTB occurs and is unacceptable early on, or persists beyond about three cycles, raising the progestogen then the estrogen dose can next be tried (*Table 5.13*). In general, gestodene-containing COCs have a good reputation for cycle control. Phasic pills might come into their own here, especially if the cycle control problem includes absent WTB.

The answer is different for BTB late in a sequence of tricycling: if this applies, *see Q 5.33*.

5.175 If cycle control is a big problem, can one prescribe two pills, for example one Marvelon plus one Mercilon-20 daily, to construct a 50-µg desogestrel product?

Preferably not. Although this might be said to be 'evidence-based', it could be more difficult to justify than with long-term users of enzyme-inducer drugs, who have been proved in studies to have lower bioavailability of the COC. If in these circumstances a thrombotic or other serious CVS event occurred, it might be more difficult to establish that there had not been another cause for the bleeding problem and hence that 'too much' estrogen was not being given by the two-pills-a-day regimen. Switching to another method would be preferable.

5.176 Later on, if there is good cycle control in an established asymptomatic COC-user, should one try moving to a lower dose?

At the time of repeat prescription, the possibility of trying a lower-dose brand (though so often not available) should be considered. Otherwise one will never know whether they might not be equally suited to a lower and probably safer dose. If no lower dose exists, both prescriber and taker of the pill can have the satisfaction of knowing that metabolic risks and hence probable risk of side-effects have been minimized within the context of marketed products.

5.177 Low blood levels of the artificial hormones usually cause BTB – but is all BTB caused by low blood levels?

No. It is true that BTB is not a totally accurate marker of blood levels, and indeed variability in BTB or WTB with the same blood level could be caused by variation at the end-organ (the endometrium). This probably explains much of the light BTB common in the first one or two cycles and the late tricycle bleeding discussed in Q 5.33.

But women find BTB annoying in any event. Why give more drug than the minimum to prevent the annoying symptom? The dose administered should ideally be only just above the woman's bleeding threshold: whether mediated by low blood level or an unusually susceptible end-organ.

5.178 Should women with BTB be advised to take additional precautions? Can they rely on their COC?

It has been suggested that attempting to find the best choice of pill by titrating downwards at follow-up, in the way described above, will lead to breakthrough conceptions. Yet pill-takers who conceive rarely report having had BTB beforehand. That conceptions rarely occur unless pills are (also) missed is, I believe, for the following reasons:

- It is a tribute to the fact that even the current low-dose pills are amazingly effective, with back-up contraceptive mechanisms (notably the progestogen 'block' to cervical mucus penetration by sperm) operating even if breakthrough ovulation should occur.
- It seems that (fortunately) BTB is an early warning – usually occurring when there is more circulating artificial steroid than the minimum to permit conception – in compliant women. (It might well be true, though, that BTB implies a reduced *margin for error*, so these women probably need reminding to be more careful than usual about not lengthening the PFI, *see Qs 5.16–5.19*).
- It is likely that the bleeding from the uterus itself temporarily enhances the anti-implantation contraceptive mechanism.
- While present, BTB probably reduces coital frequency!

5.179 How would you summarize this policy?

All we want to do is give the lowest metabolic impact to the woman that her endometrium will allow. I would stress, however, that this prescribing system is based on the hypothesis of *Fig. 5.14*, which has not yet been rigorously tested.

5.180 What should be the second choice of pill if there are non-bleeding side-effects?

See Chapter 6 (*Qs 6.21 and 6.22* and *Tables 6.1 and 6.2*).

THE PROS AND CONS OF PHASIC PILLS

5.181 What are phasic pills and what are their advantages?

Their main claimed advantage is that they tend to give a better bleeding pattern for a given (low) dose of hormones, using the given progestogen. For example, Logynon/Trinordiol gives an average daily dose of 92 µg of LNG (combined with 32.4 µg of EE). If this low dose of progestogen were used in a daily fixed-dose regimen, the incidence of BTB would probably be unacceptable.

Unexpectedly, the same has not been demonstrated for the gestodene-containing triphasics (see *Table 5.13*), when compared with their actually slightly lower-dose monophasic equivalents! However, all the gestodene combined pills are reported to give better cycle control than the LNG- or NET-containing triphasics, particularly in the early months of use.

All except one triphasic (Synphase) imitate the normal menstrual cycle to some extent, in particular by there being a higher proportion of the progestogen to the estrogen in the second half of the pill-taking cycle. Histologically, this leads to the production of an endometrium that appears more like the normal secretory phase, with more gland formation and the presence of spiral arterioles. This improved histology probably lies behind the good WTB that occurs (some patients complain it is too good!).

5.182 What about the other postulated advantage, that the approximation to the normal cycle will itself lead to a reduction in long-term side-effects?

That is unlikely I think, although not impossible. On the contrary, some of the beneficial effects – which seem to relate to the very fact that the pill cycle produces more stable hormone levels and is not the same as the normal cycle (*see* Q 5.59) – might also be reduced. As yet, we just do not know.

5.183 What are the disadvantages of phasic OCs?

These can be listed as follows:

- An increase in the time required to explain the pill packet to the user.
- An increase in the risk of pill-taking errors, maybe particularly by teenagers – although some companies have made the newer packaging much more 'user-friendly'.
- A reduction in the margin for such errors, particularly in view of the low dose being taken in the very first phase, right after the 'contraceptively dangerous' pill-free time (*see* Qs 5.16, 5.25).
- Some women complain of symptoms that imitate the premenstrual syndrome, such as breast tenderness, in the last phase of pill-taking before the withdrawal bleed.
- They are obviously not a good choice for women with (aura-free) migraines or anyone prone to headaches or mood changes or any symptom that tends to be precipitated by hormone fluctuations.
- In the UK they are extra expensive to the NHS because the pharmacist or dispensing doctor is paid a separate dispensing fee for each of the three phases – and even for the placebo phase of Logynon ED!
- A small problem with postponing withdrawal bleeds (*see* Q 5.186), and for the same reason they are not suitable for tricycling (*see* Q 5.32).
- Studies in Holland, Australia and New Zealand have all found that triphasics are definitely over-represented, among the COCs reportedly

in use, by pill-takers presenting with unwanted 'breakthrough' conceptions. The reasons might include compliance problems due to complexity of the packaging and also relatively lower innate efficacy – see bullet 3, above.

5.184 So for whom might phasic OCs be chosen?

- The main indication is for cycle control with low dose, especially to get a good withdrawal bleed. (Note, however, that neither the norethisterone- nor the gestodene-containing phasics are actually quite the lowest-dose products.)
- Upon request, if the woman likes the idea of 'imitating the menstrual cycle'; they usefully increase choice if side-effects occur with monophasic products.

5.185 What are your views specifically about BiNovum and Synphase?

- BiNovum in my view is a brand that has almost no place now that TriNovum is available. TriNovum gives a lower mean daily progestogen dose (750 µg instead of 833 µg), gives at least as good cycle control and has much better packaging.
- Synphase might be useful for women experiencing BTB in the middle of the packet of a fixed-dose brand, especially Ovysmen/Brevinor. It is the only triphasic pill that has the highest progestogen to estrogen ratio in the middle phase. However, in comparison with Trinovum there is a negligible reduction in mean daily progestogen (714 µg rather than 750 µg).

5.186 How can a woman postpone the withdrawal bleed on a phasic pill?

There is no problem with Synphase. As with fixed-dose pills (*see* Q 6.86), two packets can simply be taken in a row without the usual 7-day break. But if this is tried with one of the other phasic brands, BTB is likely (although not certain) to occur early in the new packet because of the abrupt drop in progestogen from the higher level in the last phase of the previous packet.

There are two possible solutions (see *Fig. 5.15*). Contraceptive efficacy will be maintained throughout either scheme:

- Tablets from the last phase of a 'spare' packet can be taken, thereby giving 7, 10 or 14 days' postponement according to the phasic brand in question.
- Alternatively, the woman can follow immediately with a packet of the 'nearest' fixed-dose brand in *Table 5.13* (i.e. the nearest equivalent to the

Method 1

Method 2

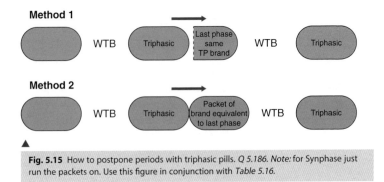

▲

Fig. 5.15 How to postpone periods with triphasic pills. *Q 5.186. Note:* for Synphase just run the packets on. Use this figure in conjunction with *Table 5.16*.

TABLE 5.16 Postponing 'periods' with phasics *(see also Fig. 5.15)*	
Name of phasic*	**Brand to follow* to delay WTB using method 2 of Fig. 5.15**
Logynon	Microgynon
Tri-Minulet	Minulet[†]
TriNovum	Norimin
BiNovum	Norimin
Synphase	Synphase

*Or the identical equivalent by another manufacturer from *Table 5.13* – the alternatives are Trinordiol, Ovranette, Triadene and Femodene/Katya 30/75.
[†]There would be a small risk of a BTB episode here, since Minulet has 25 µg less gestodene than phase 3 of Tri-Minulet.

final phase of her phasic pill). To be specific, this means using one of the brands listed in *Table 5.16*.

To avoid any possible confusion, this procedure of *Fig. 5.15* is not in the least necessary if the woman has missed pills late in her packet. In that case the advice in *Q 5.20* is all that is required to maintain efficacy. If she has a bleed, early in the new pack, she was expecting that anyway.

The combined oral contraceptive – follow-up arrangements and new routes of administration

DEALING WITH OTHER SIDE-EFFECTS AND EVENTS DURING PILL USE

CENTRAL NERVOUS SYSTEM

GASTROINTESTINAL SYSTEM

FOLLOW-UP ARRANGEMENTS: THE MONITORING OF THOSE SIDE-EFFECTS AND COMPLICATIONS PARTICULARLY RELEVANT TO COC SAFETY

6.1   What are the main aspects of pill-monitoring, once (so far as is possible) the 'safest' pill brand has been identified for the individual?

After careful selection and counselling, the list of what can (and should) be done during long-term monitoring is short – but important. In summary:

■ Start by warmly greeting the pill-taker and asking her how she is (*see* Q *11.14*). Give her space to mention her own concerns. If she has any type of bleeding side-effects, *see* Qs *5.162–5.186*. Non-bleeding side-effects are discussed below (*see* Qs *6.19, 6.20ff*).

■ Ask at each visit about headaches and particularly about any change in associated symptoms (*see* Q *5.154*). Advise in advance about all the warning symptoms in Q *6.13*, including those relevant to migraine.

■ Look for the onset of any new cardiovascular risk factors – or intercurrent disease with the same implications (*see* Q *5.139*) – especially if one is already present (e.g. arrival of age 35 in all smokers).

■ Look for the warning signs (*see* Q *6.13*), primarily:
  – a rise in BP (*see* Q *6.7* and *Table 5.11*, p. 202)
  – the onset of or change in character or worsening of migraines (*see* Qs *5.153–5.161*) – the migraine sufferer needs to be prospectively advised (i.e. more specifically than just the list at Q *6.13*)
  – sharp pleuritic pain in the chest, current or recent, is unlikely to be pleurisy – consider the rare possibility, especially in a new pill-taker, of the early symptoms of pulmonary embolism.

■ Arrange routine cervical cytology as now advised (3-yearly from age 25 to 49), with a bimanual examination only when clinically indicated (*see* Q *6.3*).

■ Advise on breast awareness (without it becoming a nerve-racking ritual) along with a good leaflet. The pill-taker should know that you will be prepared to examine her on clinical grounds, i.e. if she ever notices some change in her breasts, but routine professional breast examination has no evidence-base and no linkage whatever with any hormone methods.

■ Advise about special situations, notably immobilization, travel including long-haul air flights (*see* Qs *5.144, 6.92*), high-altitude holidays (*see* Q *5.142*), major surgery and the treatment for varicose veins (*see* Qs *6.14, 6.16*).

■ Weight is *not* routinely measured at follow-up, but BMI assessment is crucial at the start or any restart of COC-taking (*see* Q *5.122* and *Tables 5.10* and *5.11*, pp. 200–203) – and thereafter if weight changes significantly.

6.2 Which pill-takers can be seen at reduced frequency, and by whom?

In my opinion, everything depends on whether the pill-taker is one of the 'safer' women or not (*see Qs 5.138, 5.139*). The prescriber should mentally classify the pill-taker into one of the two following groups – a form of triage really – on which follow-up arrangements depend.

'AMBER LIGHT' GROUP

Women with any of the recognized relative contraindications (primarily those in WHO 3) or with any important chronic illness should normally be seen by the doctor: with a low threshold for more frequent visits, perhaps 1 month rather than 3 months after the first prescription; and it would be unlikely that the gap between checks would increase to more than 6-monthly thereafter. The reason is simple, they are the ones in whom the cardiovascular risks are focused: the heavy smokers have an inbuilt times ten or more greater risk of having a heart attack than any risk-factor-free woman (*see Q 5.102* and *Table 5.8* [p. 180]).

Even so, the COC is such a safe product that it is entirely appropriate for a family planning trained practice nurse to see the women in this category, i.e. as described immediately below, but more frequently, following an agreed protocol or patient group directions (PGD).

'GREEN LIGHT' GROUP

These ordinary 'safer' women are still seen 3 months after the first prescription, or any change of brand, for BP check and symptom assessment, as well as to answer any queries. Subsequent visits have traditionally been 6-monthly, but the frequency in this low-risk group can be further reduced: I now advise that if the BP is stable in a slim, healthy migraine-free woman after 12 months, annual checks are sufficient. WHO even suggests this annual check policy, with the prescription of 12 or 13 cycles of treatment, from the outset. But this risks missing adverse effects which occur in the early months, such as hypertension, new migraine with aura or, more remotely, venous thromboembolism (VTE) with premonitory symptoms in the leg or chest.

It is good practice and an appropriate use of scarce resources for all follow-up checks to be delegated to the practice nurse, so long as she is fully and appropriately trained in reproductive health. There must be an agreed protocol specifying when (e.g. at what BP level) she should call in the doctor.

Both nurses and doctors should recognize that pill-takers in this 'green light' group are very different from those in the first group, and are very unlikely to suffer a serious adverse effect after the first year (when the majority of the rare idiopathic VTEs tend to occur).

6.3 Ideally, shouldn't all pill-takers have a full pelvic examination at least annually?

No, this is part of medical mythology. Bimanual examinations (BMEs) can identify two main things, tenderness and enlargements. Although most of the disorders listed in Q 5.70 might in theory be picked up by a careful BME, everything mentioned is actually *less* likely to happen in pill-takers anyway, compared with, for example, the partners of intermittent condom-users! Those are the ones at the greater risk of ovarian cysts (benign or malignant), fibroids, endometriosis, ectopics, even pelvic infection. Arguably, it would be more logical to persuade them to come in, and be examined this way, if you can, rather than the pill-takers!

Obviously, BMEs should be done in pill-takers if there are clinical grounds such as pelvic symptoms in that individual; and as part of well-woman care the cervix should be screened according to guidelines.

6.4 How often should the breasts be examined?

This examination also, whether at the first or a follow-up visit, should be done solely on robust clinical grounds, including any request from the woman herself for a check, usually of some change she has noted on either side. Otherwise it is irrelevant that the woman is a pill-taker and clinicians must be prepared to defend themselves against an allegation of a 'TUBE' (totally unnecessary breast examination)!

6.5 How frequently should BP be measured, and why is it so important?

BP should be measured before treatment and subsequently checked after 3 months and then 6-monthly; if after ≥12 months it is essentially unchanged from the pretreatment visit, it can be checked annually thereafter in women free of all relevant risk factors or diseases (*see Q 6.1*). Studies have shown that (with the possible exception of one formulation requiring further study, as discussed in *Qs 6.7 and 5.101*) the COC generally causes a measurable increase in both systolic and diastolic BP. A tiny (few millimetres) increase occurs in most women and a large increase in a few (estimated at up to 1% with modern pills):

- Moderate hypertension: defined by UKMEC as BP ≥160/95 mmHg. This is WHO 4 because it increases the risks of most varieties of arterial disease and can even become irreversible. (Malignant hypertension has, rarely, been attributed to the COC.) If truly pill-induced, the hypertension is fully reversible if the pill is discontinued.
- Mild hypertension: BP 140–159/90–94 mmHg – even this should be taken seriously (WHO 3), especially if there are other circulatory risk factors (*see Qs 5.122, 6.7*).

■ Although not technically hypertension at all, I would classify as WHO 2 the situation in which the BP has gone up and though it does not quite exceed the 140/90 mmHg cut-off level for WHO 3 after appropriate resting, is found to be close to that level on repeated visits.

As generally taught, the classification as above, and any decisions arising from it, should not be based on isolated readings. Repeating the measurement after a period of rest for the woman and (if available) a second observer are ideal.

6.6 At what levels of BP should the pill be stopped?

UKMEC states, and I agree, that repeated readings ≥160/95 mmHg would always be too high, both for starting and for continuing with the COC. However, WHO is slightly more permissive, stating that a raised level that (when repeated) does not exceed 159 mmHg systolic or 99 mmHg diastolic, is WHO 3 for the COC, but that ≥160/100 mmHg is WHO 4.

6.7 When should a rather small rise in BP, perhaps not out of the normotensive range, nevertheless lead to a consideration of change of method?

Behind this question are the studies that show that hypertension acts as a marker for an increased risk of arterial disease. Studies of large populations (by life insurance companies) have shown that almost any rise in BP is associated with a small but measurable reduction in life expectancy, even in women. While it is not certain that pill-induced mild hypertension has the same significance as the idiopathic variety, it would be prudent to assume that it does. Faced, therefore, with a 33-year-old, heavy-smoking woman with a BP repeatedly hovering just below 140/90 mmHg and knowing that before pill-taking it was, say, 110/70 mmHg, one would prefer she switched to another method of birth control right away (rather than continuing to the upper age limit for a smoker of 35 years).

BP levels that are above the WHO 3 lower limit of 140/90 mmHg often indicate changing to a POP (*see Chapter 7*) but a new possibility in the younger age group would be to try one of the drospirenone-containing products (*see Qs 5.101, 6.64*).

6.8 So can the BP be used as an ongoing test of liability to arterial disease?

Possibly, yes. For years, prescribers of the pill have longed for a simple clinical test; for example, a reagent that could be added to a woman's urine in the clinic and would turn it green if she could safely continue with the COC and red if she should discontinue. It is my view that we have that test already – not perfect, but usable in the same kind of way. A rise in BP is like a red or at least pink test, implying that the woman (especially if she already has a risk factor) has now entered a category at increased risk of arterial disease.

6.9 Can patients actually on hypotensive treatment be legitimately given the COC?

This is WHO 3 (UKMEC), therefore the POP or an injectable or implant would be better choices among hormonal methods. But the COC (e.g. one with drospirenone, as just discussed) might be acceptable: given good BP control and careful monitoring in a young, non-smoking woman who accepts the extra risk, will use no other method of birth control, and after full consultation with the physician supervising control of her hypertension.

> This presupposes that the woman's hypertension is not pill-related (which would be WHO 4). It would not be acceptable for a woman whose hypertension was induced by the COC (and readily reversible by simply stopping it in favour, say, of the POP) then to be given antihypertensive drugs to enable her to stay on it. There can be few occasions when treating the side-effects of one drug by other powerful drugs can be anything but bad medicine.

6.10 What types of migraine indicate that the combined pill should be stopped?

See Qs 5.153–5.160. To recap, these WHO 4 circumstances are:

- any change in the character of non-aura migraine during use of the COC which indicates she has now developed aura (see Qs 5.154, 5.155)
- migraines that have become exceptionally severe during pill-taking, perhaps lasting more than 72 h
- migraine without aura plus the woman is now aged above 35 (UKMEC) or has other marked additional risk factor(s) for stroke
- concurrent treatment with an ergot alkaloid (rare these days).

In these categories, the estrogen of the combined pill should be stopped forthwith, and usually for ever. This is for fear that the additional thrombotic risk might result in a thrombotic stroke. But all other contraceptives are options: the POP and injectables can be started right away.

6.11 What if a woman's first-ever migraine without aura attack occurs while taking the COC? Should she stop the method?

The manufacturer's SPCs say yes to this. If there is any concern that the symptoms might be thromboembolic, in my view COCs should be stopped pending a clear diagnosis. If this rare possibility is carefully excluded, COCs may be continued or recommenced; however, on a WHO 2 basis (*see Q 5.160*), she must as usual be warned in simple terms about the important symptoms to watch out for in future (*see Q 5.154*).

6.12 What about 'ordinary' headaches that occur on the COC?

These are not a contraindication, more in the nature of a common, more or less tolerable, side-effect and one for which the woman might or might not ask help. If so, it is well worth ascertaining whether the headaches tend to occur in the pill-free week. If they do, the tricycle regimen, using the lowest acceptable fixed-dose formulation, leads – at worst – to the woman experiencing only four or five headaches a year instead of 13 (*see Q 5.32*). Moreover, there is the potential for even fewer attacks with the 365/365 regimen of Q 5.34 (unlicensed, see *Appendix A*).

As the trigger for such headaches seems often to be estrogen-withdrawal, another option worth consideration is the use of 100-µg patches of estradiol daily, through the pill-free interval (PFI).

6.13 What symptoms should lead pill-users to take urgent medical advice (potential major problems)?

Pill-users should be told to:

1. transfer at once to another effective method of birth control, *and*
2. come under medical care without delay, pending diagnosis and treatment, if any of the following should occur:

(a) severe pain in the calf of one leg – possible deep venous thrombosis (DVT)

(b) severe central pain in the chest or sharp pains on either side of the chest aggravated by breathing – could be myocardial infarction or pulmonary embolism

(c) unexplained breathlessness with or without the coughing up of blood-stained sputum – could be pulmonary embolism

(d) severe pain in the abdomen (*see Q 6.42*)

(e) any unusually severe, prolonged headache, especially if it is the first-ever attack or gets progressively worse, or is associated with the symptoms at (f) to (i) below (*see Qs 5.153–5.160*)

(f) a bad fainting attack or collapse, with or without focal epilepsy – potentially a stroke or transient ischaemic attack (TIA)

(g) weakness or paraesthesia suddenly or gradually affecting one side or one part of the body. Motor weakness and suddenness of sensory symptoms suggest a stroke or TIA: migraine aura is classically sensory not motor, and more gradual in onset

(h) marked asymmetrical disturbance of vision, e.g. a bright scotoma in a visual field, without as well as with a migraine headache following. A dark scotoma or black loss of vision is not migraine; it indicates a retinal vascular thrombosis – and emergency referral
(i) disturbance of speech (nominal aphasia) – could be aura
(j) a severe and generalized skin rash – could be erythema multiforme
   Clinical signs that might not be complaints but still demand urgent action (including stopping the COC) are:
(k) the onset of jaundice (*see Qs 6.35, 6.36*)
(l) high BP (i.e. ≥160/95 mmHg, *see Qs 6.5, 6.6*).
(m) immobilization after an accident, or emergency major or leg surgery (*see Qs 6.14–6.18*)

Potentially, the majority of the above are thrombotic or embolic catastrophes in the making. However, in the majority of cases there will quickly prove to be a much less serious explanation and the COC can be recommended.

IMPLICATIONS OF SURGERY

6.14 Should a COC-user discontinue treatment before elective major surgery?

This is WHO 3–4; it all depends on the nature of the surgery. My opinion on this is a little more cautious than some pronouncements. If it is major surgery, lasting more than 30 min and involving immobilization thereafter, i.e. mainly in bed for at least 48 h, or less major but associated with hypotension or prolonged immobilization thereafter, or any surgery involving the legs, the COC should:

1 be discontinued at least 2 (preferably 4) weeks before the operation (many coagulation factors are back to normal by 2 weeks but there is insufficient evidence to state that 2 weeks' discontinuation would always suffice)
2 not be recommended until at least 2 weeks after full mobilization. This restart can be a 'Quick start' (*see Q 6.17*): there is no need to wait for any menstrual bleeding.

The reason for this advice is the well-established increased risk of DVT postoperatively, and the potential for this to be increased by the prothrombotic changes caused by estrogens. Vessey et al [*British Medical Journal* 1986;292:526–528] estimated the risk of clinical VTE postoperatively as 0.96% on low-dose pills and 0.5% for non-takers. Given these figures, a policy of stopping the COC has the potential to prevent about 500 VTEs and up to 10 deaths in every 100 000 major operations.

For the reason that they are estrogen-free, the above rule does not apply to the POP, nor to progestogen-only injectables/implants, which can be continued without a break during major surgery. Indeed, they can all be an appropriate choice to cover the time on a waiting-list and postoperatively (*see Q 6.17*).

6.15 Should the COC be stopped for a minor operation such as laparoscopic sterilization?

This is definitely unnecessary (WHO 2) because the risk of postoperative DVT is vanishingly small after such minor surgery. The same applies to dental extraction. 'Iatrogenic' pregnancies seem frequently to be caused this way.

However, as thromboembolism occurred after 3 of 438 laparoscopic cholecystectomies in a 1993 report from Sydney (one was fatal), it would be best to avoid COC use prior to complex laparoscopies.

6.16 What about minor leg surgery, such as operative arthroscopy, or ligation of varicose veins? Or injection treatment for leg veins?

These are quite another matter. Estrogen-containing therapy should be discontinued at least 2 weeks before either such surgery or sclerotherapy, and avoided for the duration of leg-bandaging thereafter.

6.17 What contraception is suitable before and after relevant surgery? And how should the switches from and back to the COC be managed?

Progestogen-only methods are all appropriate. A good choice might be Cerazette (*see Q 7.11ff*) – or injectable DMPA (*see Q 6.14*). The first *injection* can be given at any time in the woman's pill-taking cycle, after which she just finishes the current packet. A new packet of her usual pill can be started as early as 2 weeks after full mobilization, without waiting for the expiry of the 12-week duration of the injection, whether she has amenorrhoea or if irregular bleeding is a problem. Simultaneous use of the methods is fine: after all, DMPA and the COC are quite often given together to control irregular bleeding (*see Q 8.47*).

This restart of the COC can be a 'Quick start': there is no need to wait for menstrual bleeding and 7 days of extra precautions are not needed if an anovulatory contraceptive such as Cerazette is in use. But if the method used to 'cover' the surgery has been abstinence and there is any expectation of imminent ovulation, it would be wise not to rely solely on the COC for the first 7 days.

6.18 What should be done if a patient who is a pill-taker is admitted as an emergency for major surgery or orthopaedic (fracture) treatment with immobilization?

In these circumstances the risk of DVT is high, especially if she is overweight. The COC should be discontinued at once and careful consideration given to the use of subcutaneous heparin prophylaxis. This would be particularly important for urgent major gynaecological, orthopaedic and cancer surgery.

Do not forget to ask the young girl on traction, after falling from her boyfriend's motorbike, to stop taking her (combined) pills. Indeed, the immobilization involved in treating a leg fracture after a skiing accident, even as an outpatient, can be sufficient for many continental orthopaedic surgeons to recommend heparin prophylaxis. This might be overcautious, but stopping the COC (or EE-containing ring or patch) is not: a leg fracture is at least a WHO 3 situation. Switching short term to a progestogen-only contraceptive is preferable, for all the time the leg is immobilized.

DEALING WITH OTHER SIDE-EFFECTS AND EVENTS DURING PILL USE

6.19 What general points can be made about the so-called 'minor' side-effects?

- First and foremost, avoid any hint of being dismissive or patronizing: such symptoms frequently do not seem minor to the woman affected!
- Many of them are common in the general population, hence it can be impossible to be sure that the COC is to blame in an individual case.
- The frequency of complaint depends on many factors, including anxiety about possible harm due to the therapy.

- Many side-effects can be classified under two main headings:
  - Those related to cycle control. The common problem of breakthrough bleeding (BTB) and spotting should first be evaluated as described in *Qs 5.170 and 5.171*, then managed as in *Qs 5.172–5.179*. Pill-related BTB can benefit from use of a higher-dose product, a different progestogen, or possibly a phasic pill.
  - Those that are also common in pregnancy.

6.20 Which are the common, often pregnancy-mimicking, minor (unwanted) side-effects often attributed to the COC?

Not all these are also more common in pregnancy. In some cases the link with the COC might not be causal. Beneficial minor side-effects are included within the list in *Q 5.57*. The order below is alphabetical:

Common:

- acne (usually benefited, but can worsen with levonorgestrel pills)
- breast enlargement and bloatedness with fluid retention
- cramps and pains in the legs
- cystitis and other urinary infections
- depression and loss of libido
- gingivitis
- hair loss (or gain, *see Q 6.67*)
- headaches
- nausea
- vaginal discharge (non-specific) and cervical 'erosion'/ectopy
- weight gain.

Less common:

- breast pain (see *Table 6.1, Qs 6.55*)
- chloasma (*see Q 6.67*)
- galactorrhoea (*see Q 6.55*)
- photosensitivity
- superficial thrombophlebitis.

Some more serious conditions reported in pill-takers are similarly more common in pregnancy. For example, some immune disorders; chorea, cardiomyopathy, pemphigoid gestationis, haemolytic uraemic syndrome and cholestatic jaundice; not to mention hypertension and venous and arterial thrombosis.

Subsequent questions (*see Q 6.23–6.72*) consider side-effects by body system (**excluding the circulation, because thromboembolism, hypertension and arterial disease were covered in Chapter 5**). If the woman wishes to continue with the pill method (see *Tables 6.1* and *6.2* along with *Qs 6.21 and 6.22*), suggest possible changes of formulation, which can then be tried to control her symptom(s).

6.21 Which next pill? Are there any guidelines if a patient complains of any minor side-effect and wishes to continue the method?

Beware! Before rushing to change formulations, never forget that there might be another, non-pill-related, explanation for any side-effect, and that a side-effect might be caused or highlighted because of anxiety or a psychosexual problem (see the Preface). This applies particularly to this and the next question, and the linked *Tables 6.1* and *6.2*. An emotional or psychosexual explanation becomes more probable (although not invariable) if a woman keeps returning with a wide assortment of side-effects after only taking a few tablets, and nothing ever seems to suit.

TABLE 6.1 Which second choice of pill? a: relative estrogen excess

Symptoms	Conditions
Nausea	Benign breast disease
Dizziness	Fibroids
Cyclical weight gain (fluid)	Endometriosis
'Bloating'	
Vaginal discharge (no infection)	
Some cases of breast fullness/pain	
Some cases of lost libido with no depression – especially if taking an antiandrogenic estrogen-dominant product such as Yasmin or Dianette/Clairette 2000/35 (see Q. 6.25)	

- ▓ *Treat with progestogen-dominant COC such as Loestrin 30, Microgynon 30*
- ▓ BUT *remember,* symptoms might not have a pill-related cause

TABLE 6.2 Which second choice of pill? b: relative progestogen excess

Symptoms	Conditions
Dryness of vagina	Acne/seborrhoea
Some cases of:	Hirsutism
Sustained weight gain	
Depression	
Loss of libido if associated with depressed mood (see Q 6.24)	
Lassitude	
Breast tenderness	

- ▓ *Treat with estrogen-dominant COC, such as Ovysmen/Brevinor, Marvelon or, for moderately severe acne or hirsutes, Yasmin or Dianette/Clairette 2000/35. Caution is necessary, in that estrogen-dominance might link with a slightly higher risk of VTE, see Q. 5.111*
- ▓ Remember, as in *Table 6.1,* the above symptoms might have a non-pill-related cause

On first principles, first take a history and, as appropriate, examine. If the side-effect involves abnormal bleeding, see *Table 5.15* (p. 234) and *Qs 5.170 and 5.171.* Thereafter, for both BTB and absent WTB, she might benefit from a phasic pill or a slightly higher dose.

Phasic pills might be worth changing from, however, if the symptoms are showing cyclical variation; for example, headaches, breast tenderness,

PMS-like symptoms (cyclical irritability, etc.). Monophasic pills, perhaps sustained for more than one packet consecutively (*see Qs 5.32, 5.34*) can be of real benefit here.

For all other minor side-effects there are two empirical rules and two that are more specific. The empirical rules are:

■ Reduce the dose where possible (first of the oestrogen, if possible, then of the progestogen).
■ Alternatively, switch to another progestogen.

For the more specific rules, *see Q 6.22.*

6.22 What are the more specific rules?

■ For side-effects or conditions that have become associated (mostly through clinical experience, only rarely by formal research) with a relative excess of the estrogen, prescribe a more progestogen-dominant COC.
■ Conversely, for symptoms that have become associated with the progestogen, prescribe an estrogen-dominant COC. This policy is summarized in *Tables 6.1* and *6.2*. But be aware that these tables have a rather weak evidence-base: if we are honest, we have to admit that most changes of pill to improve symptoms are ultimately on a trial-and-error basis!

CENTRAL NERVOUS SYSTEM

6.23 Is depression more common among pill-takers than controls, and how can it be managed?

For starters, the Oxford/FPA study (1985) ruled out any link between even the older higher-dose COCs and all 'serious' psychiatric illness, which primarily meant severe depression needing hospital referral.

In the RCGP study it was shown (1974) that for every 130 depressed pill-users there were 100 who were non-OC-using controls. This implies that only 30 of the 130 could really blame the COC, even with the much higher doses then given.

But it seems there are some who are free from depression when off treatment, with recurrence when rechallenged. In a proportion, altered tryptophan metabolism leads to lowered pyridoxine levels. For these it was suggested in the 1970s that pyridoxine might be beneficial (use less than 100 µg daily to avoid reversible peripheral neuropathy): in a study from Wynn's unit, 50 µg daily was given, taking up to 2 months to be effective. This work needs repeating with more modern pills. It is more common practice to try a change of progestogen or change of method, with or without antidepressant therapy.

6.24 How does the COC affect libido?

Loss of libido is reported particularly among those who are also depressed. Many extrinsic factors might explain this, including frustrated desire for a child. However, there are certainly some cases where there is a real physiological effect of the hormones and complete recovery when another method is used.

Loss of libido without depression may be linked to sex hormone-binding globulin (SHBG) levels, with lowering of androgen levels, which do affect female libido. In 2005 there was much media publicity for a very poorly controlled retrospective study by workers at Boston University Medical College. In a total of 124 women, all of whom were being treated for sexual dysfunction, the group of 62 women who were current users of the pill for at least 6 months had lowered levels of testosterone, with four times as much SHBG as 23 women who had never been on the pill. In the ex-use group ($N = 39$), who had used the pill for 6 months or more but then discontinued, levels of SHBG were lower than in current users, but over 6 months later they were still well above those in the women who had never taken COCs. The researchers postulated that this would lead to long-term loss of libido even in ex-takers of the COC, but there is very little other evidence to substantiate this. Moreover, despite the publicity given to it, this was in reality a poor study, not even providing SHBG data from a comparison group of COC-users free of concerns about their sexual function!

Contrariwise, in some women libido is actually increased on the COC because the method is so reliable, non-intercourse-related, and often reduces premenstrual tension. This might explain why, in another study, female-initiated sexual activity was found to be more common late in the pill cycle than late in the normal cycle.

6.25 How should one manage the complaint of loss of libido?

- First, the pill might be irrelevant to the problem. Thus, to begin with, discuss fully all psychosexual aspects of the relationship, and the marital and family circumstances, and offer referral for counselling as appropriate.
- Second, check whether part of the problem is soreness or dryness – which could be caused locally by thrush, or a vulval skin eruption, or suturing following delivery.
- Use of a water-soluble lubricant may help.
- Finally, changing to a different pill might help. In my experience, if depression is the main problem, and seems clearly temporally related to the pill, it is helpful to move to a lower progestogen dose or a slightly more estrogen-dominant formulation. However, loss of libido, usually

without depression, in users of pills containing cyproterone acetate (Dianette/Clairette 2000/35 [new generic marketed in UK since last edition]) or drospirenone (Yasmin) might relate to these constituents being antiandrogenic progestogens which also raise SHBG, and may improve on switching to a (less estrogen-dominant) levonorgestrel or norethisterone product.

6.26 How does the COC affect epilepsy?

The condition is not initiated by the COC. The attack rate is often reduced, although rarely it might be increased. Hormone fluctuations are unhelpful, so avoid triphasic COCs (*see Q 5.183*). Liver enzyme-inducer antiepileptic therapy is one of the few indications for at least a 50-μg dose of EE along with tricycling (*see Qs 5.38–5.41*). Moreover, regardless of therapy, if fits are commonly initiated around the pill-free time, sustained taking of monophasic pills for more than one packet consecutively, as described at either *Q 5.32* or *Q 5.34* may well help to reduce their frequency.

6.27 If epileptics and others on chronic enzyme-inducing treatments are on the pill, how should they be managed?

First, please read *Qs 5.16–5.42* before this answer.

As this situation is WHO 3, first offer another contraceptive altogether. The injectable DMPA is now the first-choice option (for its special advantage, *see Q 8.11*) along with the intrauterine methods, including the LNG-IUS (*see Q 9.149*).

As very much the second choice, if the pill is strongly preferred I used to advise shortening the PFIs as well as the increased dose mentioned above. But it simplifies compliance to eliminate most of the PFIs using the tricycle regimen (*see Q 5.32*). This also appears to improve epilepsy control, although no comparative trial has been published. After three or even (if BTB is not a problem) four consecutive packets, the woman should still shorten the PFI: arbitrarily to just 4 days. Diary cards might be helpful.

If the woman subsequently complains of BTB, exclude another cause (*see Q 5.170*) and consider taking the break earlier, either when triggered by the bleed at any time after at least seven tablets have been taken or by 'bicycling' (*see Q 5.33*).

Caution is necessary when enzyme-inducers are withdrawn, because it takes at least 4 weeks for the liver's level of excretory function to revert to normal (*see Q 5.42*).

6.28 What about headaches and migraines?

These very important CNS-related subjects have already been covered under 'risk factors' (*see Qs 5.153–5.161*) and 'monitoring' (*see Qs 6.10–6.12*).

They are important in the differential diagnosis for the conditions in the next two questions.

6.29 How can the pill affect the eyes?

If any acute visual disturbance occurs, the woman should be told to stop the pill at once, pending further investigation:

- At worst, acute loss of vision in one eye (black scotoma) could be caused by retinal artery or vein thrombosis or haemorrhage. Amaurosis fugax is the term given to a transient complete blackout of the vision of one eye, usually due to transient, often thromboembolic, retinal ischaemia. The COC should be stopped and avoided thereafter (WHO 4) along with urgent hospital referral.
- Loss of a field of vision (bright scotoma). This also must be taken seriously, even though not caused by an eye problem, because it may relate to migraine with aura or rarely a TIA.
- Blurring of vision with photophobia during a headache can be a normal manifestation during migraine without aura.
- *'Benign' intracranial hypertension* (BICH). *See Q 6.30.*

6.30 Has the COC been associated with the eye problem unhelpfully known as 'benign intracranial hypertension' (BICH)

Yes. This is a rare condition (incidence 1:100 000) of unknown aetiology, causing headache, nausea, impairment of visual acuity and field defects – through raised intracranial pressure, with papilloedema as the main clinical sign. Most patients are young women and 90% have a significantly raised BMI. Its onset can apparently be triggered by pregnancy and a number of drugs. The mechanism of the raised intracranial pressure may be (idiopathic) impairment of CSF absorption from the subarachnoid space.

Badly named, it can be very far from benign for the eyesight; indeed, urgent hospital admission is essential, for imaging to exclude a tumour or cerebral vein thrombosis. Once these are eliminated, treatment can be medical, including serial lumbar punctures and shunting to relieve the CSF pressure, or surgical by eye-saving optic nerve sheath fenestration.

There is a weak association with the COC and with other contraceptive hormones, in particular the progestogen levonorgestrel – as used in Norplant and Jadelle – which may well be coincidental. However, as the condition is certainly not 'benign' with regard to the eyesight – there is a risk of permanent visual-field loss in up to 50% if it is treated late or is recurrent – it is generally considered an absolute contraindication (WHO 4) to starting or continuing with the COC. This would of course also apply if the actual diagnosis was cerebral vein thrombosis, as applies in some cases. Exceptionally, the COC or progestogen-only methods could be used

(WHO 3 for both) if the drug associated was established not to be the COC (e.g. a tetracycline) and the BMI was below 30 – preferably with regular monitoring for papilloedema.

6.31 What about the pill and contact lenses?

An increased likelihood of discomfort or rarely corneal damage among contact-lens-users taking the COC was reported with the old hard lenses (and stronger pills). It is believed to be caused by a slight degree of corneal oedema. With modern soft lenses and low-dose pills this problem is now uncommon. If it occurs, the woman should see her optician and a brand containing the lowest possible dose of both steroids should be tried. Rarely, women have to make a straight choice between their contact lenses and this contraceptive method.

6.32 Does the pill cause or aggravate glaucoma?

There is no evidence of any effect, even among those with a family history: although, of course, intraocular pressure rarely rises significantly during the main childbearing years.

GASTROINTESTINAL SYSTEM

6.33 Does the COC cause nausea or vomiting?

Nausea can occur, particularly in the first cycle. Pill-takers can be reassured that, although it might recur after the PFI with the first pills of the next packet, nausea usually affects fewer and eventually none of the first pills in each subsequent pack. Vomiting caused by the pill itself is most unusual, but, if within 2 h, it could interfere with absorption of a tablet and hence affect cycle control and efficacy (see Q 5.26).

Both symptoms are estrogen-related and are thus not so frequent with modern pills. They are more common in very underweight women, and in them may be intolerable, starting with the very first tablet and with every COC tried. More usually, perseverance is rewarded. Use tablets with 20 μg of estrogen – or estrogen-free (i.e. the POP). Nausea can also be helped by taking the pill at night rather than in the morning.

Vomiting starting for the first time after several months of trouble-free pill-taking should not be attributed to the pill. Consider pregnancy for one thing. . . .

6.34 How often is weight gain on the COC truly due to it, and how can it be minimized?

The fear of this is one of the things that most puts young women off the pill. Yet clearly not all weight gain is caused by the pill, particularly in its modern ultra-low-dose versions; it is often blamed unfairly, as confirmed in a recent systematic review [Gallo MF et al 2006 *Cochrane Database of Systematic Reviews* (1):CD003987]. It might help to quote Endrikat et al 1995 [*Contraception* 52:229–235]. Among 228 users of a 20-µg gestodene-containing product (Femodette), after 12 cycles from baseline, as many had actually lost as had gained weight:

■ weight gain of more than 2 kg in 12.7%
■ unchanged or within ±2 kg, 73.7%
■ loss of more than 2 kg in 13.6%.

The first group (*N* = 29) would be bound to blame the pill for their weight gain, yet it is unlikely to be truly pill-attributable, as there were actually more (*N* = 31) contented (and so very likely less vocal) weight-losers!

Also very relevant to allegations about the pill and weight is that many women start the pill while still in their teens. A steady increase in weight during adolescence is the norm, regardless of pills.

There is a kind of cyclical weight gain that is estrogen-linked (*see* Q 6.21 and *Table 6.1*) and due to fluid retention. This is more noticeable in some than others, tending to be shed with a diuresis in the pill-free week. Either Yasmin or Yaz, containing the weakly diuretic drospirenone, is likely to help those with this fluid-related type of weight gain.

Moreover, mean weights among adult Northern European women (and men) do tend simply to increase year-on-year, as has been shown in several different studies of the 1990s, and if a woman happens to be taking a hormonal method over the time, it gets blamed.

Apart from appropriate advice about diet and (often most relevantly in an increasingly sedentary society) exercise, a lower-dose brand or different progestogen can be tried before necessarily trying a different method.

6.35 How should jaundice and hepatocellular damage in a COC-user be managed?

First, the pill should be stopped immediately because it has additive effects on liver metabolism. If some form of infectious hepatitis is diagnosed, the COC is temporarily WHO 4 and normally not restarted until at least 3 months after the liver function tests have returned to normal (and a small test dose of alcohol is tolerated).

Abnormal liver function tests caused by any other mechanism (e.g. cirrhosis) contraindicate the method (WHO 3–4 according to severity), although the POP is usable (*see* Q 7.51).

6.36 How often is jaundice caused by the pill? And what is the mechanism?

Rarely. Cholestatic jaundice is more common among COC-users and also in pregnancy. A COC-related past history is, in my view, WHO 4, reducing to WHO 3 if there is only a pregnancy history (cf. UKMEC, who classify the former as WHO 3 and the latter as just WHO 2).

Gilbert's disease is incidental and benign, with no impairment of liver function (WHO 2).

6.37 Does the COC cause gallstones?

The increased risk of this condition among COC-users is significant only during the early years of pill-taking. This suggests that the risk applies primarily to predisposed women. Studies of bile biochemistry have shown that contraceptive steroids can accelerate cholelithiasis.

6.38 If a woman has had definitive treatment for gallstones can she use the COC?

If the treatment was medical, the COC would, in my view, be best avoided in future (WHO 3) because of the risk of recurrence, especially if the woman was on the COC when the diagnosis was made. If the woman has had definitive surgical treatment by cholecystectomy, the COC is permitted (WHO 2).

6.39 Is acute pancreatitis linked with the COC?

Yes, perhaps, maybe through the link with gallbladder disease. Most of the sporadic cases had cofactors like obesity, alcohol abuse, hypertriglyceridaemia or lipid problems, and there have been very few reports associated with modern low-dose pills.

If a woman suffers an attack of this condition on the COC, artificial estrogen is contraindicated (WHO 4) if the triglyceride levels are high or perhaps WHO 3 if they are not. Helpfully, her triglycerides will probably fall if she transfers to any progestogen-only method.

6.40 What are the presentation and management of COC-related benign liver tumours (see Q 5.97)?

They present with abdominal pain and an upper abdominal mass, and sometimes with a life-threatening haemoperitoneum. The treatment is surgical removal. Subsequently, both the COC and progestogen-only methods should be avoided, WHO 4 (see Qs 5.97, 5.136, 7.50).

6.41 Is the COC, like cigarettes, linked with Crohn's disease?

In a 2003 guidance paper from the FSRH [*Journal of Family Planning and Reproductive Health Care* 29:127–135] it was concluded that 'a pathogenic role for the COC is unsubstantiated' in this type of inflammatory bowel disease.

- Pre-existing Crohn's is classified by UKMEC as WHO 2 for the COC.
- During severe exacerbations of any inflammatory bowel disease the documented risk of thromboembolism puts the COC into WHO category 4.
- As discussed in *Q 5.147*, Crohn's is a rare cause of poor absorption of the COC (not unless the small bowel is very extensively involved).

6.42 What is the differential diagnosis of abdominal pain that *could be* related to COC use?

- Thrombosis of major intra-abdominal vessels such as the hepatic veins or a mesenteric artery or vein. Rare: I have known only one case of the latter, whose BMI was relevantly around 39 at the time.
- Gallstones (*see Q 6.37*).
- Pancreatitis (*see Q 6.39*).
- Liver adenoma (*see Q 6.40*) or carcinoma.
- Acute porphyria (*see Q 6.43*).

Much more commonly, the pain will have an unrelated aetiology!

INBORN ERRORS OF METABOLISM

6.43 Why is the COC contraindicated in the acute porphyrias? And what advice should be given to those with latent porphyria (in their genome) but who have not suffered an attack?

There is a paucity of data about this. Both combined pills *and* progestogens alone appear to be able to provoke attacks of acute porphyria. All who have had an acute attack of severe abdominal pain (which has a 1% mortality risk) that was itself triggered by either of these hormones are, in my view, in category WHO 4 for the COC. (WHO and UKMEC have not yet assessed the porphyrias, for the COC.)

Those who are asymptomatic (no attacks) but have the inherited enzyme defect and excrete excess porphobilinogen in their urine are category WHO 3 for the COC, given Finnish reports that the low-dose COC may reduce the frequency of attacks.. The progestogen-only method of emergency contraception (*see Q 10.27*) can also be used – cautiously – provided the risks are fully explained and accepted (UKMEC says WHO 3): special caution is necessary if the woman is in her teens or early 20s because these are the ages at which first attacks of acute porphyria are most common.

The POP can also be tried with caution in latent cases if no other contraceptive is acceptable (WHO 3). Anecdotally, I have treated a latent acute porphyria case successfully with the POP after she had twice had no symptoms with the progestogen-only (levonorgestrel) emergency method.

But neither injections nor implants should ever be used (WHO 4) because, unlike tablets, they cannot be stopped immediately if a first attack actually is provoked.

6.44 Should the COC be avoided by women with non-acute porphyrias?

This is a complex subject and further advice for individual cases can be obtained from either the Cardiff Porphyria Service http://www.cardiff-porphyria.org or http://www.porphyria-europe.com. These stress that the acute hepatic porphyrias are the main problem with respect to contraceptive steroids, and that the other porphyrias are not in WHO category 4 for synthetic estrogens and progestogens: generally, after appropriate assessment and treatment they would be in WHO 2. However, estrogens have been blamed for the pathogenesis of porphyria cutanea tarda (the commonest variety), and patients who have been treated should be warned that they might relapse and need further treatment if the COC were used (i.e. it is in category WHO 3).

Some forms of porphyria result eventually in hepatic cirrhosis – which is then WHO 3 or 4, according to severity (*see Q 6.35*).

RESPIRATORY SYSTEM

Beware of the label 'pleurisy', which Vessey showed was twice as likely to be given to a COC-taker as to a non-user. If unexplained pleuritic chest pain or dyspnoea occurs (especially in a COC-taker recently returned from holiday after a long-haul flight), this is pulmonary embolism until proved otherwise (*see Qs 6.1, 6.13*).

6.45 Does the COC promote allergic rhinitis or asthma?

There is some tenuous evidence of a causal association between COC use and these conditions, particularly the former (*see Q 6.70*). But many with both complaints continue to use modern COCs with apparent impunity.

Professor Farmer, in his 1999 GP database study, showed – unexpectedly – a doubled risk of VTE in patients with asthma. This is most likely explained by diagnostic bias (asthma being a condition involving so much contact with physicians) but needs further study.

URINARY SYSTEM

6.46 What is the link between COC use and urinary tract infections?

Several studies have shown that such infections are more common in COC-users than in controls. Women on the pill might have more frequent intercourse, thus increasing their risk of so-called 'honeymoon cystitis'. But some studies have also shown an increased incidence of symptomless bacteriuria in COC-users, resolving when the pill is stopped. This suggests a causal link, so in recurrent cystitis it might sometimes be worth transferring to another method (but normally avoiding the diaphragm among female barriers, *see Q 4.51*).

REPRODUCTIVE SYSTEM – OBSTETRICS

6.47 What are the risks to the fetus if the woman continues to take the COC during early pregnancy?

In animal research, sex steroids can certainly be teratogens. Diethylstilbestrol is an obsolete non-steroidal estrogen that was proved to harm the human fetus, often with very delayed manifestations; and the hormone pregnancy tests formerly used in early pregnancy may have increased the incidence of rare congenital abnormalities.

The copious literature is, however, largely reassuring about the COC. The rate of birth defects in the Oxford/FPA and RCGP studies following COC exposure in pregnancy was no higher than expected in any group of women having a planned baby. In a major study of 1370 abnormal babies in Connecticut, there was no increase in COC use during the pregnancies compared with the mothers of normal infants. Studies of national birth defect registers in Hungary and Finland also strongly suggest that pill use in pregnancy has no effect on visible malformations, although multiple births are more common.

The rule that a pregnant woman should avoid all drugs, especially in the first trimester, remains the ideal. But the situation envisaged by the question is not uncommon – can the woman be given any kind of risk estimate? She can certainly not be promised a normal baby. Quite apart from the uncertainty about rare anomalies, at least 2% of all babies show an important abnormality. Bracken (1990) found a relative risk from COC use of 0.99 (i.e. no detectable change) for all important malformations, in a meta-analysis of 12 prospective studies. This agrees with the large population-based case–control studies.

Note that there should be no added risk at all after failed postcoital hormone treatment, which is given before implantation (*see Q 10.18*).

6.48 Is there any residual fetal risk for ex-pill-users?

Here the balance of the published work is heavily tilted towards absence of risk. In 1981 an expert scientific group of the WHO declared categorically that there was no evidence of any adverse effects on the fetus of pill use prior to conception. The only residual anxiety relates to the fact that alterations in mineral and vitamin levels have been observed in OC-users (see *Table 5.7*, pp. 174–175). These can take a few weeks to revert to normal and supplementation with vitamins (most importantly folic acid) at and just after conception has been shown to reduce the risk of neural tube defects in women with a previously affected baby.

6.49 Should women stop the COC well ahead of conception?

Some authorities advise that they should discontinue the pill and use a mechanical method of contraception for two to three cycles. This has not been proved to help, although it should certainly do no harm. Ultrasound scanning has lessened the importance of this for dating of the pregnancy. Although most authorities do not consider them important, some couples do find it reassuring that there are no detectable changes from normal in vitamin and mineral metabolism by about 2 months post pill. The fpa pill leaflet recommends waiting for one natural period before trying to become pregnant.

A woman who conceives sooner than any arbitrary time should, in the light of Q 6.48, be very strongly reassured. Avoiding drugs and cigarettes is far more important! Along with an adequate, balanced diet, the Chief Medical Officer recommends a daily dose of 0.4 mg folic acid as routine prophylaxis against neural tube defects, starting before conception.

Specialist advice should be obtained before conception if a woman on antiepileptic therapy plans a baby.

For trophoblastic disease, *see Q 5.78*.

REPRODUCTIVE SYSTEM – GYNAECOLOGY

6.50 How does the COC affect the symptoms associated with the menstrual cycle?

Beneficially in most respects (see the summary list in Q 5.57). Regular bleeding patterns are the norm but if there is irregular bleeding it is important to remember all the non-pill causes of BTB (*see Qs 5.170 and 5.171 and Table 5.15*, p. 234)!

Premenstrual syndrome (PMS) was less common overall in the RCGP study. Yet any prescriber knows that some individual pill-takers complain of a similar symptom-complex to PMS towards the end of each packet, with fluid retention, breast tenderness and depression/irritability predominating. These symptoms seem to be more common on phasic pills, and less frequent in users of Yasmin or the new (2009) Yaz. PMS symptoms are generally relieved in monophasic pill cycles compared with 'normal' cycles, especially if two or more packets are taken in succession (*see Qs 5.32, 5.34, 5.135*).

Similarly, most women notice the menstrual flow to be both lighter and less painful, but a minority who normally have light menses actually report the reverse.

BTB, absent WTB on the COC, and secondary amenorrhoea after COC use are cycle symptoms considered elsewhere (*see Qs 5.11, 5.62–5.68, 5.162–5.179*).

6.51 What is the effect of COCs on pelvic infection, functional ovarian cysts and fibroids?

These effects appear to be beneficial, overall (*see Qs 5.60, 5.61, 5.97, 5.135*).

6.52 What effect does the combined pill have on endometriosis?

This condition is helped: sometimes treated but more often maintained in suppression after initial definitive surgical or medical treatment by a progestogen-dominant COC such as Microgynon 30, on a continuous or tricycle basis (*see Qs 5.32, 5.34*).

There is also a definite clinical impression that it is less common among current users of COCs, and this has received some confirmation by the RCGP and Oxford/FPA, but any continuing protection among ex-users is not established. Most probably the potential benefit is partly negated by the regular PFIs and therefore bleeds of normal pill-taking, unlike the continuous or almost continuous regimens used therapeutically (and increasingly as a woman's choice).

The most significant gynaecological effect of the COC of course is a *benefit: protection against cancers of the ovary and endometrium* (discussed in Qs 5.58, 5.76, 5.77).

6.53 Does the COC cause vaginal discharge?

Do not attribute this to the pill without first eliminating other causes:

■ Cervical erosion (now better known as *ectopy*): this was definitely more common in the prospective studies based on COCs containing 50 μg or more of estrogen. It still occurs, although less frequently, on modern pills and requires treatment only if the woman complains.
■ On the other hand, some women (especially if taking very progestogen-dominant pills) complain of *vaginal dryness.*
■ It is still generally believed that *thrush* (*candidiasis*) is more frequent in COC-users. Yet a paper with the title *The pill does not cause 'thrush'* was published in the *British Journal of Obstetrics and Gynaecology* in 1985. The journal would never have allowed such a title if this study of over 1300 women attending three departments of genitourinary medicine in England had been the slightest bit equivocal! Other recent studies are confirmatory. This is perhaps because current low-estrogen pills have less pregnancy-mimicking effect on the glycogen content of vaginal cells. In practice, it should certainly not be assumed that modern pills are to blame in any case of recurrent thrush and the condition is therefore WHO 1 for the COC method.

■ *Trichomonas vaginalis*: COCs seem to provide some (as yet unexplained) protection against this, but none against the transmission of other STIs.

6.54 Does the COC affect other vaginal conditions?

There is a suggestion from research in the USA that the COC protects against the rare toxic shock syndrome. No effect of the pill either way has been reported on the incidence of bacterial vaginosis.

THE BREASTS

6.55 What effects does the COC have on the breasts?

For benign breast disease, *see Q 5.97*, and for breast cancer, *see Qs 5.82–5.94*. Most women notice an increase in size of their breasts and some change in texture. These effects might be acceptable but breast tenderness is not. It can occur in susceptible women with any pill formulation but seems particularly associated with the last phase of phasic brands.

Galactorrhoea among pill-takers is rare and needs investigation (plasma prolactin). A pituitary adenoma or microadenoma should be definitely excluded before labelling this as a minor side-effect (which it can sometimes be).

6.56 Should the combined pill be used during lactation?

In my view and that of the WHO, the answer is a definite 'no'. Breastfeeding is WHO 4 for the pill on several counts. First, it is an 'overkill', because practically 100% contraception can be obtained by the combination of lactation with the POP (*see Q 7.16*). Second, the COC frequently reduces the volume and quality of milk; and third, a larger dose of hormone is being given to the breastfed infant than would be the case with the POP.

MUSCULOSKELETAL SYSTEM

6.57 If given to young, postpubertal girls, will the COC cause stunting of growth? Indeed, are any other adverse effects more likely in very young teenagers than in the older young woman?

Given in high dose to young female animals, estrogen alone can lead to premature closure of the epiphyses. However, there is no evidence that a daily dose of 30 μg or even (in the past) 50 μg of EE taken with progestogen has any effect on the potential height in postpubertal girls. Menstruation normally starts when adult weight and height have mostly been achieved. Pill-taking should always be delayed until menstruation is established.

Young teenagers need good counselling, if the COC is to be prescribed at all. The risks they run are great, affecting so many aspects of emotional development, their future ability to have stable relationships, their total sexual and reproductive health (*see Qs 11.3, 11.10, 11.11*). But these are the risks of early sexual activity. No proven risks (or benefits) specific to the COC are known to be greater when it is started at 13 than at 23. So the strictly pharmacological considerations are not different from those for a woman in her early 20s. However, in amenorrhoeic teens, the estrogen content of the COC might be therapeutic, in assisting the achievement of peak bone mass.

6.58 Is the COC associated with carpal tunnel syndrome, primary Raynaud's disease, chilblains, and cramps in the legs?

Associated, yes, these have been described: but causation is less certain. Raynaud's phenomenon might be a manifestation of a contraindicating condition (for instance, a connective tissue disorder such as SLE, which might itself promote arterial disease), so the symptom must be investigated.

Otherwise, if these problems are troublesome it is worth a trial of discontinuation of the COC; but it can also be continued if the patient so wishes.

6.59 How should one assess the complaint of leg pains and cramps?

Careful assessment and examination are important. If bilateral, the symptom is less likely to be significant, but look for water retention, varicose veins, chilblains or associated Raynaud's phenomenon.

If unilateral, DVT must be excluded. If in doubt the pill should be stopped and the patient referred for further investigation. Her contraceptive future depends on an accurate diagnosis being made.

6.60 How does the COC affect arthritis and related disorders?

Most authorities in rheumatology accept that there is a reduction in rheumatoid arthritis risk of about 30% overall [Symmons DP 2002 *Best Practice & Research Clinical Rheumatology* 16:707–722]. The consistent finding is a protective effect against severe manifestations of the disease in current COC-users. This makes it WHO 1, a good choice for most with this condition.

Tenosynovitis and a form of allergic polyarthritis can occur, but causation has not been proved.

CUTANEOUS SYSTEM

6.61 Which skin conditions can be improved by COCs – and by which COCs?

Acne, seborrhoea and sometimes hirsutism can be benefited by any of the estrogen-dominant COCs (whereas there is little or no benefit when there is progestogen-dominance, *see Qs 6.21, 6.22*). In the UK, only Dianette/Clairette 2000/35 have a specific indication with respect to these conditions (see below).

6.62 What is different about drospirenone, the progestogen used in Yasmin?

Yasmin is a (2002) monophasic combined oral contraceptive marketed by Schering. Each tablet contains 3.0 mg drospirenone and 30 μg EE. Drospirenone differs from other progestogens in COCs:

- It has diuretic properties due to antimineralocorticoid activity. This might help to oppose the salt- and fluid-retaining effects of EE and so help symptoms like bloatedness (*see Q 6.64*).
- Yasmin has also been shown in a small trial, compared with Microgynon 30, to induce a very small (statistically significant) lowering of mean BP.
- Drospirenone acts as an antiandrogen, so the combination is an alternative to Dianette for the treatment of moderately severe acne and PCOS.
- Drospirenone with EE is an estrogen-dominant combination and so would not be expected to have the lower risk of VTE associated with the functionally antiestrogenic levonorgestrel (*see Q 5.111*) of, for example, Microgynon. But in the EURAS study (*see Q 5.119*), which ascertained any case of VTE (not just the 'idiopathic' cases), the actual comparative VTE risk of Yasmin was found not to be different from the other formulations.

6.63 Compared with other modern pills, does Yasmin truly have an advantage with respect to weight gain?

See Q 6.34 for the minimal effect on body mass of alternatives. A European multicentre, randomized trial did indeed show statistically lower body-weight changes as compared with the desogestrel-containing Marvelon. However, most authorities interpret this decrement in weight gain as due only to diuresis, so in long-term use there is a maintained slight (about 1%) reduction of total body water compared with controls. After allowing for this diuretic effect, over the 2 years of the study there was the same gradient of weight gain with both the products studied. This is most likely to be just the normal background increase (*see Q 6.34*) and so weight gain is probably not caused by either COC – nor indeed by Yaz (Q 6.64).

6.64 Given the above and considerations of cost, what criteria should normally be applied for using Yasmin?

Yasmin is to be welcomed as a choice for appropriate women, being an alternative to Dianette (unlike the latter, it is not marketed primarily for its acne/hirsutes benefits) and Marvelon, which is clinically recognized as possibly the best 'mainstream' pill for acne. Interestingly, Yasmin and Yaz (below) add some new WHO 4 conditions: they should not be used in patients at risk of high potassium levels (i.e. renal insufficiency, hepatic dysfunction and adrenal insufficiency). After assessing this and all the usual COC contraindications, in my view, Yasmin and Yaz are very useful COCs:

- Where there is a clear indication for estrogen/antiandrogen therapy (significant acne, which is often associated with the PCOS).
- During COC follow-up, as a useful second choice for empirical control of minor side-effects linked with fluid retention, such as cyclical breast enlargement. Pending good comparative data Yasmin appears better than other COCs for PMS symptoms, occurring either pre-treatment or on other COCs. A related new (2009) product is Yaz (Table 5.13, p.208), and after an RCT comparing with placebo this is licensed for severe PMS. With only 20 µg of EE, it is the first UK COC taken for 24 days followed by 4 placebos.
- Raised BP: the level on repeated measurement being such as to make the clinician consider a change from the current formulation of combined pill – but where the COC is still clinically usable, i.e. the BP is increased, but well below the 160/95 mmHg level which UKMEC classifies as WHO 4 (see *Qs 5.101* and Table 5.11, p. 202). Such a switch to Yasmin or Yaz, rather than another method, has a reasonable biochemical evidence base, though we need more clinical data. If the BP fails to respond adequately to a drospirenone-containing COC, Cerazette would be a good alternative.
- Lastly, what about weight? If the BMI is already >30 this is WHO 3 (non-use preferred) for the COC, anyway. The BNF recommends a less estrogen-dominant formulation with levonorgestrel or norethisterone, though the EURAS findings (*Q 5.119*) suggest no added concern with Yasmin. Otherwise, given a BMI less than 30, *anxiety* about weight gain, especially if coupled with a history of acne or of symptoms of fluid retention with other pills, would justify a trial of Yasmin or Yaz.

6.65 Where does Dianette feature now we have Yasmin? Is it to be seen primarily as an effective treatment for acne and hirsutism?

Dianette is an antiandrogen/synthetic estrogen combination (cyproterone acetate (CPA) 2 mg with EE 35 µg) for the oral treatment of moderately severe acne and moderate hirsutism in women, especially when due to PCOS (*see Q 5.66*).

These are its indications but it is also a reliable anovulant and often gives good cycle control as well. It has similar rules for missed tablets, interactions with drugs (including antibiotics), absolute and relative contraindications, and requirements for monitoring as the COC. But it is not indicated for use solely as an oral contraceptive. It can be free of charge to the woman if the prescription is marked 'for contraception' or with the symbol for 'female' (♀).

Dianette is definitely an estrogen-dominant product, as shown by its desired effect in PCOS of permitting EE to raise SHBG. So it must be expected to allow the estrogen similarly to have relatively greater effects in a prothrombotic direction than a levonorgestrel product would (see above); and indeed Vasilakis et al [*The Lancet* 2001;358:1427–1429] found a fourfold increase in VTE risk compared with levonorgestrel pills. So the CSM advice (BNF 2008) is that Dianette is contraindicated (WHO 4) in women with a past history or merely a close fanily history of confirmed idiopathic VTE, regardless of any investigations (*cf. Table 5.10*, p. 200, for ordinary COCs).

There has been no good head-to-head RCT of Yasmin versus Dianette, but indirect evidence suggests Yasmin would have almost identical effectiveness for the conditions for which Dianette is indicated.

With either product, caution is essential because so many prospective users with PCOS do have high BMIs (30–39, WHO 3). However, the added benefit due to being a therapy and not just a contraceptive might be held in many cases to justify some added risk (i.e. implying, despite the high BMI, a maintained benefit–risk difference).

6.66 What is the recommended maximum duration of treatment with Dianette?

The SPC recommends 'withdraw when resolution [of the acne or hirsutism] is complete' but repeat courses can be given if the conditions recur.

There is a concern that prolonged high-dose treatment with CPA can cause benign and malignant liver tumours in rats, and hepatotoxicity has been described with the much higher 50-mg-plus doses used by dermatologists and for prostate cancer therapy. There is some reassuring evidence, however, from the MILTS study, that the 2 mg dose as in Dianette does not increase the risk of such tumours above that for all the other COCs (which is very small, *see Q 5.96*).

Resolution of acne is usually within a year, yet in my experience patients develop a very strong 'brand loyalty' to their Dianette. The quoted SPC statement implies that we should encourage them to switch when their condition is controlled to any estrogen-dominant COC, reassuring clients that this is usually sufficient as maintenance therapy. A logical option if acne was moderately severe before the Dianette would be the new (2009) Yaz (*Q 6.64*), or Yasmin, one of which indeed might nowadays be used instead of Dianette from the outset.

It is also acceptable ultimately to return to and continue with Dianette for much longer than 1 year, assuming the woman accepts the highly unlikely, but possible, hepatic and prothrombotic risks.

Clinical tip: over 80% of moderately severe to severe acne in young women occurs as a manifestation of PCOS – so a pelvic ultrasound scan can be helpful, to enable more holistic management than just treating the skin (*see* Q 5.66).

6.67 Which skin conditions are more common in COC-users?

- *Chloasma/melasma*: this 'pregnancy mask' can develop in women on the COC after exposure to sunlight, just as in pregnancy. The condition can be very slow to fade after the pill is stopped. Mild degrees can be masked by careful use of cosmetics and tolerated if exposure to sun can be reduced. The condition can also occur/recur with the POP or other progestogen-only contraceptives, hence a non-hormonal method might have to be chosen.

- *Photosensitivity*: in prospective studies this problem tends to be reported more often in COC-takers than controls. Very rarely it might be the first manifestation of one of the porphyrias (usually non-acute type, *see* Q 6.44). Once acquired, like chloasma it tends to be permanent even if the pill is discontinued.

- *Pemphigoid (herpes) gestationis*: if this serious skin condition occurs, it absolutely contraindicates the COC (WHO 4).

- *Hirsutism*: is unlikely to be truly caused by the COC, but may be helped by an estrogen-dominant/antiandrogenic product, especially Yasmin or Dianette.

- *Loss of scalp hair*: there may be a true link but not a long-term, pill-related problem. Head hair density is always the resultant of the telogen (resting) and anagen (growth) phases. In pregnancy, and similarly in some women on the COC, a greater proportion than usual of the hair is synchronized into the growth phase. This is fine at the time but can lead to a noticeable synchronized loss some time later – as is often reported in the puerperium.

- Telangiectasia, rosacea, neurodermatitis, spider naevi, erythema multiforme, erythema nodosum, eczema, and possibly other skin disorders: all these have been described, but not established, as possibly causally associated or exacerbated by COCs, in a minority of women.

6.68 What action should be taken if such skin problems present in a COC-taker?

First, consider discontinuing the COC. Severe conditions such as erythema multiforme or pemphigoid gestationis would normally mean future avoidance of this method, even without proof of causation.

Erythema nodosum has a wide range of trigger factors and is most commonly coincidental to the COC. In a series of 128 cases, 28% had sarcoidosis, so this should be excluded. Infection (typically streptococcal) is a much more common trigger than the COC.

According to the views of the woman herself, therefore, and any dermatologist involved, if like erythema nodosum the skin condition is relatively mild, she can be cautiously rechallenged with a low-dose COC (*see Q 6.72*) – perhaps one containing a different progestogen – or with the POP. Recurrence would then suggest another method.

6.69 Does the COC cause gingivitis? Any other oral problems?

Hypertrophic gingivitis is a rare but well-recognized complication of COC use. Lesser degrees are more common, as in pregnancy. Symptoms are minimized by good oral hygiene. 'Dry socket', a painful state after tooth extraction, is also said to be more common in COC-users.

ALLERGIES AND INFLAMMATIONS

6.70 What effect does the COC have on immune mechanisms?

Several studies on immunoglobulins have suggested that artificial sex steroids can modify immune mechanisms. The effects are of a similar nature to, but less marked than, those associated with pregnancy. A study from France, however, in which antibodies to EE were reported in patients suffering from venous thrombosis, has not been confirmed.

The RCGP study, in particular among the prospective studies, showed an increase in inflammations and some disorders that are believed to have an immune basis. However, as shown in *Fig. 6.1*, these are partly balanced by a well-established protective effect against thyroid over- and underactivity, and probably rheumatoid arthritis (*see Q 6.60*). Once again,

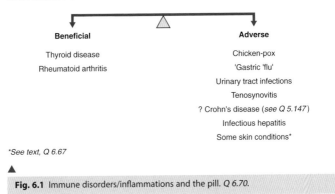

Some apparent associations of COC use with immune disorders/inflammations

Beneficial	Adverse
Thyroid disease	Chicken-pox
Rheumatoid arthritis	'Gastric 'flu'
	Urinary tract infections
	Tenosynovitis
	? Crohn's disease (*see Q 5.147*)
	Infectious hepatitis
	Some skin conditions*

*See text, Q 6.67

Fig. 6.1 Immune disorders/inflammations and the pill. *Q 6.70.*

as with both malignant and benign tumours (see *Figs 5.6* and *5.7*, pp. 159, 160), combination OCs seem to be capable of causing both beneficial and adverse effects within the same medical field. Causative associations are not all proven by any means and the magnitude of the effects described in *Fig. 6.1* is mostly small; but we badly need more information.

6.71 Does use of the COC promote transmission of HIV infection? Or make AIDS more likely after infection?

Studies among prostitutes in Nairobi were the first to suggest an increase in the likelihood of seroconversion to HIV-positive if the COC were used, but a truly causative link has not been established. Effective contraception is obviously important for any woman known to be HIV-positive, as well as regular use of condoms. For compliance reasons, the LNG-IUS or DMPA are usually better choices than the COC. They do not appear to worsen the prognosis.

6.72 Do women sometimes become allergic to the COC hormones, or in COC-users is there an increased tendency to react to other allergens?

Anecdotal data exist to suggest that either can occur. For example, in vitro studies of blood lymphocytes suggested true hypersensitivity to mestranol in two cases (one of erythema multiforme, one of erythema nodosum). However, I had a case of erythema nodosum who was able to go back on the same brand of COC without suffering any recurrence.

SPECIAL CONSIDERATIONS: WHEN TO COME OFF THE PILL?

6.73 Are there benefits to be gained from taking breaks from COC use? Is duration of use of any relevance?

From the point of view of preservation of fertility, the answer is a categorical 'no' on both counts (*see Qs 5.69, 5.70*). In relation to all the examples of circulatory disease, duration of use has now been found to have no effect (*see Q 5.102*).

Even if, intuitively, it is still felt best to limit total duration of use, breaks will be of no value; unless they are so long as to have a real influence on total accumulated duration of use (*Fig. 6.2*).

It is worth reminding any woman with this concern that during 10 years she has in fact taken 130 breaks! Not that this is true of all women now; she might have chosen to tricycle (see *Table 5.4*, p. 128, and *Q 5.32*) or fully continuous 365/365 pill-taking (*see Q 5.34*) – which with a 20-µg pill does not increase total annual dosage.

Metabolic risk markers (see *Table 5.7*, p. 174) show no apparent progression of any changes beyond 2 years' continuous use. It has even

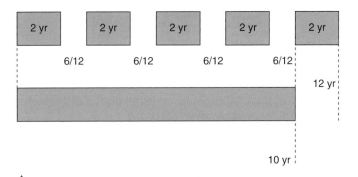

▲

Fig. 6.2 Breaks and accumulated duration of use of the COC. *Q 6.73.* The blocks represent segments of pill-taking duration (in which the only breaks taken are the pill-free weeks). Note how a woman who takes 6-monthly breaks every 2 years still accumulates 10 years of total duration in 12 years.

been argued that repeated restarting of the COC might be more harmful than the relatively steady-state situation that is maintained during sustained use.

The main problem with breaks of several months at a time was well shown in a study in which, during a planned break of just 6 months, 25% of young women had unwanted pregnancies.

6.74 What if she is hard to convince that a break will not benefit her?

Of course we should never force anyone to continue: if a woman wants to make a break, then what matters most is to arrange an effective and satisfactory alternative. But so often the notion is not hers at all, but comes from a friend or a magazine, and, if so, *Q 6.73* might help to reassure her about continuing.

6.75 What about duration of use and cancer risk (*see Qs 5.72–5.96*)?

Some studies show beneficial effects of COCs on cancer of the ovary and endometrium and others show possible harmful effects on cancer of the liver, cervix and breast. Additionally, in each of these opposite categories both the beneficial and the adverse effects described are usually found to be greater with increasing duration of use! (The definite exception is breast cancer, where age and recency of use are the important factors, *see Q 5.86*). So the advantages of increased duration of use would, again, help to balance any disadvantages. Short breaks are unlikely to be relevant since they have so little effect on total duration (see *Fig. 6.2*).

It is impossible to state with certainty whether the good effects of pill use fully outweigh the adverse effects on cancer overall (*see Q 5.74*) – although they might do so – and it is equally impossible to assess accurately the changes on both sides of the equation caused by increased duration of use (*see Q 6.76*): the pros and cons seem roughly in balance.

6.76 How much should age *per se* influence prescribing, with regard to both cardiovascular system risk and cancer?

CVS RISKS AND AGE

Here opinions have changed, triggered by the landmark decision of the FDA's Fertility and Maternal Health Drugs Advisory Committee in October 1989. Their recommendation, subsequently endorsed by the FDA itself, was for:

The removal of all age limits on the use of (combined) oral contraceptives by healthy non-smoking women – i.e. free of all risk factors.

Was this a cavalier decision, flying in the face of previously agreed practice? I think not, because:

- Healthy non-smoking pill-takers with low BMI are actually much 'safer' than we used to think.
- Modern prescribing and monitoring are more structured and careful.
- The pills themselves are believed to be safer.
- Above all, we now have a much better appreciation of the benefits of the COC to gynaecological and some aspects of general health for women, most particularly older women (*see Qs 11.37, 11.38*).

In short, even though:

- the cardiovascular risks (and breast cancer risks, see below) do increase inexorably with age, and
- the LARCS are usually even better choices,

the benefits of the COC mean the risk–benefit ratio until the average age of the menopause is little changed. But such continued provision should be only at the woman's own request and only for healthy, slim, migraine-free non-smokers!

After age 51 (mean age of menopause) fertility is so low that I recommend using a less strong contraceptive than the COC anyway (*see Q 11.46*).

The important issue of how to diagnose loss of fertility around the menopause, given how the latter is masked by the COC or other hormones, is discussed later in *Qs 7.61–7.63, 8.46, 11.41–11.43*.

RISKS OF CANCER WITH AGE

These show a general increase with age; and the 1996 CGHFBC 'model' for the risk of breast cancer shows that the pill-attributable 24% increment applied to an increasing background risk suggests proportionally more cases as the pill is used by older women (*see Q 5.92*). (The reassuring 2002 study from the CDC (*see Q 5.87*) gives insufficient information on pill-users who continue through to the menopause.)

But the COC protects against cancer of the ovary and endometrium and probably the large bowel, the incidence of which rises particularly over age 40. The extent of this balancing of the risk is difficult to quantify.

Fortunately, there are several equally effective new options for older pill-users (banded copper IUDs, IUSs, implants).

6.77 If a smoker really does give up cigarettes at age 35, can she continue to take the COC? And if so, until what age?

Studies show a marked early decline in risk of ischaemic heart disease in either gender, due to loss of the acute metabolic effects of smoking, but they suggest in men that it takes 10 years to return to the levels seen in never-smokers. If this delay is due to established early coronary atheroma in the arterial walls generated by years of smoking, one must be concerned about the prothrombotic effects of EE in any COC.

According to a 1990 report from the US, in *women* ex-smokers '. . . the increase in risk of a first myocardial infarction dissipated after 2–3 years'. This is more rapid than among the British men, but it does not establish safety if COCs had earlier been taken and continued to be taken. The ex-heavy-smoker cannot be reassured like the completely risk-factor-free woman about continuing with the pill right until her menopause (*see Q 6.76*).

To summarize, the COC is generally discontinued by smokers at age 35, in the UK: though WHO and UKMEC (in my view unwisely) allow continuing use for smokers of <15 a day. Given the risk reduction shown in studies of complete smoking cessation, according to UKMEC ex-smokers are only WHO 3 until 1 year, dropping to WHO 2 beyond 1 year of ex-use. In my view WHO 3 is the best category for truly ex-heavy-smokers regardless of time since cessation at age 35. The POP or one of the LARCs would be safer.

SOME REVISION QUESTIONS

6.78 What are the medical myths about prescribing the pill?

The list in *Table 6.3* is not exhaustive but includes some important examples currently believed by some healthcare professionals.

6.79 What are the myths relating to continuing use of the pill?

Please refer to *Table 6.4*.

TABLE 6.3 Pill myths

Myth – Do not prescribe the COC in the following circumstances:	Actuality – The COC is: (WHO 1 unless otherwise stated)
Wish to optimize fertility	Beneficial (*Q 5.70*)
Fibroids	Beneficial (*Q 5.97*)
Current amenorrhoea, after investigation	Usually beneficial (*Q 5.66*)
Past amenorrhoea, resolved	Neutral (*Q 5.68*)
Recent menarche (menstrual cycles established)	Neutral (*Q 6.57*)
History of gestational diabetes (watch weight)	Neutral (*Q 5.150*)
Thrush	Neutral (*Q 6.53*)
Recent trophoblastic disease (hCG now normal)	Neutral (*Q 5.78*)
Sickle-cell trait	Neutral (*Q 5.145*)
Thalassaemia	Neutral (*Q 5.140*)
Epilepsy (allowing for drug interactions)	Neutral (sometimes beneficial) (*Q 6.26*)
Mitral valve prolapse	WHO 2 (*Table 5.14, p. 214*)
Sickle-cell anaemia	WHO 2 (*Q 5.145*)
Any migraine (non-focal, tolerable, no change)	WHO 2 (*Q 5.161*)
Cervical neoplasia (preinvasive)	WHO 2 (*Q 5.81*)
Wish to minimize *overall* cancer risk	Not certain, but avoiding COC probably increases this risk (*Q 5.76*)

TABLE 6.4 More pill myths – current users

Myth	Actuality
1 There should be a break from pill use every few years	False (*Q 6.73*)
2 Duration of pill use should never be more than 5 (or 10) years at a time	False (*Qs 6.73–6.75*)
3 The pill should be stopped in all women reaching 35 years	Smokers (or if risk factors) (*Q 6.76*)
4 The COC should be stopped before all surgery	Only for major or leg surgery (*Q 6.14*)
5 Stop the COC if there is prolonged absence of withdrawal bleeds (to preserve fertility)	Irrelevant (*Q 5.11*)

There are also myths which many doctors share with pill-takers about 'missed pills' (see *Qs 5.19, 6.89, 10.22*)

6.80 **In what important situations do doctors commonly forget to enquire whether the patient is on an estrogen-containing pill?**

■ Emergencies: involving surgery, immobilization of a leg for fracture or confinement to bed.

■ When elective arrangements are made for a major operation or for surgery or sclerotherapy or intraluminal laser treatment for varicose veins.

■ When any potentially interacting drugs are prescribed, particularly when neurologists change antiepileptic drug regimens.

■ When arranging any laboratory test, especially of the blood. The results of many tests can be modified by the COC (see *Table 5.7*, p. 174).

NEW DEVELOPMENTS: NEW ROUTES OF ADMINISTRATION OF COMBINED HORMONES WITH ESTROGEN

There are three new routes for combined hormones currently available, at least in some countries:

6.81 **What is Evra?**

Available in the UK, Evra is a transdermal patch delivering ethinylestradiol (EE) with norelgestromin, the active metabolite of norgestimate. The daily skin dose of 150 µg norelgestromin and 20 µg EE produces blood levels in the reference range of those after a tablet of Cilest but without either the diurnal fluctuations or the oral peak dose given to the liver.

Pending more data, all the absolute and relative contraindications and indeed most of the above practical management advice in Chapters 5 and 6 about the COC apply to this product, with obvious minor adjustments. It can be seen as a bit like 'Cilest through the skin'. However in the US the FDA requires a warning in the Evra SPC, initially based on pharmacokinetics, that patch-users are exposed to about 60% more total estrogen; moreover 2 out of 3 case-control studies show an increased risk of VTE, compared with oral COCs with 30–35 µg estrogen. In other studies Evra also produced relatively more estrogen-associated side effects such as breast tenderness and nausea. The FDA concludes (2008) that 'Ortho Evra is a safe and effective method of contraception when used according to the labelling' but advises added caution for women with VTE risk factors.

About 2% of women had local skin reactions which led to discontinuation, yet the patch has excellent adhesion even in hot climates and when bathing or showering; the incidence of detachment of patches was 1.8% (complete) and 2.9% (partial). In the pooled analysis of three pivotal studies [Zieman M et al 2002 *Fertility and Sterility* 77(2 Suppl 2): S13–S18] the Pearl index for consistent users of Evra was similar to that for oral pills – and less than 1 per 100 woman-years. Interestingly, in the clinical trials one-third of the few failures occurred in the 3% weighing above 90 kg. Whether this was because of greater dilution of the dose given in more total body water, or somehow related to their extra subcutaneous adipose tissue, is unknown. But in my view this apparently reduced effectiveness contraindicates (WHO 4) Evra for such women (who are at least WHO 3 for VTE risk at that level of likely BMI anyway . . . and hence far from ideal users of this estrogen-dominant product).

Evra Summary

- Avoid use at all if body weight >90 kg, indeed in all cases with a risk factor for VTE – on safety as well as efficacy grounds.
- Warn the user that the contraceptive is in the glue of the patch, so a dry patch that has fallen off should not be reused!
- Each patch is worn for 7 days, for 3 consecutive weeks followed by a patch-free week. This regimen was shown to aid compliance, particularly in young women. Under age 20, perfect use was reported by COC-users in 68% of cycles, but in 88% of cycles by patch-users. This is probably its chief advantage.
- *Clinically*, therefore, the patch is a useful alternative to offer to those who find it difficult to remember a daily pill, especially as, if the patch-user does forget, there is a 2-day margin for error for late patch-change. Setting up a weekly text-message reminder 'Today is your patch-change day' can also be very helpful!
- As with the COC, it is essential never to lengthen the contraception-free (patch-free) interval.
- If this interval *exceeds* 8 days for any reason (either through late application or through the first new patch detaching and this being identified late), advise extra precautions for the duration of the first freshly applied patch (i.e. for 7 days). Emergency contraception should be considered if there has been sexual exposure during the preceding patch-free time, particularly if that exceeded 9 days.
- Absorption problems through vomiting/diarrhoea, and tetracycline by mouth, have no effect on this method's efficacy, but:
- During any short-term enzyme-inducer therapy, and for 28 days after this ends, additional contraception (e.g. with condoms) is advised, plus elimination of any patch-free intervals during this time.

6.82 What news is there about systemic contraception by the vaginal route?

Workers in Brazil and Israel in the early 1980s showed that a standard pill (LNG 250 μg plus EE 50 μg), as formulated for oral use, was effective when taken vaginally. Symptoms such as nausea were less frequent, although it is possible that this was partly due to achieving lower blood levels of estrogen.

Except in South America, where the above version has been marketed since 1999 as Lovelle, vaginal pills have not become popular, partly because daily compliance remains necessary as for oral pills.

6.83 So when can we expect NuvaRing in the UK?

Probably in 2009, but past experience shows this is impossible to predict! Already available in many European countries and the US, NuvaRing is a combined vaginal ring that releases etonogestrel (3-keto-desogestrel) 120 μg and EE 15 μg per day. It has proved very popular in studies, with excellent cycle control (better in a comparative trial than Microgynon 30 by mouth) and very few contraceptive failures.

NuvaRing is normally retained for 3 weeks (although there is an option of removing it for the duration of sexual activity, up to 3 h) and then taken out for a withdrawal bleed during the fourth. In many ways it therefore equates roughly to 'Mercilon via the vagina' and has all the same contraindications and a similar side-effect profile.

Alternatively, as is also true for Evra, it could be used continuously (three or four rings in a row, analogous to tricycling, *see Qs 5.29–5.32, 6.81*).

Maintenance of efficacy of NuvaRing

■ Expulsions are a small problem for some (usually parous) women, primarily during the emptying of bowels or bladder, and therefore readily recognized. After reinsertion no extra contraceptive action would normally be required.

■ As with the COC, it is still essential never to lengthen the contraception-free (i.e. ring-free) interval. If for any reason this exceeds 8 days, advise extra precautions for 7 days. Like for Evra, emergency contraception should be considered if there has been sexual exposure during any ring-free time, particularly if that exceeded 9 days.

■ Absorption problems, vomiting/diarrhoea and broad-spectrum antibiotics have no detectable effect on this method's efficacy.

■ During any short-term enzyme-inducer therapy, and for 28 days after this ends, additional contraception (e.g. with condoms) is advised, plus elimination of any ring-free intervals during this time.

6.84 When will we see the monthly combined injectable contraceptive (CIC) Lunelle in the UK?

This 'pill by injection' option appears likely to be delayed indefinitely in the UK, due to its poor uptake in the USA among other factors. Yet it proved effective, fully reversible and apparently popular in South America.

For the record, Lunelle, otherwise known as Cyclofem (25 mg DMPA with 5 mg estradiol cypionate in 0.5 ml aqueous volume) is injected intramuscularly into deltoid, thigh or buttock. Subsequent doses ought to follow every 28–30 days but must be no sooner than 23 days and no later than 33 days. Regular monthly bleeding lasting about 5 days is expected about 2 weeks after each dose as the estrogen dose falls.

PQ PATIENT QUESTIONS

SOME QUESTIONS ASKED BY USERS ABOUT THE COC

6.85 I am told thrombosis has to do with clots – I have clots with my periods, so does this mean that I can't use the pill?

Far from it! Clots with the periods just means that they are heavy, and could well improve dramatically if you went on the pill – the COC would usually do this more reliably than any POP.

6.86 Can I postpone having a pill-period?

Certainly. The bleeding you get between packets of pills is actually entirely caused by you when you take a 7-day break between packets. It is really a 'withdrawal bleed' rather than a proper period and there is no reason why from time to time you should not run two packets on to each other so there is no break and therefore no bleeding. The rules are a little different, however, for so-called phasic pills (see Q 5.186).

It is of course an option to have very infrequent pill-periods as in the so-called tricycle or 365/365 regimens (see Qs 5.32, 5.34 and Fig. 5.4 [p. 128]) – provided you accept the fact that this sometimes (not always) means taking a larger total dose of the hormones per year.

6.87 Do I always have to see periods at weekends?

Certainly not. If it happens to have worked out that your periods are tending to come at weekends on any type of COC, all you need to do is to start your next packet about 3 days early one time (meaning you only have a 4-day break), to move your withdrawal bleeding to midweek (see Q 5.52).

6.88 My 'period' is much lighter than normal, almost absent in fact, and a different colour – does this matter?

No, anything from quite average sort of bleeding through to nothing at all can be normal for the response of an individual woman's womb to the stopping of the pill's hormones. Should you have no periods at all 2 months in a row, you should take prompt advice to eliminate the possibility of pregnancy and also to discuss whether you should start the next packet. This action should be taken even if you have only missed one withdrawal bleed after a month during which you missed pills, had vomiting, severe diarrhoea or treatment with an interacting drug.

(Many other questions are asked about issues related to bleeding on the COC, whether normal, abnormal, or absent. These can be answered by reference to *Qs 5.11, 5.33, 5.40, 5.52, 5.63–5.68, 5.172–5.186 and 11.17(18–22)*).

6.89   Is it safe to make love in the 7 days between pill-packets?

Yes: but only if no pills have been missed (by forgetting, stomach upset or drug interaction) towards the end of the previous packet, and also only if you do in fact start another packet after the pill-free week (*see Qs 5.16–5.25 and 11.17(15)*). Beware, particularly when you come off the pill for any reason. You *never* have seven contraceptively safe days following any last packet of a course of the pill. This might be especially important to remember if you are stopping the pill because of sterilization (of you or your partner).

6.90   Which are the most 'dangerous' pills to be missed – presumably in the middle of the month?

Not so, the middle of the month is the least bad time to miss pills, although you should not make a habit of missing any. The worst pills to be missed are any that result in lengthening of the pill-free time (*see Qs 5.16, 5.19, 5.25*). Never be late starting your next packet! This is something lots of people don't even consider as missing a pill.

6.91   I want to switch from taking the pill every evening to morning pill-taking. How should I do this?

Ideally this should be done by taking two tablets 12 h apart on one day, *not* leaving a 36-h gap. If you want to make the change with the start of a new pack, it would be important to take the first new pill early, after 6.5 days, rather than leaving 7.5 days between the last pill of the old and the first of the new packets (see *Fig. 5.1*, p. 118, and *Q 5.16* for the reason why!)

6.92   Are there any problems in pill-taking for flight crews or long-haul air travellers?

It is easy to become confused about regular pill-taking because of passing through different time zones. The effectiveness problem is when flying due west, because the new bedtime pill might be late – hours more than the official 24 h after the preceding one. One solution is a watch that gives the time in the departure city as well as local time, and to continue to base pill-taking on the time where the journey began.

On arrival at a new destination, pill-users should always err on the side of taking a pill too early rather than late.

Suppose you fly to London from Auckland and normally take your pill at bedtime; if you then switch to taking it at the London bedtime, you could have a 36-h interval between tablets. This increases the risk of pill failure (although not much for the COC, it would be completely unacceptable for ordinary POPs, *see Qs 7.12–7.21*). With both types of pill it increases the risk of irregular or breakthrough bleeding (BTB). So what should you do?

- To recap, while on the flight or during any stopover you should continue taking your tablets at the correct hour based on your departure time zone. Nothing else needs to be done.
- Upon arrival, as the journey was westbound, after your regular COC (or POP) has been taken at 24 h on the departure time basis, take an extra tablet (use the last one in that pack) at the next London bedtime. This will be after 12 more hours in the Auckland-to-London situation, but only 8 h later if the trip was London to Los Angeles, for example. Not a problem.
- And if the journey was eastbound, taking that day's pill at the correct local time will shorten the actual pill-taking interval and this is always contraceptively safe.
- If this is done, no extra precautions are needed and, with both types of pill, the risk of either BTB or breakthrough conception should be negligible.

6.93 My skin has got worse on the pill, yet I was told it should get better – why is this?

It all depends on the severity of your acne and which pill you have been given. The recommended ones are at *Q 6.22* (see *Table 6.2*, p. 257).

6.94 Does using either the COC or the POP delay the menopause?

No. This occurs as a result of an inexorable process of egg loss, which seems to be unaffected by anything, including never having babies and pill-taking. It even occurs at the same time as it otherwise would in women who as a result of surgery have been left with only one ovary. But it can be brought on earlier by a hysterectomy.

6.95 Can I take antihistamines for hayfever and the pill?

The ones given by your GP, or that you can buy in the chemist, seem to cause no important change in the effectiveness of your pill. Other medicines might do, however (*see Qs 5.35, 5.36* and *Table 5.3* [p. 135]), and the warning sign of an interaction can be bleeding during tablet-taking. Always tell any doctor, dentist or hospital that you take the pill.

6.96 Is it true that you are more likely to get drunk if you are on the pill?

Some research published in 1984 suggested this because it showed that alcohol leaves the body more slowly in pill-users than in non-pill-users.

PATIENT QUESTIONS

Subsequently, other researchers in Australia found the opposite – that pill-takers recovered from the effect of alcohol more quickly than non-takers!

But the take-home message about which there is no argument is that all women should be extra careful about alcohol. This is because their smaller livers make it have a bigger effect than in men, both short term and long term (meaning that the risk of liver damage is greater in women).

6.97 What are the take-home messages for any new pill-taker?

Take-home messages for a new pill-taker

▥ *Your fpa leaflet:* this is not to be read and thrown away; it is something to keep safely in a drawer somewhere, for ongoing reference.

▥ *The pill only works if you take it correctly:* if you do, each new pack will always start on the same day of the week.

▥ *Even if bleeding, like a 'period', occurs (BTB), carry on pill-taking:* ring for advice if necessary. Nausea is another common early symptom. Both usually settle as your body gets used to the pill.

▥ *Never be a late restarter of your pill!* Even if your 'period' (withdrawal bleed) has not stopped yet, never start your next packet late. This is because the PFI is obviously a time when your contraceptive is not being supplied to your ovaries, so they might anyway be beginning to escape from its actions.

▥ *Lovemaking during the 7 days after any packet is only safe if you do actually go on to the next pack.* Otherwise (e.g. if you decide to stop the method) you must start using condoms after the last pill in the pack.

▥ For what to do if any pill(s) *are* more than 24 h late, *see Q 5.18ff.*

▥ Other things that may stop the pill from working include *vomiting* and *some drugs* (always mention that you are on the pill).

▥ See a doctor *at once* if any of the things at *Q 6.13* occur, especially new headaches with strange *changes in your eyesight (happening beforehand).*

▥ *As a one-off, you can shorten one PFI* to make sure all your future withdrawal bleeds avoid weekends.

▥ *You can avoid bleeding on holidays etc.* by running packs together. (Discuss this with whoever provides your pills, if you want to continue missing out 'periods' long term, *Qs 5.32, 5.34*)

▥ Good though it is as a contraceptive, *the pill does not give enough protection against Chlamydia and other STIs.* Whenever in doubt, especially with a new partner, use a condom *as well.*

▥ Finally, *always feel free to telephone or come back at any time* (maybe to the practice nurse) for any reasons of your own, including any symptoms you would like dealt with.

The progestogen-only pill

ADVANTAGES AND BENEFICIAL SIDE-EFFECTS

MAIN PROBLEMS AND DISADVANTAGES

BACKGROUND AND MECHANISMS

7.1   What are progestogen-only pills (POPs)?

In the UK these pills contain a microdose of one of four progestogens (*Table 7.1*). They are taken on a continuous daily basis, 365 days a year.

7.2   Which POPs are in current use?

See *Table 7.1*. POPs have accounted for no more than 10% of the UK oral contraceptive market, although this is set to change with the arrival of Cerazette (*see Q 7.11*). They have much to commend them, especially in the older age group.

7.3   How much is known about the POP method?

The short answer is: still remarkably little. No large cohort studies are in progress and case–control studies have not been attempted because of the low prevalence of use. Hence we are largely forced to draw on the few metabolic and clinical studies available; and otherwise to extrapolate from available data on the combined pill (adjusting in an admittedly arbitrary way for absence of artificial estrogen and presence of a particularly small dose of the progestogen).

7.4   What is the mode of action of POPs?

This is summarized in *Table 7.2*. The main action has previously been thought to be the alteration in the cervical mucus. But there is also a considerable effect on ovulation in most women and in most cycles – at least 50–60% of the time – and more in older women. Ovulation might be abolished completely, resulting in amenorrhoea, but even without this there are varying degrees of interference with the ovulatory process, as described in Q 7.5.

TABLE 7.1 Progestogen-only pills in the UK

Name	No. of tablets per packet	Progestogen	Dose (µg)
Norgeston	35	Levonorgestrel	30
Micronor/Noriday	28	Norethisterone	350
Femulen	28	Etynodiol diacetate	500
Cerazette	28	Desogestrel	75

Note: Etynodiol diacetate is a prodrug, norethisterone its active metabolite. Hence, allowing for incomplete conversion, Femulen essentially gives a slightly higher dose of norethisterone than Micronor/Noriday.

TABLE 7.2 Various progestogen delivery systems

	COC	Evra	POP (old type)	DMPA	Cerazette	Implanon
Active component	EE + one of 7 progestogens	Norelgestromin: active metabolite of norgestimate	Levonorgestrel or norethisterone (both '2nd generation')	Medroxyprogesterone acetate	Desogestrel	Etonogestrel: active metabolite of desogestrel
Administration	Oral	Transdermal	Oral	Intramuscular	Oral	Subdermal
Frequency	Daily	7-day patches	Daily	3-monthly	Daily	3-yearly
Estrogen dose	Low	Low	Nil	Nil	Nil	Nil
Progestogen dose	Low	Low	Ultra-low	High	Low	Ultra-low
Blood levels	Daily peaks & troughs	Steady	Daily peaks & troughs	Initial peak then decline	Daily peaks & troughs	Steady
First pass through liver	Yes	No	Yes	No	Yes	No
Major mechanisms						
Ovary: ↓ ovulation	+++	+++	+	+++	+++	+++
Cervical mucus: ↓ sperm penetrability	Yes	Yes	Yes	Yes	Yes	Yes
Minor mechanism						
Endometrium: ↓ receptivity to blastocyst (a weak effect, usually never utilized (see Q 5.4)	Yes	Yes	Yes	Yes	Yes	Yes

TABLE 7.2—cont'd

	COC	Evra	POP (old type)	DMPA	Cerazette	Implanon
Percentage, among consistent/correct users, conceiving in 1st year of use	0.3	0.3	0.3	0.3	<0.2	<0.1
Menstrual pattern	Regular	Regular	Often irregular	Very irregular	Often irregular	Often irregular
Amenorrhoea during use	Rare	Rare	Occasional	Very common	Common	Common
Reversibility						
Immediate termination possible?	Yes	Yes	Yes	No	Yes	Yes
By woman herself at any time?	Yes	Yes	Yes	No	Yes	No
Median time to conception from first omitted dose/removal	c. 3 months	c. 3 months	c. 2 months	c. 6 months	c. 2 months	c. 2 months

Notes:
1 For more details regarding efficacy issues, see *Table 1.2*, p. 14.
2 Cerazette is in many respects like 'oral Implanon', given that desogestrel is a prodrug for etonogestrel.
3 NuvaRing: when available, this combined contraceptive vaginal ring will have similar features to Evra (see *Q 6.83*).

It must therefore be understood at the outset that the hormonal environment of a previously cycling woman on the POP is the result of the direct effect of the exogenous progestogen and an amount of ovarian activity, which varies – both between women and between cycles. This explains the very varied menstrual pattern that is observed and is also relevant to other side-effects.

7.5 What effects can the POP have on ovarian function?

In individual women, or in the same woman in different menstrual cycles, the effects vary. Although the patterns have been described in four groups, this is for convenience. The situation is better described as a spectrum running from no interference with the ovarian cycle through to complete quiescence of the ovaries and no follicular or luteal activity.

In a short-term study (1980) of a POP with just 300 g of norethisterone (the UK's Micronor/Noriday contains 17% more NET), Swedish workers have described four main groups in this continuum (percentage of cycles in parentheses):

1. Cycles showing almost no change from normal, with apparently normal ovulation, minimal shortening of the luteal phase and progesterone levels within normal limits (40%).
2. Normal follicular phase but marked shortening of the luteal phase, with lower progesterone levels for a shorter time (21%).
3. Follicular activity with higher peak estrogen levels than usual but no ovulation and no progesterone production. Ultrasound scans of the ovaries in POP-users, most probably coming mainly from this group as described by the Swedes, show the formation of abnormal follicles or functional cysts, which might be single or multiple (23%).
4. Diminished follicular activity, low estrogen levels, no ovulation, no corpus luteum formation and no endogenous progesterone production. Ultrasound scanning confirms quiescent ovaries (16%).

> The POP is often given during lactation (*see* Q 7.53). The endocrine findings are then as in group 4, signifying the same efficacy as the COC but (except uniquely in the case of Cerazette) often shift at the time of weaning variably towards those of group 1, as expected, with an increasing risk of ovulation.

7.6 How do the changes described in the last questions show themselves in the menstrual pattern and affect the risk of contraceptive failure?

■ A majority of the women experiencing cycles of the type in group 1 above will have regular periods. They are not immune to breakthrough

bleeding (BTB), however, probably because of direct effects of the
artificial progestogen on the endometrium. Here ovulation is the norm,
the pharmacological effects on the pituitary/ovarian axis are minimal;
but this means that they are also the group with the highest risk of
breakthrough pregnancy. They are relying chiefly on the mucus and,
perhaps as a rare 'longstop' mechanism, an anti-implantation effect for
contraception (*Fig. 7.1*).

■ Groups 2 and 3, which show varying degrees of cycle disturbance, short
of complete abolition, merge with each other and are therefore together
in the middle column of *Fig. 7.1*. It is from among these women that
extra frequent or erratic, irregular bleeds will be reported: the
endometrium no longer receives adequate endogenous progesterone

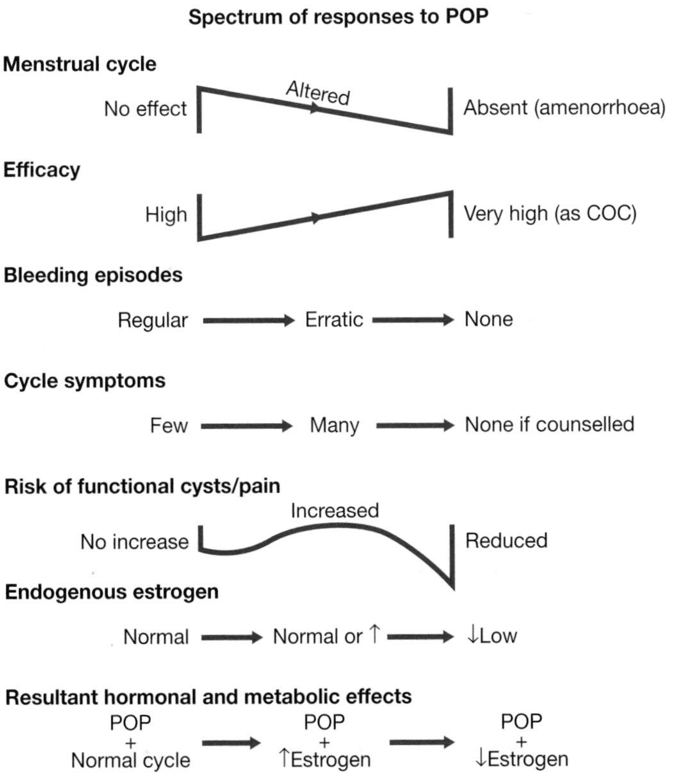

Fig. 7.1 Spectrum of responses to the progestogen-only pill. *Q 7.6. Note:* the metabolic
effects are minimal anyway in *all* the groups, across the spectrum. See also *Qs 7.5, 7.35,
7.39.*

and many of those in group 3 also have increased estrogen stimulation from the increased follicular activity. The bleeding pattern is a result of this abnormal ovarian activity and the (rather rapid) fluctuations each 24 h in the level of exogenous progestogen. It would appear that it is in cycles showing the patterns of groups 2 and 3 that symptomatic or asymptomatic functional ovarian cysts can be formed. The risk of breakthrough pregnancy is considerably less than in group 1, probably almost nil because such a cycle is anovular (although the woman could always have a group-1-type cycle in another month).

■ In group 4, at the extreme of the continuum, there is either complete amenorrhoea or intermittent, very light bleeding. The latter is caused by irregular shedding of the endometrium, receiving less estrogen than usual and just the daily exogenous progestogen administration (in a sawtooth pattern, like all oral medications, *see Q 8.5*). The risk of contraceptive failure here, with or without erratic bleeds, is nil. It is of course also the norm for POP-taking during lactation, and is common during any use of the anovulant Cerazette (*see Q 7.11*).

7.7 What, then, does amenorrhoea on the POP mean?

First, it can certainly be caused by pregnancy and this must be excluded in the usual way. Once that explanation is ruled out, paradoxically the women experiencing prolonged episodes of amenorrhoea are the ones not ovulating and so actually at least risk of conception. It is from among the group 1 POP-using women, who are experiencing regular periods and being regularly reassured thereby, that the majority of unplanned conceptions occur. *See also Q 7.65* for a discussion of the possible risks of sustained amenorrhoea.

7.8 Are any particular POPs more likely to cause erratic periods or amenorrhoea?

As has to be said about so many aspects of POP use, the possibility of differences between the POPs has been inadequately studied. The Swedish studies quoted in *Q 7.5* were not able to demonstrate any correlation between doses given or measured blood levels of the artificial progestogen and the types of ovarian reaction or the bleeding profile – even though the blood levels also showed wide patient-to-patient variation (*see Q 7.9*). So it appears that the main factor is the degree to which the end-organs, especially the ovary and the uterus, are susceptible to the effects of the POP in the blood.

7.9 In POP-takers, is there the same variability in blood levels of the steroids as described for the COC (*see Q 5.164*)?

Yes. There is the same enormous variation between women who are apparently similar, taking the same POP and having their blood levels estimated at the same time after their last tablet was ingested. But variation in target-organ sensitivity appears more important (*see* Q 7.8) in causing bleeding side-effects.

There is also (as for COC-users) the fact of variation, again about 10-fold, between the peak and trough blood levels each day within the same woman. This is shown in *Figs 5.2* (p. 119) and *8.1* (p. 333).

7.10 How does the enterohepatic cycle operate for the POP?

As in *Fig. 5.5* (*see* Q 5.35), after the artificial progestogen is absorbed, liver metabolism creates metabolites that re-enter the lumen of the bowel via the bile. But the action of the bowel flora does not result in re-formation of active progestogen. Hence, the achieved circulating levels of the POP are normally not dependent on hydrolysis by the intestinal flora and subsequent reabsorption of the progestogen; so antibiotics can have no effect on POP blood levels. However, by increasing elimination at the liver, enzyme-inducing drugs can reduce the blood levels and threaten efficacy, just as they do with the COC (*see* Q 7.28).

7.11 What is Cerazette, the desogestrel POP?

This useful product containing 75 μg desogestrel 'rewrites the textbooks' about POPs, mainly because it regularly blocks ovulation (group 4 in Q 7.5). This makes it somewhat like 'Implanon by mouth' – though advance testing the acceptability of Implanon by trying Cerazette first only gives somewhat of a 'handle' on the *non*-bleeding (hormonal-type) side-effects.

Effectiveness: There is good evidence of anovulation in 97% of cycles (i.e. Cerazette is normally in group 4 of the groups described in Q 7.5), so Cerazette only needs to utilize the (weaker) mucus contraceptive effect in about 3% of cycles. The MHRA/CSM has approved 12 h of leeway for defining a missed Cerazette tablet (cf. 3 h with all other POPs, Q 7.17–7.22). Approval was based on a study recruiting 103 women who were instructed to miss pills on days 11, 14 and 21 of the first or second Cerazette cycles. Only one woman ovulated – the expected rate – and this was unrelated to the missed tablets. The minimum time to the first post-treatment ovulation was 7 days. Given that last finding, coupled with the fact that Cerazette does not have any of the contraception-weakening pill-free weeks of the COC, the leeway for a missed Cerazette must actually be much longer than 12 h: yet the manufacturer has not applied for an extension.

Problems: As with all progestogen-only methods, irregular bleeding remains a very real problem; indeed, that is one area showing no great advantage in a comparative study with users of levonorgestrel 30 μg [Collaborative Group on Desogestrel POP 1998 *European Journal of Contraceptive and Reproductive Healthcare* 3:168–178]. The dropout rate for changes in bleeding pattern showed no difference but there was a useful trend for the more annoying frequent and prolonged bleeding experiences to lessen with continued use and at 1 year around 50% had either amenorrhoea or only one to two bleeds per 90 days. Despite this higher incidence of (more acceptable) amenorrhoea than with existing POPs, Cerazette, like Implanon, still appears to provide adequate follicular-phase levels of estradiol.

In summary, it might well become a first-line hormonal contraceptive for many women, given that:

■ It must be free of all the risks attributable to EE, plus no effects on BP were reported in the above study. Hence it can be used in many cases where the COC is WHO 4 or 3 but a pill method with comparable efficacy is desired (e.g. to cover major surgery in a young COC-user).

■ It also ablates the menstrual cycle like the COC but again without using EE. So, in those who do not get unacceptably frequent or prolonged uterine bleeds, it has potentially beneficial effects on menstrual disorders, especially dysmenorrhoea, menorrhagia and PMS.

■ It could be a good alternative anovulant method when there is a past history of ectopic pregnancy.

■ *See also Q 7.16* for the grounds to use it in women weighing >70 kg.

In the rest of this chapter and elsewhere in the book, the abbreviation POP, if used unqualified, refers to all POP products other than Cerazette.

EFFECTIVENESS

7.12 What is the overall effectiveness of the POP?

As usual, reliability depends greatly on the motivation of the woman. An overall failure rate of 0.3–4/100 woman-years can be quoted for standard POPs, the higher rate occurring when patient compliance is poor, and particularly at very young ages, as discussed in *Q 7.16*. The lower rate applies particularly during lactation (*see Q 7.53*). Cerazette had a consistent-user Pearl failure rate of just 0.17 per 100 woman-years (CI 0.0–0.9) in the pre-marketing study (in non-breastfeeders) – a result historically unprecedented in a POP trial.

7.13 What is the influence of age on the effectiveness?

In the Oxford/FPA study there was a marked influence of age on standard POPs (*Table 7.3*) – Cerazette was not available for testing. The failure rate falls from 3.1/100 woman-years for the age group 25–29 to 0.3 above the age of 40. Possible explanations are:

■ The usual influence of declining fertility with age, shown for example also for the IUD (*see Q 9.11*).

TABLE 7.3 **Progestogen-only pill – user-failure rates/100 woman-years Oxford/FPA Study (1985 report) – all women married and aged above 25, any duration of use**

All ages	Ages (years)			
	25–29	30–34	35–39	40+
0.9	3.1	2.0	1.0	0.3

NB: These figures differ from those given in *Table 1.2* – due to being different user-populations.

- Related to the first bulleted point, it is well known that the prevalence of abnormal menstrual cycles increases with increasing age, and this is likely to predispose to abnormal ovulation (and the woman's POP cycles therefore being in groups 2–4, as discussed in *Q 7.5*). Although not reported, it would be expected that the older women in the Oxford/FPA study had a greater incidence of irregular bleeding and amenorrhoea; whereas the younger women would tend to have ovarian cycles that were more 'resistant' to the effect of the exogenous progestogen, and hence more would be ovulating and at greater risk of conception. They would necessarily be relying solely on the other two main effects of the method (on the mucus and endometrium).
- Older women tend to have less frequent intercourse but this is less true now as many 40-year-olds have embarked on new relationships.
- The younger women were possibly less consistent in their pill-taking.

7.14 Do other factors affect the effectiveness of POPs? What about body weight?

The Oxford/FPA study was unable to show any statistically significant difference between the failure rate according to which particular POP brand was used, although appreciable variation was noted. Cigarette-smoking also did not appear to be of importance.

BODY WEIGHT

The Oxford/FPA study did show a trend to higher pregnancy rates with increasing weight. Although not statistically significant, this has to be taken seriously because it is not implausible biologically (see below). Moreover, there was significance in similar analyses of data for other progestogen-only methods that rely on achieving very similar blood levels.

With both the levonorgestrel-releasing vaginal ring and Norplant (*Q 8.56*), specifically in trials of the higher-silica polymer 373 (an older subcutaneous implant that had a higher failure rate overall), the pregnancy rate was positively correlated to increasing weight. The ring in particular is such a similar method that I feel that the weight effect has to be considered real for the POP also, until a larger POP study or meta-analysis settles the issue. See also the Kovacs data in Q 7.17.

The bottom line for me is that there is as yet no proof that body mass is not important in the effectiveness of the (old-type) POP. However, its influence is likely to be much less important in users of the anovulant Cerazette (Q 7.15) as also with the COC (*see* Q 5.15).

7.15 Why does the body-mass effect on efficacy show up with some low-dose progestogen methods?

Note the emphasis here on mass or weight, not BMI. Dilution of the administered drug in the greater amount of 'water of distribution' (apparent distribution volume) existing in a bigger person – whether they are tall or short – is expected, for any drug. It is the basis, after all, for usually reducing adult doses when giving drugs to children.

My explanation for the absence of a clinically important effect with the COC (*see* Q 5.15) and injectables is that they have such a high safety margin in users of whatever weight. The doses given by the progestogen-only methods of Q 7.14 (the ring and polymer 373 implant), however, are nearer the minimum for efficacy: so a factor like weight can exert a detectable influence on the failure rate, and the same probably applies to standard POPs. But it does not appear to apply to Cerazette because this is an anovulant product (with strong mucus contraceptive back-up), and hence, increased body mass should have a lesser effect on its efficacy, given good compliance.

7.16 What are the implications of the above findings with regard to efficacy?

- *In lactation:* the combination of full breastfeeding and the POP equates to almost 100% contraception (*see* Qs 7.23, 7.53). The extra effectiveness of Cerazette is unnecessary and comes at added cost. Even the young breastfeeding POP-user who is overweight would be most unlikely to conceive – until weaning begins anyway.

- *For older women:* the main implication of these findings is the remarkable efficacy of the method. As these are precisely the women who might need to transfer from the COC (see *Tables 5.10 and 5.11*, pp. 200–203), it is useful to be able to tell a woman over 40, quite truthfully, that her chances of conceiving if she is a regular taker of the old-type POP are the same as for a 25-year-old taking a modern combined pill. (The Oxford/FPA study gives method-plus-user failure rates of around 0.3 in both instances.)

- *For the young:* unfortunately, the Oxford/FPA study did not include women under the age of 25. However, extrapolating from *Table 7.3*, the expected failure rate in teenagers is likely to be quite high, say 4/100 woman-years, especially as compliance tends to be less good in the young. Some studies that included women in their twenties have shown acceptable failure rates of 1–2/100 woman-years. So, with careful selection and education of users, the POP is certainly on the list of options for the young. But Cerazette would be my preferred choice now for all normal young women who desired a POP.

■ *For the overweight* (*see* Qs 7.14, 7.15): pending more data, my own preference now is to consider high body mass (>70 kg) as a positive indication for using a single daily Cerazette. This avoids having even to raise the possibility of a higher failure rate than those quoted in Q 7.12, or the notion of taking two POPs per day – except perhaps in those well above 100 kg.

7.17 **For those users who are still ovulating, how long does the contraceptive effect on the cervical mucus last, following each dose?**

As illustrated in *Fig. 7.2*, following one tablet the effect appears maximal about 4 h later, but in this one study there was some return of sperm penetrability around 24 h. Regular POP-taking seems to abolish this, so one can assume that the cervical and uterine fluids are difficult for sperm to traverse throughout the 24 h.

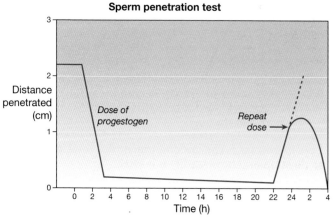

▲
Fig. 7.2 Sperm penetration of cervical mucus after progestogen. *Q 7.17. Note:* minimum reduction in sperm penetration occurs between 4 h and 22 h after a single dose of megestrol acetate (0.5 mg). Unlike the rest of the figure, the effect of a repeat dose is presumed, not experimental (redrawn from Cox 1968 The precoital use of minidosage progestogens. *Journal of Reproduction and Fertility Supplement* 5:167–172, Figure 1).

Fig. 7.2 actually derives from some work in the late 1960s using the POP megestrol acetate (0.5 mg). Similar data are available for levonorgestrel but these studies badly need repeating with more modern investigative techniques, and for Cerazette (which is still thought to use the mucus effect as back-up to its mainly anovulant action).

In a study of the POP by Kovacs in 2000 [*British Journal of Family Planning* 26:165–166], the expected effect of a levonorgestrel-containing POP in reducing sperm penetrability of the cervical mucus was undetectable in only three women: they were all very obese with body masses greater than 75 kg, confirming the greater water of dilution concept discussed in *Q 7.15*.

Scanning electron microscope (SEM) studies have shown a characteristic tight mesh of microfibrils in mucus obtained from women using various microdose progestogens – when the progestogenic effect is maximal. However, in cycling women (group 1 in *Q 7.5*), if the mucus is sampled at midcycle as little as 12 h late (36 h after the last tablet was taken) the SEM appearances are already nearly back to the normal open mesh of estrogenic mucus that sperm can readily penetrate. The contraceptive effect of the old-type POP on mucus can thus be assumed to have disappeared by 12 h if a woman is late taking a tablet – hence only 3 h of leeway in the advice at *Q 7.21*.

7.18 What endometrial effects have been described in POP-users?

As with other tissues, observations differ according to the variable amount of endogenous ovarian activity superimposed on the direct effect of the progestogen (*see Q 7.5* and *Fig. 7.1*).

That said, blockade of progesterone receptors occurs and characteristic changes have been described in the histology of the endometrium on both light and electron microscopy. Uterine glands diminish both in number and in diameter. These and associated biochemical effects are believed to reduce the likelihood of successful implantation.

7.19 How important is the endometrial effect, how long does it take to develop and how readily is it lost?

The answers to all these questions are largely unknown. The mucus effect has been more fully studied and the endometrial effect is generally considered much less important as a back-up contraceptive mechanism.

7.20 For maximum efficacy of the POP, how and when should it be taken?

As implied by *Fig. 7.2*, and the answer to *Q 7.17*, the answer to 'how?' is 'extremely regularly'. Indeed, I always tell prospective POP-users that the POP is 'a package deal'. In other words, 'here is your packet of pills, now set a dedicated alarm on your mobile!' Women who are not breastfeeding are encouraged to take their tablets at precisely the same time each day. There is very much more leeway during full lactation (*see Qs 7.6, 7.23, 7.53*). This must also be the case with Cerazette, although not so stated in its SPC.

FLYING WEST THROUGH TIME ZONES.
This might lead to inadvertent lengthening of the pill-taking interval by 8–12 h, therefore increasing conception risk – and more so with POPs than COCs. *See Q 6.92* regarding how to maintain pill efficacy when flying west.

7.21 What rule do you recommend for missed POPs (*other than Cerazette – see Q 7.23*)?

It has proved difficult to reach international agreement on the matter of 'missed-POP rules'. This is not too surprising in view of:

- the spectrum of effects of this method on different women and in different cycles (*see Q 7.5*)
- the lack of data about the relative importance of the end-organ contraceptive effects in *Table 7.2*
- the different situation applying during breastfeeding (NB: unless otherwise stated, the discussion below applies outside of 100% lactation).

There is good agreement among the authorities on one point: as the mucus effect is so quickly lost, extra precautions should begin if a woman is more than 3 h late in taking her old-type POP (27 h since the last tablet).

The difficult part of the advice is: for how long should loss of contraception be assumed? From 1985 to 1992 in the UK the fpa recommended in its instruction leaflets that an additional contraceptive method should be used just for the next 48 h. From 1993 to 2003, the fpa leaflets specified 7 days. From 2004 onwards, the leaflets, following the advice of WHO in its *Selected practice recommendations* and now UKMEC, have returned to the earlier wording for the management of a >3-h-late pill, namely:

- take one pill as soon as possible
- return to regular daily pill-taking
- abstain from sex or use additional contraception for the next 2 days.

7.22 When should emergency postcoital contraception be considered in addition, if POP tablets are missed?

For old-type POPs this decision should be based on the mucus effect, i.e. emergency pills should be offered for any unprotected intercourse that occurred:

- after the 3-h delay which might lead to loss of the mucus effect, but
- before two pills have been taken to restore it (*see Q 10.22(10)*).

A minimum 2 days of extra precautions should then follow, as advised by WHO and UKMEC.

7.23 How should the advice differ if ordinary progestogen-only pills are missed during lactation – or if Cerazette is the pill?

During lactation, ovulation in users of old-type POPs is inhibited while there is sustained amenorrhoea (*Q 7.6*); even more strongly, in fact, if the lactational amenorrhoea criteria are fully observed, since lactation even without the POP would be 98% effective (see *Fig. 2.4*, p. 39). Missing an old-type POP is then equivalent to missing a COC in mid-packet (*see Q 7.21*), therefore the 'forgiveness' time has to be much more than 3 h.

It is also now accepted that Cerazette has at least 12 h leeway for pill-taking, on its own (outside of breastfeeding), and it is probably much more in reality, given that 7-day delay before the first ovulation after cessation (*see Q 7.11*).

So what advice should we give?

It must be *more than* safe enough to recommend as normal practice in *both* cases that extra contraception is initiated (now at least only for 2 days!) after any 12 h delay.

What about emergency contraception (EC) for POP-users in lactation? If they have amenorrhoea and their offspring is not yet 6 months old, it would be exceptional to find it necessary to offer EC at all to fully breastfeeding POP-users who missed a tablet or two. Pending more data I would recommend EC as well on a 'fail-safe' basis only if *more than* two tablets had been completely missed; and be more cautious only if questioning reveals that breastfeeding is a long way short of complete.

7.24 How long does it take to establish efficacy when starting the POP?

The contraceptive effect on the mucus develops very rapidly (see *Fig. 7.2*). We do not know the minimum time needed to establish the antiovulation or anti-implantation effects. However, with a first-day start and hence taking at least seven pills before the earliest likely fertile ovulation, any POP-induced interference with it ought theoretically to be as great as it will be in later cycles. So no extra precautions are now advised with a first-day start of any POP and this seems adequate.

TABLE 7.4 Starting routines with the POP or Cerazette

	Start when?	Extra precautions?
Menstruating	1st or 2nd day of period	No
	Any time in cycle ('Quick start')	Yes[†]
During amenorrhoea	Any time ('Quick start')	Yes[†]
Postpartum		
(a) No lactation*	Day 21 (see text and Q 11.22)[‡]	No
(b) Lactation*	Day 21, or later (see Q 7.55)	No
Induced abortion/ miscarriage	Same day or next day	No
Post COC	Instant switch	No
Post DMPA	Instant switch before or at 12 weeks since last injection	No

*Bleeding irregularities minimized by starting at or after the 4th week.
[†]Provided there is reasonable certainty from the coital history that there is no blastocyst or sperm already in the upper genital tract (see Q 11.22), 'Quick start' is legitimate. It means starting *any time* plus, with the POP, just 2 days' extra precautions. Careful explanation plus follow-up to confirm that all is well are part of this package.
[‡]See Q 11.22 regarding starting artificial hormones later on, during postpartum amenorrhoea.

7.25 What, therefore, are the recommended starting routines?

See *Table 7.4* and its important footnotes.

7.26 What advice should be given to a woman who vomits a tablet and fails to replace it successfully within 2 h?

She should take extra precautions as well as taking her tablets for the duration of the vomiting and for 2 days thereafter. If intercourse took place when the mucus effect was likely to have been reduced through vomited pills, emergency contraception should be considered, as for missed POPs (*see Q 7.22*). But that would nearly always be unnecessary during full lactation, or if the pill concerned was Cerazette (*see Q 7.23*).

7.27 Should any action be taken if a POP-user requires antibiotic treatment?

No. Only yes if the antibiotic is an enzyme-inducer, meaning one of the rifamicins (e.g. rifampicin) and griseofulvin. Otherwise no action is required because, as explained in *Q 7.10*, ordinary broad-spectrum antibiotics can have no effect on the blood level of the active exogenous progestogen.

7.28 Should the POP be avoided by women using enzyme-inducing drugs?

Enzyme-inducers do lower progestogen as well as estrogen blood levels and the failure rate of any POP (including Cerazette) would therefore be expected to increase. Extra precautions should be advised during and for at least 7 days after any short-term treatment – and for 1 month after treatment lasting more than 6 weeks, or of any duration with rifampicin (*see Q 5.42*).

The drugs concerned here are identical to those listed in *Table 5.3, Q 5.36*, to which the endothelin antagonist bosentan should be added. Cerazette might be a good choice of contraceptive for a young woman being treated with bosentan, but this interaction is irrelevant to the COC since the drug is used for treating pulmonary hypertension (which is WHO 4 for the COC).

Long term, as usual a better hormonal option would be the injectable DMPA. If the POP is preferred, on a WHO 3 basis, my advice is to use the stronger Cerazette product and in addition increase the dose to two tablets per day. If the woman normally takes her enzyme-inducer drug twice daily, as many epileptics do, there are sound theoretical grounds for suggesting she takes the Cerazette tablets at the same times. Even then she should be warned that the efficacy of such a regimen is not well established and, as usual, because this is not supported by the SPCs, the 'named-patient' criteria should be observed (see *Appendix A*).

As in COC users, St John's Wort is contraindicated (see *Table 5.3*, p. 135).

7.29 Can the small dose of progestogen influence other drugs

Maybe, though we are forced by lack of data to try to extrapolate from what is known about the COC. Please read *Q 5.46*. All we can say is that lamotrigine levels *may* be slightly lowered, ciclosporin levels *may* be raised and warfarin activity *may* be increased – but the lower dose in the POP ought to lessen any effect. Awareness of these possibilities should at least help.

ADVANTAGES AND BENEFICIAL SIDE-EFFECTS

7.30 What are the advantages of the POP?

■ Acceptable efficacy, in the range of 0.3–4/100 woman-years. Higher efficacy applies to Cerazette and with all POPs in older women for whom COCs might be contraindicated.

■ No epidemiological proof, so far, of increased risk of either circulatory or malignant disease but *see Q 7.36*. Again this is not certain because of inadequate study; plus any (good or bad) effects may very well vary between women because of the variable impact of the POP on the hypothalamic–pituitary–ovarian axis.

- Avoidance of all side-effects in which artificial estrogens are implicated.
- Minimization of any side-effects in which progestogens are implicated.
- Minimal alteration in all metabolic variables that have been measured (*see Qs 7.39–7.46*).
- Good general tolerance: especially suitable for women who complain of side-effects with other hormonal methods, or in whom the latter are contraindicated.
- Most minor symptoms of the COC (such as weight gain, nausea, headaches and loss of libido) are not a problem.
- Return of women's fertility on discontinuation more rapid than after the COC.
- The tiny dose means minimal effect on lactation, and levels of the artificial steroids within breast milk seem to be negligible.
- No harmful effect from overdose, even when taken by a child.

7.31 Do the beneficial effects listed in *Q 5.57* also apply to the POP?

- Some do – most of the contraceptive benefits, for example.
- Some women report improvement in symptoms of the menstrual cycle, notably premenstrual symptoms and dysmenorrhoea. Others report the reverse (*see Qs 7.32, 7.68*). Cerazette (*see Q 7.11*) is more likely than other POPs to improve such gynaecological symptoms, and indeed might be worth a trial instead of the COC in treating some of the conditions listed in *Q 5.135*.
- Protection against pelvic infection is extremely probable through the mucus 'barrier' effect, though not yet proven for the POP (*see Qs 5.60, 8.13*).
- For the remaining items, including the cancers, listed in *Q 5.57* there is so far no evidence to suggest that the beneficial effect applies to old-type POPs. And functional ovarian cysts are more, not less, frequent (see below).

MAIN PROBLEMS AND DISADVANTAGES

7.32 What are the main problems of the POP?

- The need for obsessional regularity in pill-taking (*see Q 7.20*). This is believed to be less critical when on Cerazette and during full lactation.
- Alteration of the menstrual pattern is the main problem, except in breastfeeders. The reasons are explained in *Q 7.5*. According to that Swedish study, one can predict to some extent the type of change that the POP will produce. Women whose own normal cycles had long follicular/short luteal phases were more likely to be in group 4 on the POP (tending to have episodes of amenorrhoea). Those with regular or short cycles – who had relatively short follicular but normal-length luteal phases – were more likely to enter group 1 and have the more regular bleeding.

In general, the duration and volume of flow might change and there could be intermenstrual episodes. Alternatively, the woman might develop amenorrhoea.

All in all, cycle irregularity (especially frequent/prolonged bleeding) is the most common reason for abandoning the method – with Cerazette also. Yet a woman can be told that irregularity or oligo- or amenorrhoea mean the method is probably more effective in her particular case (*see Q 7.6*). Another disadvantage therefore is that:

- Precisely in those women with the most acceptable, regular cycles, the risk of pregnancy is greatest.
- A small number of women develop symptomatic functional ovarian cysts (*see Q 7.34*), causing pain that can sometimes be severe enough to imitate an ectopic pregnancy.
- Pregnancies in POP-users are more likely to be ectopic than are pregnancies occurring in the general population. As for the IUD (*see Qs 9.28, 9.30*), it is not thought that the POP actually increases the risk of ectopics in a population of POP-users; indeed, the reverse is true.

7.33 What is the risk of ectopic pregnancy? Why do ectopics occur in POP-users?

When compared with sexually active non-pregnant controls, studies have shown a reduced risk of ectopic pregnancy in POP-users. This is to be expected because the method often interferes with ovulation, and with fertilization. Ectopics can only happen if normal ovulation occurs, followed by fertilization, i.e. the risk relates only to a subgroup of group 1 in Q 7.5. Moreover, the effect of the POP on cervical mucus should reduce the risk of tubal damage from pelvic infection.

However, the likelihood of any breakthrough pregnancy that (rarely) actually happens being ectopic is increased. Possible explanations include the following:

- A selection effect, exactly as described for the IUD (*see Q 9.29*), if there is pre-existing tubal damage and fertilization occurs. The numerator of ectopics is reduced, but if the denominator of POP 'breakthrough' pregnancies is reduced even more, the relative frequency of ectopics among the conceptions will increase.
- Progestogens can modify tubal function. Overall, contractility and the rate of ovum transport are decreased, the latter probably from a reduction in the number of ciliated cells, but the significance to ectopic risk is not established.

Of the two, the first explanation is thought by far the more important (*see Qs 9.29, 9.30*). Like the COC, Cerazette ought to reduce the risk of

ectopics to vanishingly low levels. For a past history of ectopic,
see Q 7.51.

7.34 How frequent are functional ovarian cysts among POP-users?

In a study by the Margaret Pyke Centre, functional ovarian cysts (FOCs) as diagnosed by ultrasound occurred in as many as half the POP-users (12/21), compared with four out of the 21 controls. Most of these were asymptomatic, but seven women – all of them POP-users – complained of some pain; one required admission for rest and analgesia.

It is also clinical experience that some POP-users are diagnosed as cases of ectopic pregnancy (menstrual irregularity plus one-sided pain and a tender mass) but laparoscopy shows only a functional cyst, or evidence that one has recently ruptured.

7.35 What is the cause of functional ovarian cysts?

The precise causation of FOCs remains undefined. They are clearly due to an abnormality of ovulation (sometimes luteinization of an unruptured follicle), which is succeeded by accumulation of fluid. On the basis of the groups defined in Q 7.5, one would expect the frequency to be no different from a control population in group 1, and actually reduced in the group with quiescent ovaries: group 4. Yet they still occur in users of Cerazette: four symptomatic cysts were reported among 979 women in the study quoted in Q 7.11.

7.36 Does the POP affect neoplasia risk?

Little is known, for the reasons discussed in Qs 5.73 *and 7.3.* The UK National Case Control Study (1989) found a possible protective association with breast cancer, whereas the CGHFBC suggested an increased risk similar to that which they described for the COC *(see Q 5.85).* So the jury is still out: if there is any real influence of the POP on carcinogenesis (in the breast or elsewhere) it will be subject to two important considerations:

- Any effects will most probably be (slightly) beneficial on some cancers, adverse on others (as for the COC, *see Q 5.74),* and usually related in each case to duration of use.
- Intuitively, the effects are likely to depend in part on the amount of interaction with the woman's menstrual cycle, i.e. her 'group' in Q 7.5.

For the present, one can truthfully tell any woman that no POP study to date has shown a statistically significant increase in the risk of cancer. Even less is known about Cerazette in this respect.

7.37 What effect does the POP have on trophoblastic disease?

See Q 5.78 for a discussion of the reasons as to why, in the UK, until hCG levels are undetectable, the COC is WHO 4; and it is advised that POPs and other contraceptive hormones are WHO 3 (so that alternatives should normally be used). Thereafter, all hormone methods, including even the COC, are WHO 1.

7.38 What is the influence of the POP on benign tumours, such as benign breast disease and fibroids?

There is no evidence that any of the tumours mentioned in Q 5.97 are affected by use of any POP – but no conclusive evidence of no effect, either.

7.39 What are the effects of the POP on metabolism?

Although this has been slightly better studied than the epidemiology, there are few good studies of modern POPs. Moreover, the studies can be faulted on at least one of the following counts:

- Inadequate attention to confounding: meaning that the changes seen might be due to characteristics of the woman for whom a POP was chosen, rather than the POP itself.
- Lack of attention to the different metabolic responses to be expected, according to whether the users respond to the POP as in the groups 1, 2, 3 or 4 in Q 7.5. *Fig. 7.1* shows that the resultant metabolic effects might well vary from (in group 1) those of the normal menstrual cycle with normal ovarian estrogen plus a small effect from the POP, to the situation (group 4) where the progestogen is opposed by relatively little endogenous estrogen production.

Despite these limitations, the overall findings of the metabolic studies are very reassuring, as discussed in the next questions.

7.40 What are the effects of the POP on coagulation and fibrinolysis?

- Studies have shown that the POP, unlike COCs, has no important measurable adverse effect on blood clotting, platelet aggregation or fibrinolytic activity.
- One interesting study looked at prostacyclin and thromboxane levels. Among COC-users, prostacyclin levels were decreased (favouring platelet aggregation). There was no change in the POP group, however, and in the latter, particularly among women using levonorgestrel alone, the thromboxane concentrations were depressed. As thromboxane enhances platelet aggregation, this could even indicate a decreased risk of thrombosis in POP-users.

7.41 Presumably, the POP can therefore be used by women with a definite past history of thromboembolism, even if COC-related?

Yes, definitely, given Q 7.40 above, and backed by the epidemiological study by Vasilakis et al [*Lancet* 1999;354:1610–1611], which showed no added risk of idiopathic venous thromboembolism in users of progestogens alone. Please see also the important Box at Q 5.111, for reassurance about Cerazette, the 'third-generation' POP.

In this matter, the labelling (SPC) for norethisterone products is contradictory. In the SPC of the Noriday brand of POP (which contains only 350 µg of this progestogen), *past* thrombosis is stated to be a 'contraindication' (i.e. WHO 4). However, if you look up Primolut N in the electronic Medicine Compendium (http://www.emc.medicines.org.uk) you discover that it contains norethisterone 5000 µg and is regularly used for gynaecological indications such as menorrhagia in doses up to 15 000 µg daily. Yet, past thromboembolism is (rightly, in fact) not included as a WHO 4 contraindication. What logic is there in the manufacturer being restrictive about a past thrombosis history when the Noriday POP is prescribed, which gives a dose 45 times smaller of the identical drug? Answer: 'none' (see first sentence of this answer).

7.42 **What are the effects on blood lipids, especially high-density lipoprotein–cholesterol (HDL-C)?**

The POPs currently available seem to have little effect on all the main aspects of lipid metabolism; but in one or two studies the important subfraction HDL_2-C was slightly depressed with POPs containing either levonorgestrel or norethisterone. This was not shown with desogestrel as in Cerazette.

7.43 **What are the effects on carbohydrate metabolism?**

Once again, a consensus view is that the effects are minimal. However, some studies have shown a slight deterioration in glucose tolerance and a tendency to hyperinsulinism, particularly in users of the levonorgestrel POPs. Some studies cannot exclude the possibility that adverse metabolic findings are the result of selection of the POP by users who have arterial disease risk factors, so that use of the POP is coincidental, not causal.

7.44 **Can the POP be used by frank diabetics?**

Certainly – the POP can be the method of choice. Workers in Edinburgh have found that with POPs containing 350 µg norethisterone no increase in insulin dosage appeared necessary, and there was no change in the incidence and severity of retinopathy. They consider the POP to be an ideal choice from the metabolic point of view. In addition, only one pregnancy occurred among 50 women during the period of observation (1050 woman-months) and the woman concerned omitted a number of pills.

Generally, diabetics have exceptionally good compliance because they take their pill with each evening dose of insulin. But for younger and more fertile diabetics, the extra efficacy plus still no EE content of Cerazette would make it even more attractive.

7.45 Would you use current POPs in a diabetic with definite evidence of tissue damage, especially arteriopathy?

Yes. In my view, the uncertainty about metabolic effects, especially on lipids, makes this WHO 3 for old-type POPs but WHO 2 for Cerazette (i.e. certainly usable); but other options like an IUD or IUS might be even better.

7.46 Have any other metabolic effects been described?

■ When progestogens are administered alone, they have little if any effect on hepatic secretion of plasma proteins – compare this with the COC (*see Q 5.99*).

■ Thyroid and pituitary–adrenal function also appear to be unaffected.

■ Progestogens beneficially affect the biochemistry and physiology of cervical mucus (*see Q 7.17*), thereby probably protecting the user against pelvic infection. They also appear to improve aspects of erythrocyte metabolism in sickle-cell anaemia (*see Q 8.15*). Reassuring, but again based on small numbers.

7.47 Does the POP affect BP?

Reassuringly, apparently not. Studies have shown neither the slight rise in systolic and diastolic pressure that occurs in almost all individuals given estrogen-containing preparations and nor (and this includes Cerazette) do they appear to increase the risk of frank hypertension. COC-induced hypertension usually reverts to normal on the POP.

The same appears to apply to DMPA and other estrogen-free methods in this chapter. Though the data come from mostly small studies, progestogens seem to have an adverse effect on BP only if estrogens are also administered.

SELECTION OF USERS AND OF FORMULATIONS

7.48 For whom is the POP method particularly indicated?

Lactation (see (8), below) has hitherto been the main indication, although the working rule has been:

Wherever there are contraindications to or side-effects with the COC, and an oral hormonal method is preferred? Try the POP.

Previously there was the obstacle of reduced efficacy in making this choice in younger women, but that has disappeared with the advent of Cerazette:

1   *Women above 35 who smoke* cigarettes. On present information it is acceptable to continue use of the POP even in a smoker on her

say-so until beyond the average age of the menopause (i.e. about 51 years).

2   *Estrogen-linked contraindications* or side-effects on the COC. Some of those listed on the left of *Table 6.1* (p. 257) might improve. The POP should not be chosen preferentially for conditions such as endometriosis because it does not reliably suppress endogenous estrogen (though Cerazette might be tried for maintenance therapy).

But importantly this category of indications for the POP includes:

3   *History of or any predisposition to thromboembolism*, including known prothrombotic coagulation factor changes: since adverse effects on clotting mechanisms have not been demonstrated (*see Qs 7.40, 7.41*).

It follows, accordingly:

4   *Chronic systemic diseases* in which estrogen is the hormone that might exacerbate the condition (e.g. SLE) or where there is an extra thrombosis risk (e.g. atrial fibrillation and complicated structural heart disease (*see Qs 5.136, 5.141* and *Table 5.14*, p. 214), severe cases of Crohn's disease or ulcerative colitis (*see Q 5.147*) and, again, SLE (*see Q 5.148*)). Sickle-cell disease is another example. But (*see Q 8.15*), for this indication, DMPA might be an even better option.

5   Patients with *diabetes or obesity*. Diabetics do particularly well on the POP, especially with regard to compliance (*see Q 7.44*). There are efficacy considerations for the obese (*see Qs 7.14–7.16*).

6   Patients with *hypertension*, either related to the COC or other varieties if well controlled by treatment.

7   Patients with *migraine* (including, with appropriate caution and advice, young women with migraines which are severe or with aura) (*see Qs 5.153–5.170*).

8   During *lactation* (*see Qs 7.53, 7.54*). This is a well-established indication in which the method has the highest efficacy.

9   To cover elective major or leg surgery.

10 At the *woman's choice:* such as a reliable pill-taker who prefers a hormonal method yet wishes to use the least possible amount of exogenous hormone.

7.49   What are the contraindications to the POP?

As we have seen, a long list of conditions contraindicating use of POPs can be found in the manufacturers' SPC sheets, but most are there for medico-legal reasons, with no epidemiological basis. In general, and with the exceptions suggested below, the absolute contraindications to the COC (WHO 4) are only relative contraindications (of varying importance, most commonly WHO 2) for the POP.

As before, any list of contraindications must be, to some extent, a matter of personal judgment (*see Q 5.137*) and, with the POP, involve some informed guesswork – given the dearth of good data.

7.50 What then are the absolute contraindications to the POP, in your view?

Here (as in the next questions) the WHO categorization is used (WHO 4 in this section):

■ *Any serious side-effect occurring on the COC and not clearly due only to estrogen* – or associated with past progestogen-only use. Liver adenoma or cancer, and severe past sex-steroid-associated cholestatic jaundice would come here, because it is not clear with which of the two hormones in the COC they are primarily linked.

■ *Current breast cancer* – for fear of worsening the prognosis. This is WHO 4 pending more data, but can be WHO 3 after the woman has shown no evidence of current disease for 5 years, according to the WHO (*see Q 7.51*).

■ *Acute porphyria*, with past history of an actual attack (*see Q 6.43*). See immediately below if latent, with no history of past attack.

So it is a very short list, although, as for all medical methods, we must add:

■ Severe *allergy* to a constituent.
■ *Undiagnosed abnormal genital tract bleeding*, because the POP will confuse diagnosis.
■ Actual or possible *pregnancy*.
■ *The woman's own continuing uncertainty* about POP safety, even after full counselling.

7.51 In your view, what are only relative contraindications to the POP (i.e. when can it be used but with some added caution)?

These are in two groups:

Strong relative contraindications (WHO 3) for POP and Cerazette use
■ Past *severe* arterial diseases, or current exceptionally high risk thereof (e.g. familial hypercholesterolaemia).
■ Sex-steroid-dependent cancer, including breast cancer, when in complete remission (UKMEC states WHO 4 until 5 years of remission, then WHO 3). In all cases, agreement of the relevant hospital consultant should be obtained and the woman's autonomy respected: record that she understands it is unknown whether progestogen might alter the recurrence risk (either way).

- Recent trophoblastic disease until hCG is undetectable in blood as well as urine (UKMEC); but even with high hCG levels this is WHO 1 according to WHOMEC (*see Qs 5.78, 7.37*).
- Enzyme-inducers: although two tablets of Cerazette (one twice daily) can be taken, off licence (see *Appendix A*), another method such as an injectable, IUD or the LNG-IUS would be preferable.
- Acute porphyria, latent, with no hormone-triggered previous attack (along with caution, forewarning/monitoring); POP is fully usable (WHO 2) in all the non-acute porphyrias.
- Past symptomatic (painful) functional ovarian cysts. But persistent cysts/follicles that are commonly detected on routine ultrasonography can be disregarded if they caused no symptoms.
- Previous treatment for ectopic pregnancy in a nulliparous woman; however, this is an *indication for Cerazette*! The overall risk of ectopic pregnancy is actually reduced among POP-users, which is why the condition is classified WHO 1 by UKMEC. But since the risk can be reduced still further by methods that regularly block fertilization, it would usually be preferable to offer the COC, DMPA, Cerazette or Implanon – to better preserve the precious remaining fallopian tube.

The second group are WHO 2 relative contraindications and may be seen as *indications* when a hormone method is wanted and alternatives are unsuitable:

Weak relative contraindications (WHO 2) for POP and Cerazette
- Unwillingness to cope with irregularity or absence of periods.
- Past venous thromboembolism (VTE) or severe risk factors for VTE.
- Risk factors for arterial disease, including established hypertension and migraine with aura – more than one risk factor can be present, in contrast to COCs.
- Current liver disorder – even if there is persistent biochemical change.
- Most other chronic severe systemic diseases (but WHO 3 if the condition causes significant malabsorption of sex steroids).
- Strong family history of breast cancer – UKMEC says WHO 1 for this – even for COCs in fact! Yet intuitively it seems better in such women to avoid estrogen (and also give a lower progestogen dose).

7.52 What are the clinical implications of an increased rate of functional ovarian cysts (FOCs) with Cerazette as well as old-type POPs?

- Ultrasound studies suggest that most FOCs are asymptomatic (*see Q 7.34*).
- It is likely that altered estrogen production by functional cysts can explain some of the menstrual irregularity.

■ The main risks of FOCs are those of unnecessary surgery, especially laparoscopy, and rarely also necessary surgery for acute events such as ovarian torsion. This is why the past history of symptomatic FOCs, either before use of the POP or while taking it, should now be considered WHO 3.

In my experience, however, some women so much prefer this method to the alternatives that they are prepared to take the risk of recurrences. They should be advised to take prompt medical advice as indicated. Given the problem of distinguishing this syndrome from ectopic pregnancy, pelvic ultrasound and ultrasensitive pregnancy tests should be utilized to minimize the need for diagnostic laparoscopy.

USE OF THE POP IN LACTATION

See Q 7.23 for the enhanced-efficacy implications of the POP during breastfeeding. This is in fact the most common context in which POPs are used.

7.53 What are the effects of the POP on lactation?

The COC can reduce the volume and alter the constitution of milk. Some of the artificial steroids are transferred to the infant. By contrast, the POPs (including Cerazette) are suitable choices for lactating women. Indeed, progestogens, when administered alone by any of the means discussed in this chapter, appear to reduce neither the volume of milk nor the duration of lactation, and some reports suggest that both are increased. Careful studies on norethisterone-, levonorgestrel- and desogestrel-containing POPs show that the amount transferred to the milk is minute and most unlikely to present any hazard. Studies of the blood of suckling infants have been unable to demonstrate any progestogen because the concentration is below the limits of the sensitivity of present assays.

Last, but not least, the contraceptive combination of lactation plus old-type POP is for practical purposes 100% effective. (*See Qs 7.16, 7.23.*)

7.54 What are the implications for prescribing the POP during lactation?

■ First and foremost, the above findings need discussion. The prospective user might be interested to learn that, according to Scandinavian studies of 30-μg levonorgestrel POPs, after 2 years of lactation with regular POP-taking the infant will have received at most the equivalent of one tablet! If this is not sufficiently reassuring, of course, another method should be adopted.

■ Another advantage is that the main symptom with the POP – irregular bleeding – is unlikely during lactational amenorrhoea, except when it is first commenced postpartum (*see Q 7.55*).

7.55 When should the POP be commenced after delivery?

■ As, unlike the COC, the POP does not affect lactation or the risk of venous thrombosis, it is medically safe to start it in the immediate postpartum period. WHO calls such early use WHO 3, because of the concern that the neonate might be at some risk if exposure is in the first 6 weeks after delivery.

■ Studies have shown a greater likelihood of spotting and bleeding problems with starting early in the puerperium. So unless there are special reasons to start earlier, initiating the POP a little later – at around day 21 – is recommended by the fpa (*see Table 7.4*), as with the COC. Of course, even a 6-week time of starting would be fully effective when combined with full breastfeeding (*see Q 2.36*).

7.56 How should weaning be managed in POP-users?

Some women simply continue using the POP long term. However, I well remember a clinic in which two consecutive women described how they had unwantedly conceived another pregnancy through not being warned that they would no longer get away with occasional lateness of POP-taking once they stopped fully breastfeeding! That was before the days of Cerazette, of course.

Therefore, if efficacy is at a premium, they should be given a 'stronger' method in advance, such as a supply of the COC or Cerazette (unless that is already the POP being used in lactation), to start when breast milk is no longer the main source of their infant's nutrition, or when solid food is first introduced, or at the time of their first postpartum menses – whichever comes earlier. The resulting increased dose of hormones in the breast milk from the COC is not believed to have any relevance to the health of the baby, but the COC might very well hasten the end of lactation.

Remember that the first fertile ovulation is more likely to happen without a first warning bleed, if it is more than 6 months since delivery.

7.57 With or without lactation, which POP should be chosen?

After consideration of the contraindications (*see Qs 7.50, 7.51*), there are few guidelines:

■ During lactation, on theoretical grounds, Norgeston is possibly preferable to the other old-type POPs because such a negligible amount reaches the breast milk (*see Q 7.54*) – due to particularly strong binding to SHBG in the blood.

■ No study has shown statistically different rates of effectiveness between the levonorgestrel POPs (Norgeston, Neogest) and the norethisterone group (Micronor, Noriday, Femulen). Cerazette is in a different league (although old-type POPs are nearly 100% effective themselves, when combined with breastfeeding or other states of relative infertility such as perimenopausally).

■ A 'best buy' can also not be stated for menstrual disturbance.

The initial choice of POP for cycling women therefore depends on the degree of efficacy desired. Cerazette has now cornered the POP market for most highly fertile young women and those who are above 70 kg in weight (*see Q 7.16*); but old-type POPs would be equally suitable during full lactation, above age 40 and in other states of reduced fertility.

INITIAL MANAGEMENT AND FOLLOW-UP ARRANGEMENTS

7.58 What are the main aspects to convey during counselling?

The truth of the phrase 'forewarned is forearmed' is never so clear as in counselling about the unpredictable bleeding pattern of the POP (as indeed for all progestogen-only methods). The good efficacy, second only to Cerazette, the combined pill and injectables, of old-type POPs (especially in older women) should also be stressed – provided always that the rules for successful pill-taking are followed (*see Qs 7.20–7.28*).

As for other methods, a supplementary leaflet (e.g. that produced by the fpa) should always be supplied along with the PIL.

7.59 How should POP use be monitored?

■ A baseline BP and weight are valuable.

■ Routine cervical smear examinations are good screening practice, although (as before) not believed to have any special relevance to the contraceptive method.

■ The woman should be seen 3 months after starting the POP but all checks can then be extended to annually, with an 'open-house policy' to return sooner upon request. There need be recourse to a doctor only if problems arise, such as pelvic pain.

■ Routine examinations should be kept to a minimum.

■ BP need only be measured annually.

■ Body weight is of no relevance to monitoring.

7.60 For how long can POP use be continued?

At present the answer is 'indefinitely' as long as contraception is required, into the late 50s – in the absence of contraindications, multiple risk factors, or the occurrence of important complications.

7.61 How can the menopause be diagnosed in older POP-users?

If a user of an old-type POP develops prolonged amenorrhoea, yet was previously observing bleeding episodes, it can be difficult to distinguish between amenorrhoea secondary to the POP and the arrival of the menopause. Symptoms, especially hot flushes, can be a useful guide.

There is also evidence that the finding of a high level of FSH can have some relevance at the menopause despite continued POP-taking. Low levels, on the other hand, suggest that the woman is in group 4 of Q 7.5 still potentially fertile, and should certainly continue to use this or some alternative contraceptive method.

7.62 How do you act if the FSH is high in an older POP-user? Is there a practical protocol?

If the FSH is found to be high (at menopause levels for the laboratory), my practice above age 51 is to suggest that the woman discontinues the POP and transfers to a simple barrier method. FSH measurement is then repeated at 4–6 weeks, on two occasions if there is any doubt.

If the woman is still amenorrhoeic, has vasomotor symptoms and menopausal FSH results are again obtained, she can be advised that her chances of conception are low enough to discontinue alternative contraception – whether or not she now transfers to taking HRT.

No guarantee of total infertility can be given, however, and she is warned to return for advice should she develop any subsequent (non-HRT-related) bleeding. And women who want more complete reassurance should continue a simple method of birth control until 1 year after the last spontaneous bleed.

7.63 What if FSH measurements are still low?

If she is amenorrhoeic, the POP can simply be continued into the 50s with periodic FSH checks. But if she remains symptom-free, suggesting she is still getting enough estrogen from her ovaries, there is usually no pressure actually to establish final ovarian failure.

7.64 What about Cerazette use perimenopausally?

It is even more likely than with old-type POPs that a user of this pill will be amenorrhoeic at this age, but, even when the ovaries are non-functional, FSH levels might be maintained low, because of strong suppression of the hypothalamus/pituitary. There is medically no rush to get her off this very safe product, unlike with the COC at this age, but it is a bit of a 'contraceptive overkill'.

So, a good option is to transfer to an old-type POP and proceed as above (see Qs 7.62, 7.63). Or, if she develops unacceptable vasomotor symptoms, like any POP-user she could move to the excellent LNG-IUS plus HRT combination mentioned in Qs 9.144, 9.149 and 11.43. More controversially since we lack good studies on this, the Faculty of SRH in its Guidance 'Contraception for women aged over 40 years' [Journal of Family

Planning and Reproductive Health Care 2005;312:51–63] advises at No 56 as a Good Practice Point that a POP (and I would advise Cerazette, *see* Q 7.66) can be used with HRT to provide effective contraception. As usual, this should be on the 'named-patient' prescribing basis discussed in *Appendix A*.

7.65 Should I be concerned about hypo-estrogenism in any POP-user who develops prolonged amenorrhoea, especially with Cerazette?

This is a difficult one: even in the similar situation applying to DMPA there are insufficient data. But here there is reassurance from the pre-marketing studies about average estradiol levels, with both Implanon and Cerazette. Though both suppress the ovaries more than old-type POPs, it is believed that there is enough follicular activity through some ongoing FSH secretion and hence adequate estrogen production with all these progestogen-only methods – regardless of whether or not the users bleed.

Pending more data, therefore, my current view is that, unlike with DMPA (*see* Qs 8.23–8.25), there need be no particular concern about hypo-estrogenism or osteoporosis in long-term users of any kind of POP (or with Implanon), even if they are amenorrhoeic. But if an individual develops symptoms like hot flushes or dry vagina, proceed as at Q 7.61ff above.

7.66 If estrogen as in HRT is taken by a POP-user, won't this make her more likely to conceive?

Not when she starts off in group 4 of Q 7.5, which means she is not ovulating. She is not relying on the mucus effect for contraceptive efficacy anyway, so it cannot enhance her fertility if the mucus is improved by the added estrogen. But she might be in one of the possibly ovulating groups.

Hence, now we have Cerazette, I recommend eliminating any such concern by using only that anovulant POP when HRT is also desired, as at Q 7.64 above.

MANAGEMENT OF SIDE-EFFECTS OR COMPLICATIONS

7.67 What should be the second choice of POP if bleeding problems develop and cannot be tolerated?

- First, examine the patient for a coincidental gynaecological cause (see *Table 5.15* and Q 5.170).
- An understanding of the spectrum of individual reactions to the POP is of some help (*see* Qs 7.5, 7.6). It would appear that the bleeding problems are concentrated in groups 2 and 3. Group 1 cycles are generally the most acceptable. With good counselling, women in group

4 can also accept their long episodes of amenorrhoea. Careful assessment of the bleeding pattern therefore aids decision-making.

■ If it appears that a reduction in dose might transfer a woman from group 2 or 3 to group 1, one could, for example, switch from Femulen to Micronor/Noriday.

■ The reverse could be tried if reaching group 4 seemed likely to be achieved thereby, i.e. a trial of Femulen (the strongest old-type POP available) or Cerazette. But the bleeding irregularity might get worse, if amenorrhoea does not result.

■ With Cerazette, if the woman is prepared to persevere, improvement may still be expected through to 12 months (*see Q 7.11*). Anecdotally, taking two tablets of Cerazette daily for a while has been helpful in some cases (unlicensed use, p. 553).

If all else fails, offer a change of method.

7.68 What minor non-bleeding side-effects have been described in POP-takers?

The short answer is that POP-users report almost all of the minor side-effects reported by COC-takers, but in general less frequently. In the Oxford/FPA comparative study, headaches, psychological disturbance (including depression) and hypertension were particularly associated with COCs as causes of discontinuation of the method. However:

■ menstrual disturbance and,
■ interestingly, breast discomfort,

were reported more commonly among POP-users.

Mildly androgenic effects such as acne also occur, with no difference noted in the pre-marketing studies between the old-type levonorgestrel POP (4.2%) and Cerazette (4.1%).

7.69 Which second choice of POP should follow if non-bleeding minor side-effects develop?

The decision to change to a different POP has again to be empirical. For example, if headaches occur on a levonorgestrel POP, it might be worth transferring to one of the norethisterone group – or the desogestrel product. With support and reassurance, however, the subjective symptoms may diminish or disappear after a few months of continuing to take the same POP.

7.70 What action should be taken if a POP-user complains of low abdominal pain?

As usual, causes unrelated to contraception should be excluded. Two important possibilities must be borne in mind, although the first has a reduced likelihood with Cerazette. Importantly, both cause menstrual irregularity and perhaps a unilateral mass as well as pain:

- ectopic pregnancy
- pain due to the formation/torsion or rupture of a functional ovarian cyst: referral for ultrasound and (rarely) laparoscopy may be required (*see Q 7.52*).

7.71 Which symptoms should lead a POP-user to take urgent medical advice? Should she transfer to another method at once?

Abdominal pain is probably the only acute symptom requiring urgent advice. But neither for this nor for any of the symptoms in the 'stop COC' list in *Q 6.13* (which are mostly irrelevant because they relate to estrogen) must the woman discontinue the POP instantly. Continuing to take the POP for a few more days can do no significant harm – whereas an unplanned pregnancy might.

7.72 What should be done if a POP-user is immobilized after an accident or requires emergency (or elective) major surgery?

There is no reason for a woman using any estrogen-free preparation to discontinue the method in either of these clinical contexts.

7.73 What are the risks if a woman should become pregnant while taking the POP?

- If she has conceived, although the old-type POP does not cause ectopics, a higher proportion of conceptions than usual prove to be extrauterine: so it would be clinically important to exclude the condition (*see Q 7.33*).
- The available findings concerning teratogenesis are extremely reassuring. No cases of congenital abnormality have been reported, although there have been no good large studies. In the Oxford/FPA study there were 30 accidental pregnancies in continuing POP-users. Of these, seven were terminated, 15 ended in live births without malformations, one was ectopic and seven ended in spontaneous miscarriage (*see also Q 6.47*). Given its small dose of only one hormone, the usual 'armchair thinking' about the POP would lead one to expect an even lower rate of fetal abnormalities in breakthrough POP pregnancies than with the COC. The rate for the latter (which is more firmly documented) is itself already remarkably low.

There is certainly no need to advise switching from the POP to another method for any arbitrary time before a planned conception (indeed this is not important even for the COC, *see Q 6.49*).

7.74 **Are there any known special risks or benefits for ex-takers of the old-type POP?**

There are no data to support or refute any such ex-use effects. If they exist at all, they are likely to be clinically insignificant. Because of the known advantages of long-term anovulation, several of the ex-use benefits of the COC must be expected for ex-users of Cerazette, but its arrival on the scene is too recent for any of these yet to be demonstrable.

PQ PATIENT QUESTIONS

QUESTIONS ASKED BY USERS ABOUT THE POP

Much confusion, particularly that these 'mini-pills' are not low-dose combined pills, has to be cleared up.

7.75 Does the POP ever cause an abortion?

No. Yet, although not its usual method of action, one possible way the old-type POP operates on some occasions is by stopping implantation: the process by which a dividing fertilized egg becomes embedded in the lining of the womb. Stopping this is not now felt by most people to be causing an abortion (though it is by some) – for the reasons explained in *Qs 10.3 and 10.4*, which you should please read.

The POP is thought to use this mechanism very rarely anyway and *never* when combined with full breastfeeding (*see Q 7.23*). So if this is a major concern to you, you could use the POP only during breastfeeding, perhaps also choosing the newest and 'strongest' product – Cerazette.

Reading the question a different way, deliberately taking a large number of POPs (or combined pills for that matter) is not a recognized abortifacient method: it is most unlikely to stop a fully established implanted pregnancy (even though larger than usual daily doses do work as emergency contraceptives prior to implantation, *see Chapter 10*).

7.76 If the old-type POP is not so effective as the combined pill, why are some women recommended to use it?

This method is only a little less effective than the combined pill, especially in the older age group. Indeed, above the age of 40 or when combined with breastfeeding, it is as effective as the COC would be for a 25-year-old.

7.77 My period is overdue on the old-type POP or Cerazette. What does this mean?

First, we might need to exclude the possibility that the method has let you down. Once that has been done, the most likely explanation is that the pill is preventing egg release. So, paradoxically, you will be more effectively protected from pregnancy than is a girlfriend who is being reassured by seeing regular periods (*see Q 7.7*).

7.78 I know that COC-users do not see proper periods – is that also true of the bleeds I get on the POP?

On the old-type POP, some episodes of bleeding are caused like normal periods. In these, the special structure in your ovary known as a corpus luteum stops producing the two hormones that stimulate growth of the uterine lining, and this leads to it coming away, and hence a period. However, many POP-users, and users of Cerazette who bleed at all, have other bleeding or spotting episodes as well. These are either shorter or longer than a normal period and can be lighter or heavier. They are caused by irregular shedding of the womb lining, in turn caused by effects resulting from how the artificial hormone of the POP and the estrogen and progesterone produced by your ovary interact with each other (*see Qs 7.4–7.6 and Fig. 7.1*).

7.79 I am breastfeeding my baby and have been given the POP – won't this harm my baby?

Although a very tiny amount of the hormone does get into the breast milk, it has not been possible to show any changes in milk quantity or in quality, with either the old-type POP or with the newer product Cerazette.

There cannot be absolute proof that the POP hormone in the milk would be completely harmless: so if you are unhappy it would be important to discuss another method with your family doctor or a local clinic. However, the amount taken by the baby is very small; for example, with Norgeston your baby will take only the equivalent of one tablet if you continue to breastfeed for 2 years! It is extremely unlikely that such a minute dose would affect your baby at all (*see Qs 7.53, 7.54*).

Injectables and implants

8

INJECTABLES

BACKGROUND AND MECHANISMS

EFFECTIVENESS

ADVANTAGES AND BENEFITS

MAIN PROBLEMS AND DISADVANTAGES

SELECTION OF USERS AND OF FORMULATIONS

INITIAL MANAGEMENT AND FOLLOW-UP ARRANGEMENTS

INJECTABLES

BACKGROUND AND MECHANISMS

8.1 What are injectables?

The two available in the UK are progestogenic steroids given on a regular basis by deep intramuscular injection (*Q 8.43*) for contraception. Experience with them dates back to the early 1960s. According to the UN (2003), DMPA is used by about 13 million women worldwide.

8.2 What injectables are available in the UK?

■ *Depot medroxyprogesterone acetate (DMPA, Depo-Provera):* this is available in aqueous microcrystalline suspension and is normally given in a dose of 150 mg every 12 weeks. Other regimens have also been tried and proved effective.

■ *Norethisterone enantate (NET-EN: Noristerat, Norigest):* this is available in a vehicle of benzyl benzoate and castor oil, the dose being 200 mg every 8 weeks. Other regimens are not now recommended.

> DMPA is an example of a pregnane progestogen, which is more closely related to natural progesterone than are either estrane progestogens such as norethisterone or gonanes such as levonorgestrel – all derived from 19-nortestosterone.

8.3 What is the status and availability of injectables worldwide and in the UK?

DMPA has been repeatedly endorsed by WHO, the International Planned Parenthood Federation (IPPF) and virtually every other relevant authority. It is currently available for long-term contraceptive use in more than 130 countries. It is, in fact, the first-choice reversible method in South Africa and was approved for similar licensing in the US at the end of 1992. In 1984, the UK Minister of Health agreed to the recommendation by the CSM that the method could be used long term for contraception by selected women after full counselling about its long-term (and slow-to-reverse) nature. It now has the status of a first-line option in the UK and is one of the LARCs promoted as being much more cost-effective than the COC by NICE (2005). Yet it is still chosen currently by a very small minority – less than 2% of women use injectable contraception in the UK. This low usage is largely provider-led: the option is offered so infrequently. But most of those who do use it are very satisfied customers!

NET-EN is used, chiefly in Germany and a number of developing countries, even less widely. It is also available in the UK, a product licence for antifertility use having been granted. Although it is only officially for short-term use, longer-term use is acceptable in selected patients after counselling. But the oily injection is more painful than DMPA and its duration of action is only 8 weeks. Most of what follows relates to DMPA.

8.4 What is the mode of action of injectables?

The primary action of the progestogen dose given by both injectables is, like the COC, to prevent ovulation. As with other hormonal methods, this is supplemented chiefly by contraceptive actions at the mucus level (*see* Q 7.4 and *Table 7.2*). The anovulation effect is so strong it almost never needs to operate at the endometrial level, by preventing implantation, though it probably has that potential. More frequent injections, say every 10 weeks, can be offered to a user who wishes to ensure, for her own ethical reasons, that that mechanism of action never could happen.

8.5 Do injectables provide a steady dose?

No – see *Fig. 8.1*. Although the levels fluctuate far less than with any oral method (COC or POP), there is a much higher level initially, declining

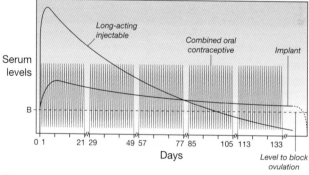

Fig. 8.1 Blood levels of progestogen hormone in users of three delivery systems. *Q 8.5.* This is a schematic representation for DMPA. After an injection there is a relatively high level (B indicates the level to block ovulation), then a decline as time passes. Oral contraceptives (the POP would be similar, without a 7-day break) show wide fluctuations – a sawtooth pattern. Implants result in remarkably constant blood levels (adapted from Population reports K2, May 1983. Population information program. Johns Hopkins University, Figure 1).

exponentially thereafter. The release of hormone at a relatively constant or so-called zero-order rate is one of the advantages sought in newer injectables, and also rings and implants.

8.6 What is known about individual variation in blood levels?

This exists, as for the oral methods. However, the inter-individual variation is rather less marked because variable absorption from the gut and variable first-pass metabolism (*see Q 5.35*) are not involved. Blood levels seem to decline more rapidly in thin women (*see Q 8.9*). NET-EN has a shorter duration of action than DMPA.

8.7 What effects do injectables have on ovarian function?

As ovulation is generally inhibited, the 'spectrum effect' described in Q 7.5 for the POP is not observed with these agents. However, minimal follicular activity occurs, especially towards the end of the injection period and more in some women than others. Importantly, this follicular estradiol keeps serum concentrations in the range normally found in the early to middle follicular phase (90–290 pmol/L). This prevents clinical hypo-estrogenism (whether as symptoms or signs), probably in the majority of users. However, there is some concern about a few who in long-term use are found to have abnormally low estradiol levels (*see Qs 8.19, 8.23*).

EFFECTIVENESS

8.8 What is the overall effectiveness of injectables?

Among available reversible contraceptives the use-effectiveness of these methods is greater than that of the COC because the factor of the user's memory is almost eliminated. The range of efficacy quoted for DMPA is 0 (0.3 according to WHO)–1/100 woman-years, and for NET-EN 0.4–2/100 woman-years.

8.9 What factors influence the effectiveness of injectables?

As usual, the rate of failure is marginally higher in younger, more fertile women. With either compound, but especially NET-EN, it is essential not to massage the injection site (*see Q 8.43*) because this shortens the duration of action, increasing the failure rate in early studies. Local infection of the injection site can also be a factor (*see Q 8.16(12)*). It is important to insert the complete dose without spillage and ensure it is truly intramuscular even in an obese woman.

For the ticklish problem of overdue injections, *see Q 8.52ff*.

8.10   What are the recommended starting routines for injectables?

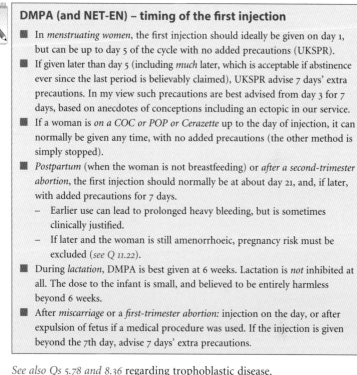

> **DMPA (and NET-EN) – timing of the first injection**
>
> ■ In *menstruating women*, the first injection should ideally be given on day 1, but can be up to day 5 of the cycle with no added precautions (UKSPR).
>
> ■ If given later than day 5 (including *much* later, which is acceptable if abstinence ever since the last period is believably claimed), UKSPR advise 7 days' extra precautions. In my view such precautions are best advised from day 3 for 7 days, based on anecdotes of conceptions including an ectopic in our service.
>
> ■ If a woman is *on a COC or POP or Cerazette* up to the day of injection, it can normally be given any time, with no added precautions (the other method is simply stopped).
>
> ■ *Postpartum* (when the woman is not breastfeeding) or *after a second-trimester abortion*, the first injection should normally be at about day 21, and, if later, with added precautions for 7 days.
>   – Earlier use can lead to prolonged heavy bleeding, but is sometimes clinically justified.
>   – If later and the woman is still amenorrhoeic, pregnancy risk must be excluded (*see Q 11.22*).
>
> ■ During *lactation*, DMPA is best given at 6 weeks. Lactation is *not* inhibited at all. The dose to the infant is small, and believed to be entirely harmless beyond 6 weeks.
>
> ■ After *miscarriage* or a *first-trimester abortion*: injection on the day, or after expulsion of fetus if a medical procedure was used. If the injection is given beyond the 7th day, advise 7 days' extra precautions.

See also Qs 5.78 and 8.36 regarding trophoblastic disease.

8.11   Do interactions with other drugs pose any problem with injectables?

There is certainly no problem with *non-enzyme-inducing antibiotics*, because the drug is not recycled from the gut.

   Drugs inducing liver enzymes (*see Q 5.38*). *DMPA is one of the first-choice methods for all women using such drugs who wish to use a hormonal method, and this is definitely preferable to special regimens with the COC or POP.*

   NB: This is a change in the clinical advice about this since earlier editions of this book, caused by data that have recently been made available (though they were already on file with the company, Pharmacia). This supports *not* shortening the injection interval or increasing the dose.

   The reason is that in studies the hepatic clearance of DMPA is found to equate to hepatic blood flow. In other words, the liver is normally eliminating all the medroxyprogesterone acetate (MPA) hormone in each unit volume of blood that flows through it, and an increase in enzyme activity in the hepatocytes cannot make the liver do better than the 100% clearance already occurring!

Hence, the bottom line on enzyme-inducers now is: Depo-Provera is a logical first choice method. (Yet, as this work was based on a small number of cases, for the most potent enzyme-inducers (rifampcin, rifabutin) personally I would be happier to shorten the injection interval to 10 weeks).

8.12 Might injectables affect the action of other drugs?

Please *see Q 5.46*, which describes this type of interaction with the COC, where the main clinically relevant interactions are:

- ■ lowered lamotrigine levels
- ■ increased ciclosporin levels
- ■ increased INRs with warfarin.

Pending further data (there are none for DMPA at present) we have to assume the possibility of similar effects with injectables, and therefore follow the same advice as given in *Q 5.46*, including, with warfarin, more frequent INR tests during early DMPA use and dose adjustment as required. Awareness is the main thing.

NB: With warfarin there is here a specific increased risk of large haematomas after injections, so the method is WHO 2, or WHO 3 if there is no recent INR available in the range 2–3. It would be more usual to advise another method (e.g. Implanon, *see Qs 8.56ff*).

ADVANTAGES AND BENEFITS

8.13 What are the beneficial effects of injectables?

CONTRACEPTIVE BENEFITS

1 *High effectiveness:* definitely greater than the COC. Moreover, uniquely, its efficacy remains unaffected by enzyme-inducing drugs (*see Q 8.11*).
2 *Minimizes 'forgettability':* a problem that exists with all pill methods.
3 *Highly convenient, non-intercourse-related.*
4 *Fully reversible:* although with some delay.

NON-CONTRACEPTIVE BENEFITS

Most of those in *Q 5.57* are believed to apply.

5 In many women there is a reduction in the disorders of the menstrual cycle, though benefit cannot be reliably predicted:
   (a) less heavy bleeding, often culminating over time in amenorrhoea (which can be a health benefit in reducing the risk of gynaecological disorders as listed in *Q 5.58* – but with the caveats in *Qs 8.23–8.25*)

    (b) less anaemia; indeed, the haemoglobin has been noted to rise regardless of the bleeding pattern, suggesting a direct haemopoietic effect as well as less quantity of loss

    (c) less dysmenorrhoea

    (d) fewer symptoms of premenstrual tension (not invariably – in some women similar symptoms (*see Q 8.16(11)*) occur early in each injection interval)

    (e) no ovulation pain.

Given the common side-effects of frequent or prolonged bleeding (*see Q 8.16*) none of the above improvements can be reliably predicted for the individual woman.

  6 Less pelvic inflammatory disease (PID): like other progestogen-containing contraceptives. Confirmed by a WHO study (1985).

  7 Fewer extrauterine pregnancies, because ovulation is inhibited.

  8 Possibly fewer functional ovarian cysts overall, for the same reason (*see Q 5.61*), but this has not been well studied.

  9 Reduction in the growth of fibroids but, once again, only if oligo- or amenorrhoea is achieved.

 10 A possible reduction in the rate of endometriosis, which indeed can be treated by high-dose oral MPA or by DMPA (unless they fail to produce amenorrhoea).

 11 Overdose extremely unlikely and would not be fatal.

 12 Beneficial social effects, especially because the method is under a woman's control.

 13 Protection against endometrial cancer (*see Q 8.31*).

It is not known how many of the other benefits described for the COC (*see Q 5.57*) apply also to injectables (namely, a reduction in risk of benign breast disease, thyroid disease, rheumatoid arthritis, TSS, trichomonal vaginitis and, above all, ovarian cancer). On theoretical grounds, most are likely benefits, only waiting to be firmly established.

BENEFITS NOT (NECESSARILY) SHARED WITH THE COC

 14 Definite beneficial effects on frank sickle-cell disease (*see Q 8.15*).

 15 Reduction of aggression, mood swings and epileptic attacks: especially in patients with severe learning disabilities, DMPA is reported as very beneficial if the timing of these problems is regularly premenstrual or menstrual. Extended use by, for example, 'tricycling' (*see Qs 5.32, 5.34*) of the COC or using Cerazette or Implanon can be a way of obtaining a similar benefit, providing amenorrhoea is achieved (*see Q 5.32*).

 16 Lactation is not suppressed and might even be enhanced due to increased production of prolactin – but the POP is lower-dose and equally effective (*see Q 8.39*).

 17 Complete freedom from side-effects due to estrogen. Its mortality rate approaches very close to zero.

> These improvements are variable, and dependent on the bleeding pattern experienced by individual women.

8.14 In view of the above advantages, why has there been so much adverse publicity over the years about injectables?

Mainly because of:

■ Unfounded excessive anxiety about cancer as a result of irrelevant studies on different species (e.g. dogs). The balance of the evidence is actually favourable (*see Q 8.31*).

■ The possibility of abuse (by providers, 'pushing' the method on women or, worse, giving it without their knowledge or consent). This is a potential problem with any injection, but one that is not best solved by banning a good product.

■ The impossibility of removing the injection if side-effects occur.

Yet, overall, safety is clearly greater than with the COC, which itself is amazingly safe. Wherever injectables have been made available as a realistic choice, continuation rates are better than for most other methods.

8.15 What is the effect of DMPA on homozygous sickle-cell disease?

A careful trial in the West Indies demonstrated a highly significant improvement in the haematological picture, and a reduction in the number of painful crises, in patients treated with 3-monthly injections of DMPA. It is suggested that this could be the method of choice for both SS and SC disease.

There are theoretical reasons for believing that all progestogen-containing contraceptives would be similarly beneficial, including the POP, Cerazette, implants (*see Q 8.57*) and even perhaps the COC – although, with the last, the artificial estrogen content has its own potential disadvantages (*see Q 5.145*).

MAIN PROBLEMS AND DISADVANTAGES

8.16 What are the main disadvantages of injectables?

1 First and foremost, the fact that the *injection cannot be removed* once given. This must always be mentioned to the potential user: the method is irreversible for at least 2–3 months (depending on the injectable used) and early side-effects would therefore have to be tolerated for a long time.

2 *Disturbance of menstruation*, when it occurs, can be so marked and variable over time that it has been called 'menstrual chaos'. With reassuring counselling, *amenorrhoea* (from the outset or it may follow an early phase of bleeding) is usually very acceptable (*see Q 8.42*).

3 Possible risks of *long-term hypo-estrogenism* (*see* Q 8.23).

4 *Delay in the return*, but no actual loss, *of fertility* (*see* Q 8.38).

5 *Weight gain:* with most other contraceptives the method is often blamed unfairly, but not so with this one. Most women gain weight – up to 2–3 kg in the first year – and a few do so rapidly after the very first dose. This possibility must always be discussed with users in advance. The increase is not associated with fluid retention and diuretics are useless.

6 *Depression* (*see* Q 8.49) and other mood changes. This might be said to be the last of the 'main' problems in this list.

7 Possible unconfirmed *adverse effects on the fetus* (*see* Q 8.54).

8 *Galactorrhoea* can occur, with a raised prolactin (usually within the normal range).

9 *Mildly androgenic effects* such as acne can happen but are surprisingly uncommon.

10 *Enuresis*, rarely, has been reported as recurring in women who were enuretic at adolescence. It is unlikely that the link is causal but it might be attributable to a relaxing effect of the progestogens on smooth muscle.

11 *Subjective 'minor' side-effects.* These are many and varied, as with all hormonal methods. Some can be truly attributable to the method and in some cases they might be placebo reactions. The following have been reported:

   (a) loss of libido, vaginal dryness (relatively rare, but biologically plausible, *see* Qs 8.23 *and* 8.25)

   (b) lassitude

   (c) variable mood changes (already mentioned)

   (d) bloatedness

   (e) dizziness

   (f) breast symptoms (increase or decrease in size and tenderness)

   (g) leg cramps

   (h) headaches

   (i) acne – not frequent, because MPA is a progesterone-based molecule.

12 Local complications:

   (a) *haematoma of the injection site* (particularly in patients using anticoagulants, which are therefore a strong WHO 3 contraindication to the method, especially as the needle of an obvious alternative, Implanon, is inserted far more superficially and only once in 3 years)

   (b) *infection of the injection site.* I am aware of a legal action alleging that a frank abscess caused failure of the method. Therefore, if this rare event occurs, a repeat dose should be given immediately.

8.17 What are the effects of injectables on metabolism?

Although many studies have been reported (particularly on DMPA), they tend to be cross-sectional and poorly controlled, especially for cigarette-smoking, and might not be standardized for the time since the last injection was given, individual variation, the presence or absence of ovarian activity, and so on. Too often the studies tell us more about the users than about DMPA.

8.18 What are the effects on blood coagulation and fibrinolysis?

To summarize much research, there is no proven effect of any significance on either of these. In the WHO Collaborative Study (1998) there was a small and non-significant increase in the odds ratio for venous thromboembolism (VTE). This could have been related to selective use of the methods by women at greater risk, and to diagnostic bias.

For the present, it remains good practice to use either DMPA or NET-EN where there is a past history of VTE (WHO 2).

8.19 What are the effects on blood lipids, especially high-density lipoprotein–cholesterol (HDL-C)?

Available data about blood lipids are scanty and difficult to interpret. Most researchers have reassuringly found no effect or even a decrease in triglycerides or total cholesterol with both injectables. A few DMPA studies show a less encouraging increase in low-density lipoprotein–cholesterol (LDL-C) and decrease (of up to 15%) in HDL-C levels with DMPA. In a prospective study of NET-EN, HDL-C declined more markedly, by about 25% after the first injection, but did not change further with up to 4 years of use.

These results are hard to interpret because so many DMPA-users smoke, but they could also be at least partly related to the lower endogenous estradiol production in users of injectables. Their relation to amenorrhoea and the overall clinical significance for arterial disease are not clear (*see Qs 8.20 and 8.21* and, with regard to contraindications, *Qs 8.36 and 8.37*).

8.20 What are the effects on carbohydrate metabolism?

Some reports find an increase in insulin levels with both these injectables, which would cause some theoretical concerns, but most report no change. The development of overt diabetes in women using DMPA for contraception has not been reported.

UKMEC classifies established diabetes as WHO 3 if of more than 20 years' duration or if there is diabetic tissue damage. In my view, given the lipid changes of *Q 8.19* above, diabetes with evidence of established arterial disease, like other atherogenic states, is WHO 4 for DMPA.

8.21 Do any other surrogate tests suggest a risk of arterial wall disease?

Yes, a small study by Sorensen et al 2002 [*Circulation* 106:1646–1651], of 12 DMPA-users and 9 controls, used magnetic resonance imaging (MRI) to evaluate arterial function in the brachial artery. The results (after 1 year) suggested that endothelial function might be slightly impaired in the DMPA-users, in a manner that has been proposed as a possible surrogate marker for risk of arterial disease. The recency of this technique and its non-clinical end-point makes us wary of drawing conclusions or changing practice through this study alone (*but see Q 8.23ff*).

8.22 Are there any other metabolic effects?

In general, only minimal effects have been shown. Because all progestogens appear capable of causing attacks of acute porphyria, and especially because injectables cannot be rapidly reversed, they are absolutely contraindicated, even in latent acute porphyria (WHO 4, *see Qs 6.43 and 8.36*). Other porphyrias such as the commonest, porphyria cutanea tarda, are WHO 2 and not a problem.

Injectables do not appear adversely to affect liver function. They are metabolized by the liver but can be used safely by women with a history of jaundice or hepatitis B carrier states (WHO 2). If there is chronic cirrhosis with mild liver function test abnormality, this also would be WHO 2. But injectables should preferably not be used at all if liver function tests are currently grossly abnormal (WHO 3) – if any hormonal method were suitable, the POP would be preferred.

8.23 What is the present information on hypo-estrogenism and progestogen-only injectables?

For DMPA the evidence-base is still incomplete – and data are all but absent for NET-EN. The discussion below relates to DMPA only.

For years there has been some cause for concern, as follows:

■ It has been known since the 1970s that DMPA is a powerful suppressant of FSH as well as LH levels, so that estradiol levels in long-term users of DMPA are always on the low side, as in the follicular phase of the cycle; although after 5 years of use most are above those of postmenopausal women and do not suggest true functional insufficiency. However, in some individuals very low levels are found – well under 100 pmol/L (compare this with 150–200 pmol/L as the target bone-sparing threshold level in low-dose estrogen replacement after the menopause).

■ Estradiol levels can be very low whether women are seeing bleeds (bleeds from the endometrium in DMPA-users not being 'periods' anyway) or have complete amenorrhoea. Contrariwise, other long-term users with complete amenorrhoea have enough ovarian follicular activity for perfectly adequate estradiol levels – up to over 300 pmol/L – to be measurable.

■ It is also well established that premature menopause (idiopathic or after bilateral oophorectomy) increases the risk of acute myocardial infarction (AMI) and osteoporosis thereafter, unless the missing estrogen is replaced.

So the big question is: does prolonged hypo-estrogenism in some women through use of DMPA (with or without oligo-/amenorrhoea) lead, by analogy with premature menopause, to added risk of bone density loss or frank osteoporosis, or possibly arterial disease in those already predisposed, such as smokers?

8.24 What do we know, then, about the osteoporosis risk in long-term users of DMPA?

After more than 20 years of research but no randomized controlled trials or adequate comparative studies, there remains uncertainty – not about the fact of these variably low follicular-phase estradiol levels in DMPA-users, but about their implications for bone health. We know that:

■ Mean bone density is lower in DMPA-users than in controls in cross-sectional comparisons.

■ This finding is, like the estrogen levels, unconnected to the bleeding pattern (it may or may not occur in women experiencing either amenorrhoea or irregular bleeding).

■ Bone density increases again along with the restoration of more normal estradiol levels upon discontinuation – suggestive of a real DMPA effect, but also reassuring for reversibility (Cundy T et al 1998 *Obstetrics and Gynecology* 92:569–573). The effect might prove comparable to prolonged lactation, where some bone density loss occurs but with reversal after cessation.

■ From limited evidence, the bone mineral density in adolescent DMPA-users is lower than in controls using implants (or COCs). This has raised concern that normal *peak bone mass* that is normally fully developed by age 25 might not be achieved in young users.

Yet:

■ Long-term DMPA-using women examined after their menopause versus lifetime never-users have *not* been shown to differ in their bone densities, again suggesting recovery of bone mass after stopping.

■ No excess of limb or vertebral fractures has ever been shown in long-term DMPA-users.

Based on the above, WHOMEC therefore simply states that DMPA is WHO 2 for adolescents and for women over age 45.

American and UK drug regulators have been more cautious, however – see below.

8.25 How should prospective and long-term users of DMPA be managed, pending more data?

The CSM circular (18 November 2004) was later endorsed by the excellent publication by NICE on *Long-Acting Reversible Contraception (LARC)* [2005, RCOG Press, available at: http://guidance.nice.org.uk/CG30/niceguidance/pdf/English] and had one main recommendation, namely *'careful re-evaluation of risks and benefits in all those who wish to continue use for more than 2 years'*. I fully agree with the Faculty of SRH interpretation of this as a *regular 2-yearly reassessment in long-term users*, as summarized below:

Clinically, in the UK, the following is now advised:

UK protocol for choice and duration of use of DMPA

1 DMPA is WHO 4 if *strong risk factors* for osteoporosis already exist, such as:

   - known current osteoporosis or osteopenia
   - long-term corticosteroid treatment
   - severe malabsorption syndromes
   - secondary amenorrhoea, due to anorexia nervosa or marathon running.

   But the category could become WHO 3 if a bone scan shows no osteopenia, the risk factor has ceased, and the young woman has been obtaining either natural estrogen during normal cycling or EE via the COC.

2 **Both smoking, a known risk factor for reducing bone density, and a clear FH (family history) of osteoporosis are WHO 2 for DMPA**

3 **DMPA is WHO 2 (UKMEC), i.e. benefits outweigh risks, if** *under age 19* due to the above unconfirmed concern that it may prevent achievement of peak bone mass. Since WHO 2 means 'broadly usable' this aligns with the UK guidance (November 2004), to use DMPA first-line 'but only after other methods have been discussed' and are unsuitable or unacceptable.

4 **DMPA is also WHO 2** *above age 45* because of the possibility of incipient ovarian failure by then and as 'gentler' methods are available, such as the POP, which would be equally effective at this age. (Above 50 would be WHO 3–4.)

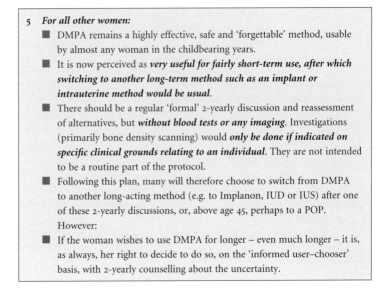

5   *For all other women:*

- DMPA remains a highly effective, safe and 'forgettable' method, usable by almost any woman in the childbearing years.
- It is now perceived as *very useful for fairly short-term use, after which switching to another long-term method such as an implant or intrauterine method would be usual*.
- There should be a regular 'formal' 2-yearly discussion and reassessment of alternatives, but *without blood tests or any imaging*. Investigations (primarily bone density scanning) would *only be done if indicated on specific clinical grounds relating to an individual*. They are not intended to be a routine part of the protocol.
- Following this plan, many will therefore choose to switch from DMPA to another long-acting method (e.g. to Implanon, IUD or IUS) after one of these 2-yearly discussions, or, above age 45, perhaps to a POP. However:
- If the woman wishes to use DMPA for longer – even much longer – it is, as always, her right to decide to do so, on the 'informed user–chooser' basis, with 2-yearly counselling about the uncertainty.

Notes:

- *African Caribbean women:* It is well established [Family Planning Masterclass, pp.87–88] that they have a higher mineral bone density at all ages. White women have a 2.5-fold greater risk of osteoporosis.
- *High BMI*: Due mainly to peripheral conversion in fat depots of androgens to estrogens, women with a BMI above 30 are another group less likely to be osteopenic than are very-low-BMI women, especially if the latter smoke or are of Asian origin.

These are other relevant factors in discussion both about initiation of DMPA in teenagers and its continuation on request for perhaps a longer rather than shorter time.

When all is said and done, there is more to DMPA than bones! And it is clearly a safer method overall than the EE-containing COC. . . .

8.26   Would you have similar concerns about long-term oligo- or amenorrhoeic users of any POP (including Cerazette), of Implanon or of the LNG-IUS?

It is recommended as an alternative in the protocol above, but are there not similar bone density concerns with long-term Implanon?

The answer is 'no' – the data are reassuring *so far*: in a non-randomized comparative study described below, Q *8.72*, after 2 years, bone densities among users of Implanon remained similar to those among users of the copper IUD. By analogy, therefore, there are no worries so far on this account with Cerazette ('oral Implanon'), either – or with the LNG-IUS (below).

8.27 What is thought to be the explanation for the difference between DMPA and other progestogen-only methods?

With DMPA the problem seems to be long-term suppression of FSH, presumably related to the relatively high blood levels achieved especially in early weeks (see *Fig. 8.1*, Q *8.5*), and, as we have seen, the occurrence of some bleeding is no guide to estrogen levels. By contrast, with Implanon and all POPs, although they also often block ovulation and corpus luteum formation, there seems generally to be sufficient FSH release to maintain enough follicular activity thereby supplying adequate estrogen for (presumed) arterial and (measured) bone health.

And with the LNG-IUS, after the first year, 85% of users are cycling normally (*see* Q *9.143ff*) – almost all are oligo- or amenorrhoeic but this is due to local effects of the LNG at the level of the end-organ, the endometrium.

8.28 But what do we know about the risk of heart attacks and other arterial diseases in long-term DMPA-users?

A report about current DMPA or POP use by WHO [*Contraception* 1998;57:315–324] reassuringly showed no statistically increased risk of VTE, or AMI or stroke: but a doubling of the risk of haemorrhagic stroke if there was established hypertension. It is unclear if this risk was a function of the hypertension alone, i.e. not increased by the contraceptive methods.

A clinically important real difference in AMI risk might only be detectable in ex-users, and many years later, because women (fortunately) have so low a risk of AMI in the childbearing years. Given also the lipid changes in Q *8.19* it is clear that more data are needed in this area, focusing on delayed effects in long-term and ex-users.

8.29 What effects do injectables have on BP?

Studies show no consistent and certainly no significant change in either systolic or diastolic BP in women using either injectable. But the limited WHO evidence in Q8.28 suggests that women who do have hypertension may have an increased risk of cardiovascular events if they use DMPA.

Interestingly, neither WHO nor the IPPF in their latest guidelines recommend regular BP measurements, aside from the first visit to assess pre-existing hypertension. In the UK it is usual to check BP rather frequently, yet 2-yearly checks would be more than adequate.

8.30 Do injectables affect neoplasia in animals?

Given enormous doses of DMPA, beagle bitches (which are by nature prone to breast lumps) can develop malignant tumours of the breast. Two out of 12 rhesus monkeys given 50 times the human contraceptive dose in a 10-year trial developed endometrial carcinoma. No cases were observed in monkeys treated with the human dose or 10 times the human dose.

The animal models (beagle bitches or rhesus monkeys) are believed by most authorities to be manifesting species-specific reactions that are not applicable to the human, and the doses used have been irrelevantly high.

8.31 What are the latest data about DMPA and cancer in the human?

The 1991 publications by WHO from good hospital-based, case–control studies in developing countries [including *International Journal of Cancer* 49:182–195] still provide the best data to date. The findings were:

- *Endometrial cancer:* a protective effect, in fact a fivefold reduction in risk. There was also an ex-use protective effect detectable for at least 8 years after cessation of DMPA use. It seems the reduction in risk is as great for DMPA as for the COC.
- *Epithelial ovarian cancer:* a protective effect as with the COC was (surprisingly) not demonstrated but there is certainly no increase in risk either. It might be that protection would be shown only in a population of DMPA-users at high risk of ovarian cancer (not so far studied).
- *Primary liver cancer:* no increased risk, and this was in countries (Thailand and Kenya) where hepatitis B is endemic.
- *Cervical cancer:* no increased risk. This is the finding of a larger and better WHO study than the earlier one reported in 1984, which showed a small association with DMPA use. It confirms the suspicion at the earlier time that the association was due to confounding by factors such as sexual activity and smoking.
- *Breast cancer: see Q 8.32.*

Overall, these results are very favourable to this much-maligned method.

8.32 Does DMPA increase the risk of breast cancer?

In the large WHO (1991) hospital-based, case–control study from five centres, reported in *The Lancet* [338:833–838], there was no link with breast cancer in the total population (869 cases, 11 890 controls), nor any increased risk with increased duration of use. The only statistically increased risk was for use in the first 4 years after initial exposure, mainly in women under 35.

There was no increase in risk among women who started DMPA more than 5 years previously.

On the one hand, DMPA might – perhaps – be bringing forward the appearance of cancers that would have become manifest later. On the other hand, it is possible that the association in the WHO study is entirely caused by detection bias; recent users (who would necessarily be younger) or their physicians being more likely to discover breast lumps in the first 4 years of DMPA use.

The 1996 CGHFBC study differs slightly, giving similar results for DMPA to those for the COC (*see Q 5.84*), i.e. a possible but *non-significant* increased risk in current users, which diminishes reassuringly to nil after 10 years in ex-users. More data are needed and the jury is still out.

8.33 Can DMPA be used in cases of trophoblastic disease?

In the UK it is advised by UKMEC that DMPA is WHO 3 and ideally best avoided until hCG is undetectable (*see Q 5.78*). Thereafter there is no objection to this method (WHO 1), which can be a very suitable means of preventing pregnancy, as is usually recommended for at least 6 months after hCG testing is negative.

8.34 Is there any evidence that injectables affect the development or growth of benign tumours?

The growth of uterine fibroids is usually inhibited, presumably because of hypo-estrogenism. Other benign tumours appear to be unaffected.

SELECTION OF USERS AND OF FORMULATIONS

8.35 For whom are injectables particularly indicated?

1 First and foremost, if a systemic, non-intercourse-related method is chosen by the woman and *other options* (particularly those containing estrogen) are *contraindicated, or disliked*. This includes:

(a) *chronic systemic diseases:* the great effectiveness of DMPA as a contraceptive often helps to outweigh the continuing uncertainty as to what effect (either way) an injectable might have on the disease. With that proviso, and given the reversibility problem, DMPA might be a possible choice (WHO 3 or WHO 2) for almost all the conditions listed as absolute (*see Q 5.136*) or relative (*see Q 5.138*) contraindications to the COC – including after VTE or with a known prothrombotic abnormality of coagulation (WHO 2), including those that are acquired in SLE and related conditions (*see Q 5.148*)

(b) to cover relevant elective surgery (*see Q 6.17*)

(c) forgetful pill-takers.

2 Women wanting hormonal contraception and on long-term enzyme-inducers, since they do not affect the efficacy of DMPA (*see Q 8.11*).

3 Women in whom *long-term progestogens are indicated anyway*, e.g. sickle-cell disease (*see Q 8.15*) and some with fibroids and endometriosis.

4 Past history of a *tubal ectopic pregnancy*: because, like the COC, it is an anovulant and will prevent pregnancy in any location (*see Q 8.13*).

5 *Epilepsy:* the frequency of seizures can sometimes be reduced.

6 At the woman's choice.

8.36 What are the absolute contraindications (WHO 4) to DMPA?

■ Past *severe arterial* diseases, or current very high risk thereof (because of the above evidence about low estrogen levels, coupled with reports of lowered HDL-C).

■ Current osteopenia, osteoporosis or any severe risk factor(s) for osteoporosis, including chronic corticosteroid treatment (>5 mg prednisolone/day).

■ Any serious adverse effect of COCs not certainly related solely to the estrogen (e.g. liver adenoma or cancer – but UKMEC classifies these as WHO 3).

■ Recent breast cancer *not* yet clearly in remission (see below).

■ Acute porphyria, even if latent, no history of actual attack (progestogens as well as estrogens are believed capable of precipitating attacks – and the injection is not 'removable').

■ Undiagnosed genital tract bleeding.

■ Actual or possible pregnancy.

■ Hypersensitivity to any component.

■ The woman's own continuing uncertainty about the safety of an injectable, even after full counselling.

8.37 What are the relative contraindications to DMPA?

Here is my list, but, as usual, the judgments of other authorities such as WHO and UKMEC may differ, to some extent. See introductory remarks at *Q 5.137*. All below are WHO 2 unless otherwise stated:

■ According to degree, except as first bullet above, arterial disease risk generally is WHO 2. This category includes hypertension once it has been diagnosed and controlled.

■ Familial hyperlipidaemia (UKMEC) and longstanding diabetes mellitus (*see Q 8.20*) are WHO 3, since other progestogen-only methods such as the POP would be preferred.

■ Short-term or lower-dose steroid treatment, recovered anorexia nervosa with normal menstrual cycling (see above – if bone density scanning is satisfactory these are usually WHO 3).

■ Under 18 or over 45 years of age are WHO 2 with respect to bone health (see above), but there are additional considerations above 45, including the diagnostic problem of any irregular bleeding (WHO 3 above age 50).

■ Active liver disease, including cirrhosis, with abnormal liver function tests – caution required (WHO 3) – but category WHO 2 with normal biochemistry.

■ Recent trophoblastic disease is WHO 3 (UKMEC) until hCG is undetectable in blood as well as urine, then WHO 1.

■ DMPA is usable in all non-acute porphyrias (WHO 2).

■ Sex-steroid-dependent cancer, including breast cancer, in complete remission is WHO 3 (after 5 years according to WHOMEC). The POP or LNG-IUS are lower-dose and more reversible, but seek the advice of the oncologist looking after your patient.

■ Unacceptability (despite reassurance) of possible menstrual irregularities, especially cultural/religious taboos – e.g. Islam and Orthodox Judaism – associated with abnormal bleeding.

■ Obesity: although this is protective against estrogen lack and further weight gain is not inevitable.

■ Past *severe* endogenous depression, especially if apparently hormone-related.

■ Planning a pregnancy in the near future – *see Q 8.38*.

■ Bleeding tendency. This is WHO 3 with respect to deep haematoma risk, minimized by extra care when injections are given. With the INR in the correct range (2–3) *warfarin treatment* may be only WHO 2 for DMPA and also in my opinion for Implanon if inserted by an expert in the correct, almost avascular, superficial location.

8.38 What effects do injectables have on future fertility?

Return of fertility is slow, especially with DMPA, but complete. In the largest study (*Fig. 8.2*), of parous women in Thailand, the mean time to conception was 9 months after the last injection. Now, the last injection has a significant antifertility effect for about 15 weeks (the 12-week injection frequency we use in the UK being set to prevent not the average but rather the most DMPA-resistant woman from conceiving). So the true delay after stopping the method is a mean of only 5.5 months, comparing very favourably with discontinuation of the COC (mean delay 3 months, *Fig. 8.2*). Underweight women regained their fertility faster.

The same study showed that 91% of DMPA-users had conceived by 2 years from discontinuation, as just defined, compared with 95% of former COC-users – not a statistically significant difference and confirming the lack of any permanent fertility loss.

Secondary amenorrhoea does persist in a minority and should be investigated and treated if it lasts for more than 9 months after the last

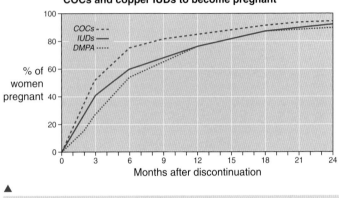

Fig. 8.2 Cumulative conception rates for women discontinuing DMPA, COCs and copper IUDs to become pregnant. *Q 8.38. Note:* researchers assumed that users 'discontinued' DMPA 15 weeks after their last injection (source: Pardthaisong T 1984 *Journal of Biosocial Science* 16:23–34).

injection (*see Qs 5.63–5.68*). This is very responsive to treatment by standard ovulation-induction methods.

8.39 What are the effects of injectables on lactation?

■ Both injectables appear to increase the volume of breast milk.
■ Most studies suggest no important change in its composition.
■ The amount of hormone transmitted to the infant in breast milk is very small, less than 0.5% of the maternal dose.

Although no long-term effects on infant growth and development have been reported, the amount of exposure to an artificial hormone is obviously greater than with the POP. In view of this minimal uncertainty, in my view it would be preferable for most lactating women in the UK to use the POP, transferring to the injectable as one option when the child is weaned. (The combination of POP plus full lactation is already almost 100% effective contraception.)

If DMPA or NET-EN *is* used in lactation, it should ideally be given 5–6 weeks after delivery, this delay being helpful to minimize bleeding problems. But it is sometimes right to give an injectable much earlier than this.

8.40 Which injectable should be chosen?

■ The natural first choice is DMPA, because its effects are better known and it is marginally more effective. The injection is less uncomfortable and only needs to be given four times a year. Moreover, NET-EN is still not licensed for long-term use.

■ Possible reasons for selecting NET-EN include:
- more bleeds, reduced likelihood of complete amenorrhoea if that state is rejected by the prospective user
- shorter time until spontaneous reversal of the effect, if unacceptable side-effects were to develop after the first injection
- more rapid return of fertility after the last injection
- less risk of marked weight gain
- if DMPA proves unsatisfactory, as an empirical second choice.

INITIAL MANAGEMENT AND FOLLOW-UP ARRANGEMENTS

8.41 What should be done at the first visit prior to giving an injectable?

■ A good medical history should be taken with special reference to the absolute and relative contraindications, especially those related to arterial disease and osteoporosis (*see Qs 8.36, 8.37*).

■ Record the weight. This is more important than with all other hormonal methods, none of which has been established as causing the weight gain for which they are so regularly blamed.

■ Record the BP. The evidence suggests it is not especially relevant to the method (*see Q 8.29*) but it is desirable as a baseline.

■ Discuss breast self-examination/awareness with a good leaflet – not leading to a nerve-racking ritual. Offer to examine the breasts only if she has any concern.

■ Carry out a pelvic examination only if there are clinical grounds – i.e. rarely – and take a cervical smear only if due. A bimanual examination might be clinically indicated after childbirth to exclude the possibility of retained products.

8.42 What is the minimum information that should be conveyed at counselling?

Failure to counsel adequately has been the main cause of adverse publicity in the UK. The following should be discussed:

■ *Impossibility of rapid reversal* if any side-effect was unacceptable.

■ *Amenorrhoea:* as Dr Wilson of Glasgow has declared, reassurance that a 'monthly clean-out' of the 'bad blood' is not necessary for good health might make all the difference between happy acceptance and chronic anxiety and dissatisfaction.

■ *The possibility of frequent irregular bleeding:* reassure the woman that medical advice is available if this should occur (*see Q 8.47*).

■ *Weight gain:* this is not inevitable. If potential users are forewarned in a very positive way, experience shows they can sometimes succeed in resisting the DMPA-caused weight increase by lifestyle change, including taking more exercise.

■ *Delay in fertility return:* women should be told that on average it might take 9 months from the time of the last injection to conceive (*see* Q 8.38) but even longer is possible.

■ *Theoretical long-term risks:* the cancer balance seems on present evidence to be rather favourable to the method (*see* Q 8.31). The issue of *osteoporosis* in my view should be raised at this stage primarily if there are contraindicating WHO 4 or WHO 3 risk factors (*see* Qs 8.36, 8.37) – otherwise it can wait for 2 years!

■ Answer her questions and *supply the fpa's leaflet:* in addition to the licensed product information leaflet in the pack.

8.43 How are the injectables given?

By deep intramuscular injection. In the UK this is usually from the preloaded syringe into the upper outer quadrant of the buttock, outer thigh or (less often, because there is less muscle there) into the deltoid. Avoid major nerves and aspirate with care before injection of the dose. Warfarin treatment is WHO 2 or WHO 3 if a recent satisfactory INR test is not available.

The DMPA ampoule should be very thoroughly shaken to remove any sediment. NET-EN should be warmed to body temperature. The site of either injection should not be massaged.

See also Q 8.9. If any of the dose is spilled, the amount lost should be carefully estimated and normally replaced by another complete injection.

8.44 What are the requirements for successful monitoring and follow-up?

■ Careful planning of the date for the next dose. Try to avoid the complexities of Q 8.52 by explaining that if a planned date proves inconvenient, it is far better she requests the next dose a week or two early than be late. DMPA may always be given *early*: UKMEC says up to 2 weeks early, though up to 4 weeks early would not be unsafe.

■ Equally important is the ready access between injections to medical advice by telephone or in person, to deal with any anxieties arising.

■ BP needs checking at most 2-yearly (*see* Q 8.29) and weight at each visit in the first year; but thereafter, if stable, mainly at the patient's request.

■ Cervical screening is performed according to local policies.

8.45 To what age can use of injectables be continued?

The implications and management of prolonged use is discussed in Qs 8.23–8.25.

At around age 45 (when the method is WHO 2 for all), a review is appropriate. DMPA becomes at least WHO 3 by then, or possibly at an earlier age, if there are any arterial cardiovascular or osteoporosis risk factors. If the user is worried about efficacy, she can be informed that the POP becomes 'at least as strong as the COC' above 45.

DMPA is a 'contraceptive overkill' above the mean age of the menopause (50–51).

8.46 How can the menopause be diagnosed?

Juliato et al in *Contraception* 2007;76:282–286 showed that FSH may give a tentative hint, if elevated above age 50. DMPA then still has to be discontinued and alternative contraception practised (*see Q 11.42ff*). Transferring to another method at about age 45 is therefore normally preferable, as just suggested.

MANAGEMENT OF SIDE-EFFECTS AND PRACTICAL PROBLEMS

8.47 How should non-acceptable, prolonged or much-too-frequent bleeding be managed?

First, check that it does not have a non-DMPA-related cause, by examination for retained products of conception, polyps, *Chlamydia* or carcinoma. An ultrasound scan might be required. If the uterus is firm and non-tender, with a normal closed cervical os, it is unlikely that the bleeding has any cause other than as a side-effect of the injectable. *Drugs?* enquiry should be made, but, by rights, with DMPA *no interacting drug should cause bleeding* (*see Q 8.11*).

- Advise that this bleeding has a better prognosis than with implants, usually being an early problem that is then generally followed by amenorrhoea after 3–6 months.
- If it does not resolve, the next injection may be given early (but not less than 4 weeks since the last dose). More frequent injections, e.g. 10-weekly, often speed up the appearance of amenorrhoea.
  However:
- Clinical experience suggests that giving additional *cyclical* estrogen is more usually successful. The rationale for providing estrogen cyclically is to thicken an atrophic endometrium and then produce some 'pharmacological curettages', i.e. withdrawal bleeds designed to clear out the existing endometrium that is bleeding in an unacceptable way – in the hope that a 'better' endometrium and a more acceptable bleeding pattern will be obtained post treatment. The woman should be pre-warned that this is unlikely to be so good as during the short-term COC, but that it might be one she will find 'OK'.

■ Possible treatments are:
  – EE 30 μg (as such, or more usually within a pill formulation such as Microgynon 30) given for 21 days followed by 7 pill-free days, usually for three cycles. If an acceptable bleeding pattern does not follow when this is discontinued, in selected cases courses of estrogen may be repeated. Or:
  – if the woman has a WHO 4 contraindication to EE, one might try an alternative that, in a pilot study, was effective in stopping a single bleeding episode with *Implanon* (*see* Q 8.70), namely doxycycline 100 mg bd for 5 days. The benefit, which is likely only to be short term, is believed to be mediated through certain enzymes in the endometrium. It is probably independent of the antibiotic's beneficial effect on chlamydial endometritis: but one should test for this first, as usual with irregular bleeding.

Iron treatment is very rarely indicated to correct anaemia (*see* Q 8.13(5)). The actual amount lost even over many days is usually not great. But irregular bleeding remains the most common reason for discontinuing the method. The problem is most pronounced postpartum, often helped by delaying the first dose.

8.48 How should amenorrhoea be managed?

■ Pregnancy should be eliminated as the (very rare) cause.
■ The woman should be counselled as in Q 8.42. I find it helpful to say, also, 'there's no blood coming away because there is no blood to come away'. The establishment of prolonged amenorrhoea can often be the best solution for women with bleeding problems. It is duration of use not the presence or absence of amenorrhoea that is relevant in the protocol of Q 8.25 above.
■ One cycle of the COC (or a natural estrogen) will usually cause a withdrawal 'period' and this helps to reassure some women.

8.49 What about other minor side-effects?

Management can only be empirical, for example, switching to the other injectable or another method. Weight gain is the most common complaint: dieting is possible but difficult. Diuretics are useless. Pyridoxine treatment can be tried if depression is reported (*see* Q 6.23), but there have been no good studies – moreover, the depression is not uncommonly related more to factors within the user herself than to her contraceptive.

8.50 What symptoms should lead an injectable-user to take urgent medical advice?

There are none known that are specifically related to the method, unlike with the COC or POP. There are sporadic reports of massive uterine 'flooding', not necessarily causally related.

8.51 Are prolonged immobilization or major surgery contraindications to injectables?

There is no need to discontinue either DMPA or NET-EN before any kind of surgery. Indeed, an injectable can be a very satisfactory option to replace the combined pill for women at high risk of pregnancy while on the waiting list for major surgery (*see Q 6.17*).

8.52 How should one handle the problem of overdue injections? How can one maintain contraception without avoidably risking fetal exposure to the drug?

Being overdue is a common but difficult practical problem. Even if the woman is not amenorrhoeic, any bleeds she has give unreliable information about when she ovulates. Waiting 'till the next period' risks the woman conceiving during a potentially very long wait (*see Q 8.38*)!

According to WHO and UKMEC, there is a full 2 weeks of leeway for late injections with both injectables, so the late DMPA dose might simply be given at 14 weeks. The manufacturer of DMPA is much more cautious. Due to sporadic reports of failures, my own current advice is a compromise, with a bit more caution beyond 13 weeks than UKMEC. See Box below (subtract 4 weeks or 28 days from all numbers if the injectable is NET-EN).

> **Protocol for late injection, assuming continuing unprotected intercourse**
>
> ■ From day 85 to day 91 (13th week), give the injection. No pregnancy testing, and no added precautions. (The SPC advises the latter when only 5 days late; but just giving the next dose must be acceptable, given that in many countries '3-monthly', which is every 13 weeks, is the usual injection frequency!)
>
> ■ From day 92 to day 98 (14th week), give the injection, plus advice to abstain or use additional contraceptive protection for the next 7 days. Hormonal emergency contraception (EC, *Q 10.6ff*) is an option for discussion, but the risk of ovulation is low. Pregnancy testing is unnecessary (too early to be positive).
>
> ■ Beyond day 98 (end of 14th week), EC may be indicated: this depends on the woman's coital history. With or without EC, the next injection is best postponed, but not for long: if possible, make a deal with her that she will either abstain or use condoms with greater care than ever before, UNTIL there has been a total of 14 days since the last sexual exposure. If a sensitive (20 IU/L) pregnancy test on an early morning urine is then negative, this adequately excludes an implantation.
>
>   – the next dose can be given as usual plus the usual advice for 7 further days of abstinence or barrier contraception; and
>
>   – a follow-up pregnancy test in a further 2 weeks is wise.

> ■ NB: If the woman and her partner are not prepared to abstain or use condoms for the necessary days to reach 14 since her last sex, a useful compromise is to provide the POP (e.g. Cerazette) for that time and then proceed as above. (The teratogenic risks to a fetus exposed to the POP have been established as very low.)

In all circumstances, counsel the woman regarding possible failure and the need for later pregnancy testing if there is doubt.

What should NOT happen is the woman who is over 2 weeks late with her injection being told to 'go away until you have your next period'!

8.53 Beyond 14 weeks, what about the option of just giving the next dose, along with due warnings to the woman?

In rare cases, if a continuing sexually active woman at high risk of conception without her DMPA absolutely refuses to follow the policy just described (*see* Q 8.52), it might sometimes be acceptable (given a negative ultrasensitive pregnancy test at the time) to give the next dose anyway, plus a supply of condoms for the next 7 days. There should certainly be recorded warnings of the (low) risk of fetal harm along with 100% follow-up. Beyond 14 weeks this would normally be *without* giving postcoital levonorgestrel.

8.54 What are the risks if a fetus is exposed to injectables?

■ There is no evidence of an increase in ectopic or miscarriage rates.

■ There is some concern that offspring of women exposed to DMPA during pregnancy, especially in the 4 weeks after an injection, are at increased risk of low birth weight and subsequent infant mortality. But it has been suggested this could be due to confounding, e.g. by social class of the users.

■ Masculinization of the female fetus, particularly transient enlargement of the clitoris, and a possible increase in the incidence of hypospadias in males exposed to MPA and similar hormones have been reported. But no serious fetal malformation risks have been established with the very low doses used for contraception in DMPA and NET-EN. Meaningful conclusions about what must be very low potential teratogenic risks are unlikely ever to be reached because proceeding to term after exposure to injectables is such a rare event.

Every effort must of course continue to be made to prevent all fetal exposure (*see* Q 8.53).

8.55   Are there any known risks or benefits for ex-users of injectables?

There are no established teratogenic effects on pregnancies among recent ex-users of injectables. The only known problem is prolonged amenorrhoea and delayed return of fertility (*see Q 8.38*). There is a definite ex-use (as well as during-use) protective effect against carcinoma of the endometrium.

SUBDERMAL IMPLANTS

BACKGROUND AND MECHANISMS

8.56   Subdermal implants – is this route of contraception still worth offering, since Norplant?

It is sadly true of Norplant that the media, combined with legal action, destroyed public and professional confidence in the USA and UK in what, since 1993, had been a very satisfactory option for many women. But the implant route is far from defunct; it is being used by over 11 million women worldwide (according to WHO estimates).

Implants contain a progestogen in a slow-release carrier, made either of dimethylsiloxane (as in Norplant with six implants and the very similar two-rod Norplant II, now called Jadelle) or ethylene vinyl acetate (as in Implanon). Implanon is now the only marketed implant in the UK. Its main features are summarized in *Table 7.2*, pp. 294–295. See also FSRH Guidance (2008), progestogen-only Implants: www.fsrh.org.

8.57   What is Implanon? And what are its pharmacokinetics?

It is a single 40-mm rod, just 2 mm in diameter, inserted far more simply and quickly than Norplant (*Fig. 8.3*). The implant contains 68 mg of etonogestrel – the name for the active metabolite of desogestrel previously known as 3-keto-desogestrel. This is dispersed in an ethylene vinyl acetate (EVA) matrix and covered by a 0.06-mm rate-limiting EVA membrane.

After the insertion of Implanon, etonogestrel is rapidly absorbed into the circulation. Ovulation-inhibiting concentrations are reached within 1 day. Maximum serum concentrations (between 472 and 1270 pg/mL) are reached within 1 to 13 days. The release rate of the implant decreases with time from about 60–70 µg to a steady 30–40 µg per day. As a result, serum concentrations decline over the first few months. By the end of the first year, a mean concentration of approximately 200 pg/mL (range 150–261 pg/mL) is measured, which slowly decreases to 156 pg/mL (range 111–202 pg/mL) by the end of its licensed duration of use (3 years). Lower

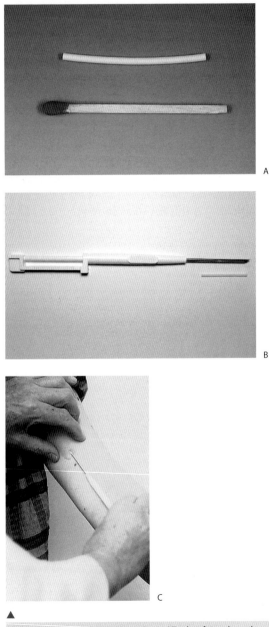

Fig. 8.3 Implanon. *Q 8.57. Note:* picture (C) taken from *above* the patient.

levels are noted in women of higher body mass (*see* Q 8.61). The ovulation-inhibiting blood level is about 90 pg/mL.

8.58   What is the mechanism of action of Implanon?

Implanon works primarily by ovulation inhibition, supplemented mainly by the usual sperm-blocking mucus effect of progestogens. Releasing as it does the chief active metabolite of desogestrel, in some ways it may usefully be considered as 'Cerazette through the skin', though it is in practice more effective than the latter.

If a woman develops regular cycles on Implanon, as with Cerazette this suggests that the anovular effect is no longer operative and she is now relying only on the mucus effect. This fact might affect management, if avoidance of pregnancy is more than usually crucial or there is another factor that might affect efficacy (such as very gross obesity, Q 8.61).

8.59   How is Implanon inserted? And by whom?

To answer the second question first: it is fully accepted (see LARC Guideline on NICE website) that Nurse Practitioners are entirely appropriate in this role. The best person to insert is someone who has been well trained and thereafter maintains his/her expertise by ongoing experience. In the UK, the best training is obtainable through the Faculty of SRH. The manufacturer (Organon) can provide names of Faculty-approved trainers.

- ■ Implanon is inserted under local anaesthesia, subdermally but very superficially under the skin over the biceps, medially in the upper arm 6–8 cm above the elbow crease, from a dedicated sterile preloaded applicator by a simple injection-and-withdrawal technique – aided by the blunt bevel of its cleverly shaped wide-bore needle.
- ■ Current teaching, contrary to the SPC, is to insert superficial to the biceps muscle and *anterior* to the groove between the triceps and biceps, well away from the neurovascular bundle. (This policy follows cases like one of my own, a difficult removal (under ultrasound control) when a too-deep Implanon was partially imbedded in the neurovascular bundle and pulsating in time with the artery . . .)
- ■ If the insertion follows removal in a woman who wishes to continue the method, it is best not to reinsert in exactly the same site, but rather 1–2 mm anteriorly, along a new line parallel to the previous implant.
- ■ Although this implant is much easier than Norplant both to insert or remove, specific training (on a 'model arm', then live) is essential: and cannot be adequately obtained from any book.

EFFECTIVENESS AND REVERSIBILITY

8.60 How effective is Implanon?

In the pre-marketing trials, Implanon had the unique distinction of an apparently zero failure rate. In 2003 the manufacturer's estimate of true failures from among all reported was a mere 13 worldwide, with about 1 million units sold. The first-year failure rate in 'perfect use' (which of course is almost identical to 'typical use') is now estimated as <1 in 1000 insertions (shown as <0.1% failures at 1 year in *Table 1.2*, p. 14).

Nearly all 'failures' that have been reported either had had the insertion during a conception cycle or were failures to insert at all (hence the advice always to palpate the Implanon in situ just after insertion) or were caused by drug interactions (*Q 8.62*).

8.61 What is the effect of high body mass on efficacy and should this affect management?

- In the pre-marketing studies, blood levels were definitely lower in heavier women. Yet, presumably because of the very high margin of efficacy of Implanon, failures have not been shown subsequently to correlate with BMI. So UKMEC classifies BMI >30 as WHO 1.
- *Clinically:* Implanon may be offered without restriction to very overweight women, among whom both the COC and Evra have a high VTE risk and the latter has a proven high failure rate. Although they have more subcutaneous tissue in the arm, they are fortunately not more prone to 'lost' implants, provided there is correct subdermal placement.
- *Earlier replacement?* Because of those lower blood levels, the manufacturer's SPC says 'consider' this in the third year of use by 'heavier' women. Assuming the reduced effect relates to dilution in a greater amount of total body water (*see Q 7.15*), I would consider reimplanting sooner only in young presumed highly fertile women *weighing more than 100 kg*. Note this is based on weight not BMI. An alternative would be additional contraception (e.g. condoms). The trigger for either action would *only* be if she began to cycle regularly in the third year (suggesting reliance solely on the mucus effect).

8.62 How do enzyme-inducer drugs affect Implanon?

The SPC states that hepatic enzyme inducers may be expected to lower the blood levels of etonogestrel, but there have been no specific interaction studies. Therefore, women on short-term treatment with any of these drugs are advised to use a barrier method in addition and (because reversal of enzyme induction always takes time) for 28 days thereafter.

During *long-term enzyme-inducer drug treatment*, Organon makes only one recommendation: transfer to a non-hormonal method and removal of the Implanon. This seems a bit wasteful and may be resisted by satisfied users; moreover, those in monogamous relationships may reject the long-term use of barriers. So, despite the absence of specific trials, one might instead consider compensating for the enzyme induction. Fitting a second Implanon or a supplementary daily Cerazette are options on a 'named-patient' basis, p. 553. Theoretically, a preplanned early replacement policy should also maintain effectiveness. As a guide, in *normal* users, at 12–18 months the mean etonogestrel blood levels are still around twice those needed to suppress ovulation. The return of regular cycles is a useful practical hint that the method might be less effective (*see Q 8.58*): seemingly confirmed by a case report [*Journal of Family Planning and Reproductive Health Care* 2007;33:277–278] of an HIV-positive woman on an enzyme-inducing antiretroviral drug who started having regular cycles from the 23rd month and conceived an ectopic pregnancy at 30 months. Nevertheless, if an early replacement is planned, it would be safest to record the woman's understanding that, as a means of compensating for enzyme induction, this practice is only theoretical and unlicensed (p. 553).

Therefore, since long-term users of enzyme-inducer drugs do so well with DMPA or the LNG-IUS (or a copper IUD), these are better options. Antibiotics, unless enzyme-inducing, pose no interaction problems.

Regarding the possible effects of Implanon on other drugs, specifically lamotrigine, ciclosporin and warfarin: *see Qs 5.46 and Q 8.12.*

8.63 How is Implanon removed and are its effects fully reversible?

Reversal is normally simple – and there is no evidence of it causing subsequent reduced fertility.

■ The effects are rapidly reversible. Compared with DMPA this is an advantage which is not intuitive and so is worth emphasizing. After removal, serum etonogestrel levels were undetectable within 1 week; hence advise that return of fertility is essentially immediate.

■ Under local anaesthesia, steady digital pressure on the proximal end of the Implanon with a 2-mm incision over the distal end leads to delivery of that end of the rod, removal being completed by grasping it with mosquito forceps.

■ Again, *training* for removal is crucial, using the 'model arm' and then live under supervision.

■ *Removal problems:* can be minimized by good training, in both the insertion and removal techniques. *Difficult removals* correlate with initially too-deep insertion. Beware particularly of the thin or very muscular woman with very little subcutaneous tissue. Insertion can then easily allow the tip of the rod to enter the (biceps) muscle, with deep migration following.

■ Specialized ultrasound techniques are required to localize a 'lost' Implanon and removal may need to be done by a visiting expert, possibly under ultrasound control: therefore Organon should be contacted for advice in all such cases.

■ Research is in progress at the Margaret Pyke Centre and elsewhere to evaluate a new radio-opaque Implanon with an improved inserter system.

ADVANTAGES AND INDICATIONS

8.64 What are the indications for, and the particular advantages of, Implanon?

The main indication is the woman's desire for a convenient and completely 'forgettable' yet at all times rapidly reversible method, as effective as, but without the finality of, sterilization, which is independent of intercourse: especially when other options are contraindicated or disliked.

Advantages include the following:

■ There is a long duration of action with one treatment (3 years), and high continuation rates.

■ There is no initial peak dose given orally to the liver.

■ Blood levels are low and steady, rather than fluctuating (as with the POP) or initially too high (as with injectables); this, with the previous point, means metabolic changes are minimal and believed negligible.

■ Implanon is estrogen-free, and therefore definitely usable if there is a history of VTE (WHO 2) or *migraine with aura* (WHO 2) – *see Q 5.158*.

■ Median systolic and diastolic BPs were unchanged in trials for up to 4 years.

■ Being an anovulant, special indications include past ectopic pregnancy and as a possibility to treat menstrual disorders, although the outcome is not reliably beneficial (bleeding patterns are unpredictable – see below).

■ Long-term health benefits (e.g. on gynaecological cancers) are possible, similar to those already established for the COC and DMPA: but the method is too new for there to be any evidence either way to date.

DISADVANTAGES AND CONTRAINDICATIONS

8.65 What local adverse effects have been reported?

■ Infection of the site.

■ Scarring (very rare).

■ Expulsion.

- Migration and difficult removal (see above)
- Local itching.

Minor systemic side-effects are dealt with below (*Q. 8.71*).

8.66 What are absolute contraindications (WHO 4) to the insertion of Implanon?

Contraindications are similar to those of Cerazette, which contains the same progestogen.

- Any serious adverse effect of COCs not certainly related solely to the estrogen (e.g. *liver adenoma or cancer*: UKMEC is more permissive, WHO 3).
- *Recent breast cancer* not yet clearly in remission (if so, *see Q 8.67* below).
- *Acute porphyria with history of actual attack* precipitated by hormones; otherwise WHO 3.
- Known or suspected *pregnancy*.
- *Undiagnosed genital tract bleeding.*
- *Hypersensitivity* to any component.

The manufacturer adds 'severe hepatic disease' and 'active venous thromboembolic disorder', which are both classified by UKMEC as WHO 3. There is actually no evidence that Implanon (like all other progestogen-only methods) can increase VTE risk.

8.67 What are the relative contraindications?

First, those which in my view are WHO 3:

- *Acute porphyria, latent*, with no previous attack. The Porphyria Centres tend to classify this like DMPA as WHO 4, being doubtless unaware how quickly Implanon can be reversed in the event of a severe attack. However, it would indeed be WHO 4 if expertise in removal was not readily available. Implanon is usable in all the *non-acute porphyrias*.
- Current *severe liver disorder* with persistent biochemical change.
- *Recent trophoblastic disease* until hCG is undetectable in blood as well as urine; then WHO 1.
- *Sex-steroid-dependent cancer*, chiefly breast cancer, in complete remission (WHO advises after 5 years). In all cases, agreement of the relevant hospital consultant should be obtained and the woman's autonomy respected. Record that she understands it is unknown whether progestogen alone in Implanon alters the recurrence risk.
- *Enzyme-inducers* – discussed above (another method such as DMPA, IUD or LNG-IUS would normally be preferable).
- Past symptomatic (painful) functional ovarian cysts – *might* recur using Implanon, especially in the third year with lower blood levels.

Weaker relative contraindications (WHO 2):

- *Past VTE or severe risk factors for VTE*: in practice, this would more often be an indication (see above).
- *Risk factors for arterial disease*: more than one risk factor can be present.
- *Current liver disorder*, with normal biochemistry.
- Most other chronic severe systemic diseases: indeed most are WHO 1.
- Unacceptability of irregular menstrual bleeding – which remains a problem with all progestogen-only methods, certainly including Implanon.

THE COUNSELLING AND INSERTION VISITS

8.68   What is the current advice concerning the timing of Implanon insertions, and therefore the implications for counselling?

- In the woman's natural cycle, day 1–5 is the usual timing; if any *later* than day 5 (in which case there should have been no sexual exposure up to that day), UKMEC recommends additional contraception for 7 days. My personal recommendation is for condom use for seven days when Implanon is inserted on day 3 or later, as with the COC: for fear of an unusually early ovulation in that cycle.
- If a woman is on an anovulant method (COC or Cerazette or DMPA), the implant can be inserted at any time with the current method discontinued immediately (or overlapped with the DMPA or to the end of the current pack, as preferred).

Clinical implications:

Insertions only during the above tiny natural-cycle window for women who are not abstaining are a logistic and conception-risk nightmare! Not to mention complicating any arrangements for several clients at a training session. . . . So, a useful practice tip is *routinely* to recommend use of an anovulant method (i.e. one of those at the second bullet above), at counselling, for use from then until the Implanon insertion. The best of the options is the COC, if acceptable, since the other two so often cause irregular bleeding in early weeks of use. If the COC is chosen, it *may* help to run on packets (as in 'tricycling'), so the implant is placed during already-established amenorrhoea.

Timing in other circumstances:

- Following delivery (not breastfeeding), insertion on about day 21 is recommended. If later and still amenorrhoeic, pregnancy risk should be excluded (*see Q.11.22*), and 7 days' added precautions advised.

■ If fully breastfeeding, insert after day 21 or in WHO's view after 6 weeks, with no need for added contraception for 7 days. A study from Thailand showed that even just after insertion, when the mean release rate was highest at 67 μg of etonogestrel per day, the amount ingested by the infant would never be greater than a negligible 10–20 ng/kg/day.

■ Following first- or second-trimester abortion or miscarriage, immediate insertion is best on the day of surgically induced abortion (or the second part of a medical abortion); or it can be up to 5 days later.

    If insertion is delayed by more than 5 days later, an added method such as condoms is recommended for 7 days.

■ If an IUD or LNG-IUS is in use, insert at any time and leave the intrauterine method in situ until the next period starts or for a minimum of 7 days (*see Q 9.13*).

At the counselling visit:

■ Explain whatever applies from the above and recommend an anovulant method, preferably the COC taken continuously, until the insertion visit.

■ Explain likely changes to the bleeding pattern and the possibility also of 'hormonal' side-effects (see below). This discussion should, as always, be backed by a good leaflet, such as the fpa one, and be well documented.

ONGOING SUPERVISION AND MANAGEMENT OF SIDE-EFFECTS

8.69 What is important during follow-up for Implanon?

First, no treatment-specific follow-up is actually necessary (including no need for BP checks). The SPC recommends one visit at 3 months, but the user can be told to cancel this if all is well. More important is an explicit 'open-house' policy, so the woman knows she can return at any time to discuss possible side-effects whether general (*Q 8.71*) or local (*Q 8.65*).

A 'credit card' or other reminder is important, so she does not forget to arrange a replacement implant if she wishes to continue the method beyond 3 years.

Avoid always any provider pressure to persevere if the woman really wants the implant removed (the standard for the maximum waiting time for removal should be no more than 2 weeks).

8.70 What about bleeding problems, their incidence and management?

In trials comparing Implanon with the old six-implant Norplant, the bleeding patterns were in fact more irregular with the former.

■ Amenorrhoea is significantly more common, as expected for an anovulant method. Reassure re this (*Q 8.48*) in advance.

■ About a quarter of women report infrequent bleeding and spotting.

■ Normal cycling is reported by a small proportion of users, increasing in the third year.

■ However, the combined rate for the more annoying 'frequent bleeding and spotting' and 'prolonged bleeding and spotting' is of the order of 20% at 6 months. Some improvement can be expected up till then, but irregular bleeding patterns with Implanon tend to remain irregular.

CLINICAL MANAGEMENT

With reassurance, most women are happy to accept one of the patterns in the first three bullet points above. For the fourth group, perseverance up to 6 months may help, but is rewarded less often than with DMPA.

After eliminating unrelated causes for the bleeding (as for DMPA, *Q 8.47*), including the possibility that someone has prescribed an interacting drug:

■ The best short-term treatment is cyclical estrogen therapy to produce some endometrial proliferation and 'pharmacological curettages' (i.e. withdrawal bleeds), on a similar basis to the regimen above for DMPA (*Q 8.47*). This may most easily be provided by three cycles of Mercilon or Marvelon, after which the bleeding may (or sometimes may not!) become acceptable.

As before (*Q 8.47*), the plan should be explained to the woman, who should also understand that it is not certain to work. Courses may be repeated if an acceptable bleeding pattern does not follow.

Alternatively:

■ If the woman has a WHO 4 contraindication to EE, an option that was shown to be effective short term is doxycycline 100 mg bd for 5 days. In a pilot study [Weisberg E et al 2006 *Human Reproduction* 21:295–302] this was more effective than placebo in terminating a single episode of prolonged bleeding. The benefit is believed to be mediated through matrix metalloproteinase enzymes in the endometrium, probably independently of an effect on chlamydial endometritis: but one should test for *Chlamydia* first, as usual with all irregular bleeding. Unfortunately, clinical experience so far suggests that bleeding tends to recur, soon after a doxycycline course ends.

■ Some clinicians report success from use of an added Cerazette tablet daily for a few weeks at a time (unlicensed use, see p. 553).

8.71 What are the reported minor side-effects with Implanon?

■ *Reported* but *not proven*, minor side-effects were:
 – acne (but sometimes this improved . . .)
 – headache

- abdominal pain (possibly related to functional cysts?)
- breast pain
- 'dizziness'
- mood changes (depression, emotional lability)
- libido decrease
- hair loss.

■ *Weight gain*: in the pre-marketing RCT, the mean body weight increase over 2 years was 2.6% with Implanon and 2.9% with Norplant, while in a parallel study, similar users of an IUD showed weight increases of 2.4% in the same timescale. Unlike DMPA, causation of the weight gain that some individuals attribute to Implanon has not been established.

8.72 What, if any, are the effects of Implanon on bone density?

Since Implanon suppresses ovulation and does not supply any estrogen, the same questions as with DMPA arise over possible hypo-estrogenism However, it appears that, like Cerazette and other POPs, the suppression of FSH levels with Implanon is less complete, allowing higher follicular estrogen levels.

In a non-randomized comparative study, no bone density changes or differences in the means, ranges or standard errors were detected between 44 users of Implanon and 29 users of copper IUDs over 2 years, which is reassuring. Pending more data, women who discontinue DMPA on the basis of the bone density protocol at *Q 8.25* above may very reasonably transfer to using Implanon – they can be told it is 'rather like having Depo-Provera every 3 years . . .'.

8.73 What are other possible routes for contraceptive hormones?

Subcutaneous DMPA (DMPA-SC) is given in a dose of 104 mg every 12 weeks, with the potential to self-inject. It is marketed in North America as depo-subQ provera 104. Despite the one-third lower dose than standard DMPA, there were no pregnancies in 720 women over 1 year, including among the 44% of study subjects who were overweight (26%) or obese (18%); 55% were amenorrhoeic at the end of 1 year [Jain J et al 2004 *Contraception* 70:269–275; www.depo-subqprovera104.com]. There is a suggestion that it *may* affect bone density less than DMPA 150 mg.

For completeness, one should also mention the rectal, transnasal and sublingual routes, all of which are in current use for other drugs. There are at present no known plans for routine contraception by those routes.

PQ **PATIENT QUESTIONS**

QUESTIONS ASKED BY USERS

Most questions asked are about DMPA, or Depo-Provera, as it is much better known by the general public than implants are.

8.74 What are in practice the most effective purely hormonal contraceptives currently available?

Implants and injectables. The COC and the POP and the patch all fail far more often – through human error.

8.75 Do injectables cause cancer in women?

This currently seems very unlikely and one cancer (of the lining of the womb) is now proved to be less frequent (*see Qs. 8.30–8.33*).

8.76 But is it safe? How does the safety (freedom from health risk) of Depo-Provera compare with 'the pill'?

Overall, because it doesn't contain estrogen, its safety is believed to be greater than that of the combined pill. No deaths have ever been clearly blamed upon it (*see Q 8.14*).

8.77 Why are some people so opposed to Depo-Provera?

Mainly because of its potential for abuse and the fact that if side-effects occur – even though they are fewer overall than with the pill – the drug's action cannot be reversed once given. You have to wait for the last injection to wear off (*see Q 8.16*).

8.78 So is it a 'last resort' method?

No! In the UK its licence used to require it to be used only after very special counselling along with the special package leaflet. But it is now approved as a 'first-line' option.

8.79 Can I be too young to be given Depo-Provera?

Some doctors are reluctant to give it to very young teenagers who are just beginning their normal menstrual cycle. Up to age 18 it is used a bit cautiously (WHO 2). But if a young person does not want to or should not take the COC or Cerazette, injectables or the implant Implanon would normally be preferable to inserting an IUD or Mirena for a teenager.

8.80 Won't I put on a lot of weight?

Depo-Provera unfortunately does seem to increase people's appetites. But forewarned is forearmed! Experience shows that if you watch your diet it is possible to avoid gaining much weight, especially if you also start taking more exercise. Putting on weight is less likely if you start off being on the thin side.

8.81   Can I be too old to be given Depo-Provera?

Over the age of 45, injectables are stronger contraceptives than are really required and there is an increasing risk of disease of the arteries and of osteoporosis. Many other good choices are now available, so other methods are usually preferable, especially in smokers (*see Qs 8.19 and 6.50*).

8.82   Where (on the body) is the injection given?

Usually into the upper outer region of the buttocks, on either side, but it can sometimes be given into the shoulder or thigh muscles.

8.83   Why can't the injection be given right after having my baby?

It *can* be, but if given too soon it tends to cause more bleeding problems in the weeks after childbirth. These are less if it is given at about 5–6 weeks but because it does not have any thrombosis risks it can also be given much earlier, if you are prepared to accept some extra irregular bleeding.

8.84   How long does the injection last? And what if I forget to have the next one?

Officially they last for 12 weeks, and each injection should be on time. If you are overdue a dose, abstain from sex or use condoms, although if you forget that too, up to 14 weeks something can still be done about it (*see Q 8.52*). Although some women can become pregnant if they are just a few days overdue, others (and we do not know who they are in advance) go on being contracepted by the previous injection for much longer (*see Q 8.85*).

8.85   How far ahead should I discontinue injections if planning another baby?

You should plan for up to 1 year after the last injection because it is quite usual (and nothing to worry about) for conception to be delayed that long. But in fact you might well conceive much sooner.

8.86   Excess bleeding – will it harm me in any way if I can live with it? And what if my periods stop altogether?

The short answer to the first question is 'no'. You ought to be examined to eliminate any cause not related to the Depo-Provera. A blood test is sometimes done to check that you are not anaemic. Some treatments can be tried to stop the bleeding (*see Q 8.47*). Otherwise, if you can live with an unpredictable bleeding pattern, it will do you no harm. If you choose to have intercourse during bleeding, that too is medically harmless.

Usually after about the second injection the bleeding stops completely – and this too is OK, not a medical problem at all if you are happy about it (*see Q 8.47*).

Intrauterine devices and systems

9

PAIN AND BLEEDING

PATIENT INFORMATION AND FOLLOW-UP ARRANGEMENTS

BACKGROUND AND MECHANISMS

9.1 How would you define an intrauterine device?

This is any solid object that is wholly retained within the uterine cavity for the purpose of preventing pregnancy. Such devices are usually inserted via the cervical canal and might have marker thread(s) attached, which are visible at the external os. There are three main types with frames: inert, copper-bearing and hormone-releasing (often called 'systems'). There are now also two frameless (implantable) varieties: copper-bearing (GyneFix being the sole representative thus far) and hormone-releasing.

9.2 Should they be abbreviated IUD or IUCD?

Underlying this question is the possibility of confusion of 'intrauterine device' with 'intrauterine death' of a fetus. Hence, many gynaecologists prefer IUCD for intrauterine contraceptive device. But this leads to problems in translation and, moreover, IUD is now well established in the world literature. An amusing compromise adopted by an expert committee of the World Health Organization (WHO) in the 1970s was the following: to use IUD (without full stops) for intrauterine device, and I.U.D. for intrauterine death! This agreed notation will be used here.

9.3 What is the history of IUDs?

An oft-quoted but poorly substantiated story describes the first IUD as a stone or stones placed in the uterus of camels in North Africa to prevent pregnancies during long caravan journeys. One version of the story, however, suggests that the stones were actually put in the vagina, making the method more akin to a chastity belt than an IUD! Over 2500 years ago, Hippocrates is credited with using a hollow lead tube to insert pessaries or other objects into human uteri. (The translations differ as to whether this was for contraception or other purposes.) Casanova recommended a gold ball; and as recently as 1950 one woman apparently used her wedding ring as a do-it-yourself IUD!

Cervicouterine stem pessaries were used from the late nineteenth century. They were made from material as exotic as ivory, glass, ebony and diamond-studded platinum, and were used for many purposes – including contraception. Some were shaped like collar-studs or had V-shaped flexible wings inserted into the lower uterine cavity. When the devices fractured, as they sometimes did, leaving just the intrauterine part in position, it was learnt that the latter (rather than the surface cap covering the external os) was the contraceptive. The first completely intrauterine device was a ring made of silkworm gut, described by Dr Richter of Braslaw. Later, silver wire was wound around the silkworm gut by Grafenberg and it is of interest that later versions were made of German silver, an alloy that contains copper. Now made of coiled stainless steel, the design is still one of the most widely used in the world (because it is so popular in China).

Many of the early devices were used as abortifacients as well as contraceptives, and the resultant haemorrhage and pelvic infection led to widespread condemnation by the medical profession. This retarded acceptance of the method, which was only really achieved in 1962 at the first International Conference on IUDs in New York City. The Lippes loop was presented to this conference by its inventor, and became the standard inert device (*Fig. 9.1*) against which many newer devices were compared: many now being bioactive, bearing copper (*Fig. 9.2*) or releasing hormones (*Fig. 9.13*, p. 451). The lay terms 'loop' and 'coil' are unhelpful and not used here.

The intrauterine method received a body blow in the mid-1970s with severe illnesses and even deaths linked to the now infamous Dalkon Shield device: this was the biggest single factor in the IUD's subsequent undeserved reputation – that of causing severe pelvic inflammatory disease (PID) and later tubal factor infertility. This still prevents many potential users in the UK, and even more in the US, from giving the intrauterine approach a fair hearing when it is proposed – it has too much 'baggage' with it from the past. Yet the latest IUDs are much improved and very different from those of 30 years ago; and as for the LNG-IUS (*see Q 9.143ff*), I see no reason to retract a statement of mine in the 1990s that it is 'the greatest advance in the contraceptive field since the combined pill'.

The FSRH Guidance (2007) Intrauterine contraception (133 references) is highly congruent with this chapter: www.fsrh.org.

9.4 How prevalent is use of the IUD?

It is estimated by WHO that over 150 million IUDs are in use worldwide, over 60 million of them in one country – China. In the UK, IUDs are fitted in a mere 4% of women in the childbearing years. This is far fewer than might be predicted from the method's advantages (*see Q 9.18*). So, as it is, as has been well said, it is long past 'time to forgive the IUD'.

9.5 What are the effects of IUD insertion on the genital tract?

Many cellular and biochemical changes have been described, but it is now clear that any IUD in situ long term acts chiefly by interfering with gametes and fertilization.

- All types of IUD lead to a marked increase in the number of leucocytes, both in the endometrium and in the uterine and tubal fluid. All the different types of white cell involved in a typical foreign body reaction are represented.
- Inert and copper devices lead to elevated levels of prostaglandins.

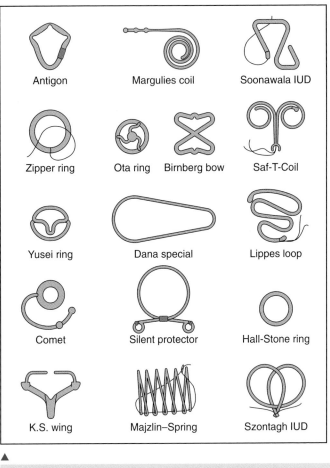

Antigon   Margulies coil   Soonawala IUD

Zipper ring   Ota ring   Birnberg bow   Saf-T-Coil

Yusei ring   Dana special   Lippes loop

Comet   Silent protector   Hall-Stone ring

K.S. wing   Majzlin–Spring   Szontagh IUD

▲

Fig. 9.1 Past inert IUDs. *Q 9.3. Figs 9.2, 9.12* and *9.13* show current bioactive IUDs.

- Copper enhances the foreign body reaction and leads to a range of biochemical changes in the endometrium, affecting enzyme systems and hormone receptors.
- Copper ions are also toxic to sperm and blastocyst.
- Progestogen-releasing IUDs alter endometrial histology with a decidual reaction and glandular atrophy, and inhibit estrogen and progesterone receptors. They also markedly reduce the sperm penetrability of uterine fluid and cervical mucus. In the first year of use they do also inhibit ovulation in a significant minority of cycles.

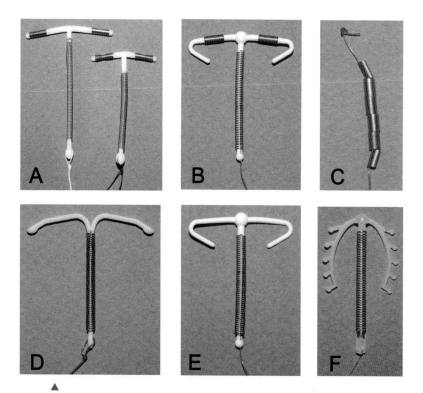

Fig. 9.2 Copper IUDs. **A**: T-Safe Cu 380A QL (Quick-Load) (FP Sales) or TT 380 Slimline (Durbin) and related Mini TT 380 Slimline with shorter stem and narrower 'armspan' (Durbin); **B**: Flexi-T 380 (FP Sales); **C**: GyneFix (Durbin, FP Sales); **D**: Nova-T 380 (Schering); also UT 380 Short (Durbin) with short stem; **E**: Flexi-T 300 (FP Sales) with short stem; **F**: Multiload Cu375 (Organon) or Load 375 (Durbin). *Q 9.3*. Images reproduced by kind permission of Dr Anne MacGregor. Images B–F are not exactly to scale of A.

9.6 Are there any known systemic effects of copper IUDs (outside the genital tract)?

An increase in some circulating immunoglobulins has been reported, but neither this nor the minute amount of copper entering the systemic circulation in users of copper IUDs is thought to be of clinical significance (except perhaps in Wilson's disease, *see* Q 9.85). Absorption of hormones or any other chemicals that are carried by bioactive devices must always be presumed, but systemic effects even of the progestogen-releasing IUDs are small (and depend on the release rate).

Inert and copper IUDs have no effect on the pituitary or ovary. However, uterine shedding starts 2–3 days before circulating levels of estrogen and progesterone have reached the levels usual at the start of the menses in non-IUD-users.

9.7 So what is the main mode of action of IUDs?

The main effect is now believed to be by the blocking of fertilization. The inflammatory cells of the fluid in the whole genital tract (including the tubes) appear with all IUDs to impede sperm transport and fertilization. Actual phagocytosis of the sperm has been reported. Copper is also directly toxic to the sperm and ova. In various studies of long-term IUD-users, viable sperm have very rarely been found in the uterine cavity, the tubes or in aspirates of the pouch of Douglas, in clear contrast with the findings in sexually active controls.

However, an implantation-blocking effect is a back-up contraceptive mechanism. The remarkable effectiveness of copper IUDs when inserted postcoitally, up to 5 days after ovulation, indicates that they can still be exceptionally effective when the action cannot be by blocking fertilization. To work by this mechanism, IUDs seem only to require to be present in the uterus for the last 9 days of each cycle. This implies the need for caution whenever IUDs are removed (*see* Qs 9.13, 9.14).

The progesterone- or progestogen-releasing IUDs (*see* Qs 9.143–9.149) markedly impair the sperm penetrability of cervical and uterine fluids, as well as sometimes stopping fertile ovulation, and they also have an anti-implantation effect. All these effects, though strong, take time to build up: too slowly for the LNG-IUS to be a reliable postcoital contraceptive (*see* Qs 9.146, 10.5, 10.33).

9.8 So how do IUDs mainly act when they are in situ long term?

They mainly act before fertilization; the postfertilization effects are potential but rarely utilized by in situ IUDs or IUSs. However, a prospective long-term user cannot be guaranteed that her IUD or IUS will never in an occasional cycle block the implantation of a blastocyst. If she has ethical problems about that possibility, she should perhaps only use anovulant, barrier or natural methods (or sterilization) (*see* Q 10.2).

9.9 Why are inert devices now no longer used in the UK?

Their market was taken by the copper IUDs. As the surface area of inert devices is reduced, so the bleeding and pain side-effects are minimized but the failure rate increases. By virtue of its additional contraceptive actions (*see* Q 9.5), copper enables smaller devices to be used without loss of efficacy. The major advantage of inert devices (long-term use through to the menopause) is disappearing with the steady increase in permissible duration of use of copper IUDs, now at least 10 years for the *banded* devices.

From this point in this chapter, the term IUD if unqualified will refer to a copper-bearing IUD.

EFFECTIVENESS

9.10 What is the overall failure rate?

For all current devices this is low, in the range of 0.2–2.0/100 woman-years, including pregnancies that are due to unrecognized expulsions (estimated at about one-third of the total) – in the first year (see *Table 1.2*, p. 14).

Three IUD designs stand out as the most effective currently available. These are:

■ T-Safe Cu 380A and its various clones (others in the UK are the TT 380 Slimline (also a Mini-version) and the T-Safe Cu 380A QL *or* 'Quick-Load')
■ GyneFix, which, like T-Safe Cu 380A, utilizes copper bands
■ the levonorgestrel-releasing (LNG)-IUS discussed later (*see Q 9.143ff*).

Based on no less than 16 000 woman-years of use in multicentre WHO and Population Council studies, the first of these is now the 'gold standard' among copper devices. At 7 years of use the cumulative failure rate was 1.4/100 women, putting it in the same league as female sterilization! The LNG-IUS is equally effective, but all other IUD designs, being unbanded, appear to be less so. The former market-leader, the Nova-T 200, had a much higher failure rate and its distribution ceased in October 2001. It has been replaced by the confusingly named Nova-T 380, with more copper wire but still not apparently quite as effective as the 'gold standard' (*see Qs 9.93, 9.94*) and the user has to have more reinsertions (*see Q 9.21*).

9.11 What factors influence failure rates (and other problems) of IUDs?

■ By far the most important factor is the insertion process: and *that* is affected by the competence of the doctor or other professional in inserting the device into the correct high fundal position. The few appropriate comparative studies that have been done show that the difference between doctors, for all the problems (summarized in Q 9.20), is greater than the difference between devices. Therefore, also long-lived (i.e. banded) copper IUDs are better, since they require fewer reinsertions with their associated problems (*see Q 9.21*).
■ The second most important factor in comparative studies is the age and hence relative fertility of the population. Above 35, the first-year failure rate (of 0.1–0.5/100 woman-years with any device) is so good that IUDs become the method of choice for many older women (*see Qs 9.19, 9.21*).
■ Duration of use (*see Q 9.133*).

9.12 Are the various aspects of device design almost irrelevant then?

No. Attention to the shape and size of a device and of its introducer, and the insertion technique, can all influence efficacy. The ideal design would maximize delivery of any bioactive agent such as copper to the most important (high fundal) zone, and minimize the:

- likelihood of malposition (especially too low in the cavity)
- likelihood of expulsion
- liability to, and seriousness of, translocation and perforation (*see Qs 9.42, 9.44*).

Also, if possible:

- the severity and duration of bleeding and pain (*see Q 9.76*)
- any liability to exacerbate pelvic infection (*see Q 9.61*).

9.13 How can insufficient caution when removing an IUD cause iatrogenic pregnancy?

The answer follows from Q 9.7. If one of the major actions of IUDs is to block implantation, removal at any time before the last 9 days of the cycle can enable the blastocyst to arrive at a non-IUD-bearing uterus. Pregnancy could therefore result even if a woman were being sterilized at the time of removal, and this has in fact been reported. A more serious risk would be a clip-induced ectopic, due to trapping the blastocyst in the tube. These events are rare because of the strong pre-fertilization effects of in situ IUDs (*see Q 9.5*) but they are entirely preventable (see below and *Q 11.16*).

9.14 How can such pregnancies be avoided?

Either by removal during a period or, more usually, by following a '7-day rule', i.e. advice in advance to abstain or use a barrier method for 7 days before any IUD is removed; 7 days is believed to allow sufficient time – namely that between ejaculation and the latest likely implantation – for the IUD to have its antinidatory effects in that cycle. The 7-day rule is particularly important before sterilization, for fear of that iatrogenic tubal ectopic. It is also wise before any attempted replacement of an IUD.

Occasionally an IUD needs to be removed midcycle although it has been recently relied upon (*see Q 9.66*). Postcoital hormone treatment should be considered in such cases (*see Chapter 10*).

9.15 How can excessive caution about the time of insertion of IUDs cause iatrogenic pregnancies?

By slavish adherence to the myth that it is best to insert only during or just after the menses! If women are told to wait until after their next period, not a few return pregnant. Several US-based studies have shown that IUDs can be inserted with relative safety on the day they are requested, provided the woman's history indicates she will not have an implanted pregnancy. For many women this 'Quick start' approach is even more appropriate than for the COC (*see Q 5.42*).

Especially relevant was a US study based on about 9000 IUD insertions [White MK et al 1980 *Obstetrics and Gynecology* 55:220–224] that showed a statistically significant doubling of the rate of expulsion if copper-T IUDs were inserted on days 1–5 of the cycle as compared with days 11–17. Because the patients were unaware of the expulsion (usually partial) in nearly 40% of the cases, extra pregnancies are likely if IUDs are inserted only during the menses.

Finally, of course, deliberate postcoital IUD insertion up to day 19 of a 28-day cycle (adjusted for cycle length) is very effective (*see Chapter 10*).

9.16 What is the likely explanation for a high expulsion rate when IUDs are inserted very early in the cycle? And what might be done about it?

The main increase in expulsion rate occurs when IUDs are inserted during the menstrual flow (day 1–5 in the paper quoted above) and this is most probably linked with extra myometrial activity at that time due to prostaglandins. The intraluminal pressure can rise above 100 mmHg and the fundal cavity is also narrower then (see *Fig. 9.8*, p. 425) than at midcycle.

Sometimes there is no practical alternative to fitting an IUD or IUS menstrually or just premenstrually. In particular, if there is a history of dysmenorrhoea I now suggest that the prostaglandin inhibitor treatment routinely given as premedication for the insertion (a prostaglandin synthetase inhibitor (PGSI) such as mefenamic acid or ibuprofen) is continued – until and during that next period.

9.17 So when are IUDs best inserted?

The answer is: not during heavy days of the menses but at any time from their ending phase through until about midcycle. At the Margaret Pyke Centre we target days 4–12 of a normal cycle. Beyond that, if intercourse has been continuing, postcoital insertion in good faith is still permissible up to 5 days after the calculated ovulation day (*see Q 10.14*) but with caution and counselling, appropriate screening, consideration of antibiotics, good records and follow-up.

ADVANTAGES AND BENEFITS

9.18 What are the advantages of IUDs?

■ Effective:
  – highly, comparable to female sterilization, indeed better than some methods of the latter

- postcoitally (not the LNG-IUS)
- postabortally.
- Safe:
  - mortality about 1:500 000
  - no known, unwanted systemic effects (not LNG-IUS).
- Independent of intercourse.
- Does not require any day-to-day actions, such as taking a pill.
- Motivation is chiefly required around the time of insertion and never subsequently if side-effects are acceptable – it then being truly a 'default' method, for over 10 years duration of use in the case of T-Safe Cu 380A.
- Relatively cheap and easy to distribute.
- Does not influence milk volume or composition.
- With sympathetic providers the method is under a woman's control and (a point of occasional relevance) if the threads are removed, can be undetectable by her partner.
- Continuation rates high.
- Reversible (*see Q 9.137*).

What a remarkable list of advantages, amounting to transcervical sterilization without a general anaesthetic or hospital visit! Add to them a hint – unproven so far – from five out of six case–control studies that *copper IUDs might actually be protective against endometrial cancer* [see Grimes DA 2000 *The Lancet* 356:1013–1019], and, although it has been around too short a time to prove the point, there is actually more reason to expect a reduction of this risk in users of the LNG-IUS, through its endometrial suppressive action.

It makes one wonder why we do not at least offer this choice, as a routine, to all parous young women and also to many more who, although nulliparous, are in mutually faithful relationships. See below!

9.19   For whom are IUDs indicated?

The answer is: upon request for contraception, unless the absolute contraindications apply (*see Qs 9.84, 9.85*) or if the relative contraindications are unacceptable to the woman herself after discussion in the light of alternatives. More specifically, in view of the threats to fertility to be discussed (which are not due to the intrauterine method but to the prevalence of STIs in most societies), and the fact that these are not only more serious when there is no family but also more probable in the very young: IUDs are still not first-choice methods for most young women until they have had children. But nulliparity in monogamous relationships is no more than WHO 2 and IUDs are often a good choice for such women above age 35 – especially those with the view that their career will be likely to take precedence over ever having a child.

Modern intrauterine contraception can substitute well for female sterilization (*see Q 11.49ff*). Unless the man volunteers for vasectomy, which does add greater efficacy, the IUD (or IUS) might be so acceptable that it remains in use until final removal 1 year after the menopause.

MAIN PROBLEMS AND DISADVANTAGES

9.20 In summary, what are the main problems and disadvantages of intrauterine contraception using copper?

These can be listed briefly as in the Box below (please read this in conjunction with Q 9.21). *Note: these are **not** in order of frequency and are far more related to the skill or otherwise of the inserting clinician than any problems with the method itself.*

Problems that may occur during intrauterine contraception using copper

1 *Intrauterine pregnancy*: increased risk of miscarriage, hence of infection
2 *Extrauterine pregnancy* (but no increase (actually a reduction) in overall population risk, *see Q 9.29*)
3 *Expulsion or partial expulsion*, with risks of pregnancy (see (1))
4 *Malposition* of the device, which could cause items (1), (3), (7) and (8) in this list, as well as being one cause of 'lost threads'
5 *Perforation* with risks of pregnancy, also risk of IUD penetration of bowel/bladder and adhesion formation – and the resultant risks of surgery
6 *Pelvic infection/salpingitis*: although IUDs are definitely **not** the initiating cause (*see Q 9.48*).
7 *Pain*
8 *Abnormal bleeding*: this can be increased in amount, duration, and/or frequency

Rare problems are considered at Qs 9.72, 9.87, 9.112 and 9.126. But with respect to carcinogenesis, whether of endometrium or cervix, all available data are reassuring.

9.21 Are the problems in the Box at *Q 9.20* interconnected? Please give examples.

Very much so, and it is instructive to see how:

■ *Insertion*: first and foremost is capable (either directly or indirectly) of causing any one of problems (1) to (8). The importance of this factor cannot be over-emphasized: its impact must be minimized by skill: through good training and maintained experience.

> **IUD/IUS slogan 1**
> The insertion process can be relevant to the causation of every category of IUD problem.
>
> **IUD/IUS slogan 2**
> Most IUD problems are less common with increasing duration of use.

Therefore, why use a 5-year device when a 10-year one will fit?

- *Pain*: can be a symptom of (1) to (6) in the Box at Q 9.20. Hence these should first be excluded before terming it a side-effect (i.e. something that the woman might or might not be able to live with). Beware the stoical woman or the one who tries too hard to avoid troubling the doctor!

- *Bleeding*: might sometimes mean directly or indirectly numbers (1), (2), (3) or (4) and even (6) (chlamydial endometritis can cause bleeding). So this too is not necessarily just a side-effect.

- *Fertility*: can be impaired (indirectly or directly) by any of (1) to (6) (*see Qs 9.23, 9.31, 9.48*). Hence the general view that young nulliparae should think twice before using this method.

- *'Lost threads'*: can signify any of (1), (3), (4) and (5) (*see Q 9.32*).

- Malposition of the device: can cause numbers (1), (3), (7) and (8) in the Box at Q 9.20, as well as 'lost threads'.

- *Increasing age*: has been found to increase the risk of (2) (ectopics), possibly because more years of sexual activity means more chance of an initial or recurrent infection to damage a tube, and of (8) (heavy periods). These risks are regardless of whether there is also an IUD present. But age definitely reduces the risk of (1), (3) and (6) (*see Qs 9.11, 9.37, 9.52*).

- *Duration of use*: reduces most problems, i.e. (1), (3), (6), (7) and (8). This is partly because most problems are insertion-linked (see above) and therefore occur primarily in the first year of use (*see Qs 9.133, 9.134*).

INTRAUTERINE PREGNANCY (IUD IN SITU)

9.22 Does intrauterine pregnancy pose problems for IUD-users? Is there an increased risk of teratogenesis?

There is absolutely no evidence for an increased risk of any of the more common fetal abnormalities, whether the device is present at the time of conception or during organogenesis – at least for the inert and copper-containing types. Proof of this is (as usual) impossible, especially as 2% of all babies have an abnormality, and most particularly for the rarer disorders.

There are as yet no adequate data concerning any possible effects of a high local dose of progestogen on a continuing pregnancy (*see Q 9.145*).

9.23 Should the device be removed and, if so, surely this will increase the risk of miscarriage?

Counter-intuitively, the 'obvious' course of action – which is to leave the device alone so as to avoid disturbing the pregnancy – has been shown to result in a high rate of miscarriage (above 50%). Moreover, more often than expected this occurs in the second trimester, with dangerous complications, particularly haemorrhage and sepsis; septic second-trimester abortions were 26 times more frequent in one study. There is also evidence that the risks of antepartum haemorrhage, of preterm delivery and of stillbirth are increased if the IUD remains present.

Such problems are not restricted to the Dalkon Shield, although first reported for that device. Tatum (the inventor of the first T-device) produced good evidence that removal of a copper device in the early part of pregnancy reduced the spontaneous abortion rate from 54% to 20%. So the slogan is:

> **IUD/IUS slogan 3**
> If an intrauterine method fails and the woman wishes to proceed to full-term delivery, do not leave the device in situ.

9.24 How should removal of the device be managed?

1 Begin by counselling the woman and warning her that she is at increased risk of miscarriage whatever is done, but that the risk can usually be reduced considerably by gentle removal of the device.
2 Arrange an ultrasound scan. Occasionally the device can be identified above the pregnancy sac and it might be judged that removal would cause excessive trauma/rupture of the membranes. But far more commonly the device is below the sac (displacement having been the probable cause of the method failure, in fact).
3 Removal should then be performed, at the earliest possible stage in pregnancy, whenever the threads of the device are still accessible. In rare cases of heavy bleeding or leakage of liquor thereafter, the woman might need immediate admission. However, she can usually continue as an outpatient, with appropriate advice about the subsequent occurrence of any pain or more bleeding than the slight show to be expected at IUD removal. If the threads are (already) missing, consider the possibility of perforation, not only of expulsion; and in all cases categorize/supervise the pregnancy as 'high risk' (*see Q 9.23*).

See also Q *9.27*: the vital importance after delivery of establishing where the IUD is . . .

9.25 What if the outcome after counselling is to be a legal abortion?

Clearly, the removal of the device is then best performed at the time of termination. In my view there should be routine *Chlamydia* testing and antibiotic cover for all such procedures. The latter is essential:

■ If the woman is first seen with an IUD-associated incomplete abortion.
■ If medical induction of the termination is planned with mifepristone and/or prostaglandins (PGs). This is because of anecdotes, especially in the second trimester, of severe infections, implying that the presence of the foreign body increases the sepsis risk. Indeed, the IUD should be removed at the outset of treatment, whether by mifepristone or PG pessary, and not left to come away with the products of conception.

9.26 Should an ultrasound scan be done after all failures of an IUD or IUS, even if the woman does not go on to full term?

In my opinion, yes, because the pregnancy might have resulted from the device being malpositioned or even placed in one horn of a bicornute uterus.

9.27 What if the original IUD is never found following spontaneous or induced abortion? Or at full term?

It is unbelievable how often the original presence of an IUD is forgotten, especially after delivery. If the IUD is thought about at all, unnoticed expulsion is assumed. There should be a thorough search for it in the placenta and membranes, and its presence or otherwise recorded. If not, a women might find herself, at a later stage, with two intrauterine IUDs (in situ failure) or with one in her uterus and one still at large – free in the abdomen (a perforation therefore explaining how the original conception occurred). See *Table 9.2*, p. 396. Many legal cases have resulted, and they are indefensible. One can nearly always exclude either an embedded or perforated device with plain abdominal X-rays as a supplement to ultrasound scanning (*see* Q *9.34*).

EXTRAUTERINE PREGNANCY

9.28 What is the risk of extrauterine pregnancy when an IUD-user becomes pregnant, and is the rate really increased?

No! to the second question. First and foremost, it is now clearly established that copper IUDs do *not* increase the overall risk of ectopics in a population, as compared with suitable non-IUD-using controls.

The rate of ectopics is fundamentally dependent on the rate of pelvic infection (*see Q 9.49*) in that community. Because in situ copper IUDs drastically reduce fertilization rates (*see Q 9.7*), even women with damaged tubes (who will be at definite risk of an ectopic when they come to try for a pregnancy) might well escape this while using an IUD.

The risk among current users of the Progestosert (progesterone-containing) IUD appears to have been truly higher; but the more potent LNG-IUS seems to block fertilization so well that in the Population Council study [Sivin I et al *Contraception* 1990;42:361–378] no ectopics at all occurred during a massive 3371 woman-years of use! However, they do very rarely occur even with the IUS.

9.29 But surely ectopics are more common among IUD conceptions?

Precisely, but this does not invalidate the above answer. As a working rule, the ratio increases roughly 10-fold. Thus, approximately 1 in 10–20 IUD-associated pregnancies will be extrauterine if the background rate is 1 in 100–200 pregnancies among non-IUD-users. My assessment of the literature is as follows: IUDs do not prevent extrauterine pregnancy (through the antifertilization effect) quite as well as they prevent intrauterine pregnancy (with the *added anti-implantation effect*). Hence there will be such a great reduction in the denominator of uterine pregnancies as to lead to an increased proportion of ectopics, even though the numerator of ectopic pregnancies is also reduced. It might help to use real numbers (*Table 9.1*, which, for simplicity, assumes an unreal population having 100% fertility by the end of 1 year).

TABLE 9.1 Ectopic pregnancy risk with IUDs			
	Annual conceptions (no.)	Ectopics (no.)	Ratio
Ordinarily, in a society, let the ectopic rate be 1 in 100 pregnancies.			
Assuming zero infertility, if 1000 women use no contraception:	1000	10	1:100
If the same 1000 women use a copper IUD with a first-year failure rate of 1/100 woman-years:	10	1	1:10
Reduction:	990	9	

Although, in row 3 of the table, 1 in 10 among the IUD conceptions is ectopic, this is actually a 10-fold reduction in the expected number and rate in the population. The numerator of the first ratio (10/1000) is truly lowered, 1 instead of 10, or a 90% fall in the rate in the population. So it is clearly a myth that IUDs 'cause' ectopics. But the denominator of total conceptions is so massively reduced (by 99%) as to allow there to be relatively more ectopics among the few conceptions.

The ectopic problem is caused by pre-existing tubal damage and should not be blamed on the IUD. Very probably, even the one woman who has an ectopic while using the IUD was due to get one (along with the other nine women) in the future, anyway, once her IUD was removed and she tried to conceive.

A similar explanation holds for the apparently increased rate of ectopics among conceptions with the POP, which nevertheless also protects against ectopics overall as compared with non-contracepting controls.

9.30 What are the implications for management?

The main point is that, even if only by the above selection mechanism (relatively more ectopics being allowed to happen relative to the intrauterine pregnancies), once an IUD-user actually is pregnant she could well have an ectopic. So the slogan is:

> **IUD/IUS slogan 4**
> Every IUD-user with a late or unusually light period and pelvic pain has an ectopic pregnancy till proved otherwise.

In practice, every IUD-user in whom pregnancy is suspected, even before there is a positive pregnancy test, should have a pelvic examination with gentle lateral cervical movement to detect adnexal tenderness; and each IUD-user should be warned prospectively, backed by a leaflet, that marked pelvic pain should always receive prompt medical attention, particularly if her period is late.

Beware also of the IUD-user who has just been sterilized. She could have a clip-induced ectopic if she was not advised appropriately (*see Qs 9.13, 9.14*), i.e. not to rely on the IUD for 7 days before surgery (although actually this risk would be even higher if she was operated on late in the cycle while using no effective contraception at all).

9.31 Is past tubal pregnancy a contraindication to the modern banded copper IUD, or to the LNG-IUS?

In my view this is a relative contraindication (WHO 2) – and stronger (WHO 3) in young nulliparous rather than parous women. Although the

IUD method definitely reduces the overall risk of ectopics in a population, as we have seen clearly in *Table 9.1*, it sometimes *selectively* fails to prevent them. The woman concerned should ideally use a method that will provide maximal protection to her one remaining tube. This is why I differ from WHO, which (on a population basis) classifies past ectopic as WHO 1 for the IUD and IUS.

A poor choice would also be the old-type progestogen-only pill (*see Q 7.33*). Good choices would be the combined pill, Cerazette, an injectable or Implanon (*see Q 8.60*). The common factor is that all these are anovulants and therefore equally good at stopping both tubal and intrauterine conceptions.

If a copper device is nevertheless chosen, as the WHO 2 category permits, the T-Safe Cu 380A or the GyneFix should be used, because ectopics (like all conceptions) are much less frequent with these banded products. The LNG-IUS would be another option with this history: in the randomized European trial [Andersson K et al 1994 *Contraception* 49:56–72] an ectopic was more than 10 times less likely in the LNG-IUS group than among users of the old Nova-T 200.

'LOST THREADS'

9.32 What is the differential diagnosis of 'lost threads' with IUDs?

The first possibility is that the threads are in fact present but not being palpated by the user. This could be because of her inexperience or because the threads have retreated to just within the external os. If the threads are truly absent, then the differential diagnosis is as shown in *Table 9.2*.

9.33 What are the 'do's and don'ts' of the management of 'lost threads'?

The first message from *Table 9.2* is another IUD 'slogan', namely:

> **IUD/IUS slogan 5**
> The IUD-user with 'lost threads' is either pregnant already or at increased risk of becoming pregnant.

The device under the liver (after perforation) is just as bad at preventing pregnancy as the one in the toilet after unrecognized expulsion. . . . And if the threads have gone because the IUD was not optimally positioned, this might leave part of the cavity unprotected and so increase the conception risk.

TABLE 9.2 Differential diagnosis of 'lost threads' with IUDs

Main diagnoses A: Not pregnant	Clinical clues	B: Pregnant	Clinical clues
(1) **Device in uterus** Threads cut too short, or caught up around device during original insertion or avulsed at a previous removal attempt; or device itself malpositioned	(a) Periods likely to be those characteristic of IUD in situ (b) Uterus normal size	(4) **Device in situ + pregnancy**	(a) Amenorrhoea (b) Pregnancy test likely to be positive, with clinically enlarged uterus (sufficient to pull up thread)
(2) **Unrecognized expulsion**	(a) Recent periods as woman's normal pattern (b) Uterus normal size	(5) **Unrecognized expulsion + pregnancy**	(a) Amenorrhoea, following one or more apparently normal periods (i.e. unmodified by IUD) (b) Signs of pregnancy variably present (may be too early on first presentation) or pregnancy test positive
(3) **Perforation of uterus**	As (2) plus (rarely) mass or actual IUD palpated on bimanual examination	(6) **Perforation of uterus + pregnancy**	As (5) plus (rarely) mass or actual IUD identified on bimanual examination

- All such women therefore need to be advised to use an alternative contraceptive method until the protective presence of an IUD has been established.
- Consider also the possible need for postcoital contraception, especially if recent expulsion is diagnosed (*see* Q 10.22).
- In general, X-rays and any form of intrauterine manipulation should be arranged in the follicular phase of the menstrual cycle, for fear of disturbing a pregnancy that might go to term.
- Above all, women with this problem need full explanations and supportive counselling throughout the management, which is described below (*see* Q 9.34).

9.34 What is the recommended protocol for the management of 'lost threads'?

I recommend the very practical scheme in *Fig. 9.3*, amplified below. Diagnosis and treatment are simultaneous in most cases, with minimum use of hospital facilities. Exclude implanted pregnancy. Take a careful menstrual history, do a bimanual examination and, if indicated, perform the most sensitive pregnancy test available. If the woman is pregnant, the management is primarily that of the pregnancy itself. Note, however, that if an IUD is not recovered in the products of conception or, much later, at full term in the placenta, an X-ray should be taken before assuming expulsion (as opposed to perforation or malposition).

In the absence of pregnancy, proceed as follows:

1   First, insert and open the jaws of *long-handled narrow artery forceps* (Spencer–Wells or equivalent) within the endocervical canal – without reaching the level of the internal cervical os. In a (1992) study of 400 women with 'lost threads', the Margaret Pyke Centre found that almost 50% of the IUDs were identified/retrieved this way, meaning that the woman had had a wasted trip because this could so easily have been done by the referring doctor.

2   If the threads are readily located and the IUD/IUS is judged to be correctly located (and undisturbed by the procedure in 1), no further action need be taken; but disappearance of the threads might be a sign of malposition. So it is often advisable (after discussion with the woman) to remove and replace the device. An ultrasound scan is very helpful here but, if not available on site (as it increasingly is), this can be deferred until later in the sequence, because it might be unnecessary if the device is removed successfully.

3   *Try the use of thread-retrievers.* The most established of these in the UK is the Emmett retriever, which is available presterilized and disposable. It has a handle to which is attached a thin plastic strip with multiple

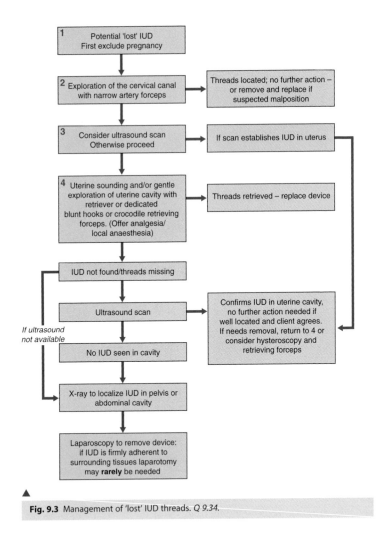

Fig. 9.3 Management of 'lost' IUD threads. *Q 9.34.*

notches designed to trap the threads, when the edge is used like a curette against each surface of the fundus. The MI-Mark Helix was found to be significantly less effective than either this or the (no longer available) Retrievette, in the Margaret Pyke Centre study above.

What about analgesia? Ideally (and this is policy at the Margaret Pyke Centre) a prostaglandin inhibitor such as mefenamic acid should be routinely given about 30–60 min before any intrauterine manipulations

– as for all IUD insertions. A few women, especially nulliparae, require a paracervical block with local anaesthetic (*see Q 9.108*). If the cervix is stenosed, pretreatment with EE (30 mg daily for 5 days) can soften and dilate the canal. Misoprostol 200 mg vaginally as a single dose the night before has been tried (unlicensed use) but was not particularly helpful in my own small series.

4 Next, try *small, blunt IUD-removal hooks* (Grafenberg pattern). In skilled hands these metal devices can be used to hook down either a thread or part of the device itself, but they can also cause trauma at the internal os. Blind traction on a partially perforated device can be dangerous (*see Q 9.47*).

5 *Various resterilizable IUD-retrieving forceps* (e.g. the Patterson alligator forceps), with short jaws opening wholly in the uterine cavity, can next be tried with success. Otherwise, and usually after imaging (if not already done), try suction using a Karman curette, and hysteroscopy. All require good analgesia but local anaesthesia is nearly always sufficient. General anaesthesia should very rarely be required for any device that is in utero.

6 Arrange *appropriate imaging*. An ultrasound scan can be arranged at this point, if it has not already been done. In fact, the scan should have been done earlier if the device was not readily located by sound or retriever at (3), so as to avoid unnecessary discomfort. Confirmation of correct intrauterine location within a non-pregnant uterus can be helpful for a woman who wishes to continue using the same device, but if there is any suspicion that it is malpositioned (e.g. too low or rotated), appropriate steps should be taken for its removal as above. If the scan shows unequivocally that the uterus is empty, an X-ray is then required to differentiate between expulsion and perforation (*see Qs 9.37–9.47*). If the latter is confirmed, refer to an expert (2) laparoscopist (see *Fig. 9.3*).

9.35   What if ultrasound facilities are not available?

In some clinical settings it might then be useful to arrange an X-ray with a uterine marker. The most practical marker is another IUD, preferably of a different pattern from that originally fitted. There are three possible X-ray findings:

■ *Only the newly inserted device visible*: this implies unrecognized expulsion of the first device.

■ *IUDs shown on the abdominal radiograph in close proximity*: if a lateral view also shows that the IUDs are contiguous, this means that the first device is actually in utero. This should be a rare finding if the X-ray is arranged only after stages (1) to (5) above. However, it is well worth removing the second IUD, as this might bring down part of the original device.

■ *The IUDs might be clearly separated on the X-ray*: this establishes the diagnosis of complete perforation (translocation) (*see Qs 9.42–9.47*).

9.36 Some IUDs, especially the Chinese steel spring one, do not have threads anyway, how are they removed?

After excluding pregnancy (i.e. usually by a normal LMP), and at minimum giving a PGSI premedicant (but considering a full paracervical block if dilatation will be required, *see Q 9.108*), blunt hooks nearly always work. Patterson forceps should be available as back-up. *See Qs 9.104 and 9.125* for a discussion on estrogen pretreatment if the woman is hypoestrogenic (e.g. postmenopausally).

EXPULSION

9.37 What influences the frequency of partial or complete expulsion?

In past studies the rate varied, but is quoted as about 5% for *all* current Cu-IUDs and the LNG-IUS. The rates are influenced by:

■ Characteristics of the woman (age, parity and uterine shape) – also the wrong timing of insertion in relation to the menses (*see Qs 9.15–9.17*, sometimes indicating a course of PGSIs (*see Q 9.16*)).
■ The size and nature of the device.
■ *Above all*, the skill of the person performing the insertion (*see Q 9.21*).

9.38 When do expulsions most commonly occur?

During the menses, most particularly one of the first three menstruations after insertion. About one-third of first-year pregnancies among IUD-users occur after unnoticed expulsion. This should not happen if women are taught to check for the presence of the threads (and the absence of any part of a partially expelled device) after each period and prior to relying on the device for that cycle. Among users for more than 3 years, the expulsion rate with most devices approaches nil. If lost threads are reported but intercourse has been continuing, consider emergency contraception (*Q 10.22*)

9.39 What effect do age and parity have on the expulsion rate?

Young nulliparous women have higher expulsion rates for all devices than parous women. After the first child there is a negligible effect of increasing parity on the expulsion rate. However, IUD expulsion rates seem to decline in a fairly linear fashion with increasing age. In studies either of parous or of nulliparous women, the rates of expulsion are about half over the age of 30 than in women below that age.

9.40 What is the effect of the size and shape of the uterus?

If the cavity of the uterus is significantly distorted, either congenitally or by fibroids, there will be an increase in uterine activity (and cramps) after insertion and an increased likelihood of both malposition and expulsion. Ideally, therefore, such women should avoid framed IUDs, although the GyneFix is often usable. Careful sounding, as described in Q 9.112, during the insertion might lead to a change of plan, but, in practice, quite gross distortions of the uterine cavity can be difficult to identify clinically (see *Fig. 9.10* (p. 435) and Q 9.91). If in doubt, a good pre-insertion ultrasound scan of the contours of the uterine cavity is invaluable, and this should always be done if fibroids are identified.

9.41 What is the effect of the size and shape of the device itself?

Different expulsion rates between devices certainly exist. For example, the rate for the now obsolete Copper 7 (particularly for partial expulsions) was considerably higher than that for the T-shaped IUDs, even after controlling for other variables. In an RCT, the Flexi-T 300 had a higher expulsion rate than the T-Safe Cu 380A.

Aside from insertion skill, expulsion rates are probably most correlated with the precise fit of any framed device within the uterus of different women.

PERFORATION

9.42 What problems are associated with uterine perforation?

- *Pregnancy*: most perforations first present as a pregnancy with 'lost threads'.
- *Adhesions or penetration*: if the device is bioactive (copper or progestogen-containing) it leads to adhesion formation or might penetrate the wall of bowel or bladder. 'Closed' devices (e.g. rings) are particularly associated with bowel strangulation.

Yet the uterus always heals so completely that any IUD or IUS may be used in future if requested (WHO 2).

9.43 Should perforated devices be removed? Should it be considered an emergency?

In countries with developed medical services the benefits of removal always outweigh the risks. There are usually no specific symptoms, so removal can be elective but prompt after diagnosis (see Q 9.34).

While waiting for hospital admission the patient should be warned to use alternative contraception, and that any abdominal pain, particularly if there is associated diarrhoea, must be reported promptly. Serious complications involving the bowel have been reported (including one death from peritonitis in a user of the Copper 7).

9.44 What is the frequency of uterine perforation following IUD insertion?

The true incidence is difficult to establish but is commonly quoted as 1–2 per 1000 insertions. It is probably even lower for T-shaped IUDs that are positioned by a 'withdrawal' technique. Only one perforation in 1815 insertions of such devices was reported by Chi in 1987 (*see also Q 11.24*).

9.45 What factors affect the perforation rate?

The rate is affected by the usual three kinds of variable:

■ *Features of the woman*: the main factor here is recent pregnancy, puerperal insertions having a higher rate (*see Q 11.24*).
■ *Features of the device and its inserting system*: linear devices, such as the Lippes loop, that were inserted by a 'push' technique (rather than the 'withdrawal' techniques now more commonly used) were more likely to perforate. An important safety factor is to avoid loading any IUD into its inserter too far ahead of the insertion, so that the plastic loses its 'memory' (*see Q 9.114*). The sharp stilette of the GyneFix has obvious potential for this risk.
■ *Features of the inserting clinician*: this is again by far and away the most important factor. As Lippes himself observed: 'IUDs do not perforate. For this to happen we need a practitioner.' Almost all perforations are produced at insertion even though the diagnosis might be long delayed (and frequently emerges only when the empty uterus permits a pregnancy). Perforations are more common:
   – when the operator is inexperienced
   – when the position of the uterus is misdiagnosed (especially unrecognized retroversion), and probably:
   – when a holding forceps or tenaculum is not used (*see Q 9.112*).

9.46 What is the best way to remove perforated devices?

When a device was clearly palpable vaginally in the pouch of Douglas, I was able to remove it by simple colpotomy. Laparoscopic removal is far more usual. Even if there are adhesions, the device can usually be grasped intra-abdominally under vision at one end or the other and pulled through its own 'tunnel'. However, great care is necessary because devices can sometimes be adherent to the actual wall of bowel or bladder, and, these days, IUD or IUS removal is best undertaken by a specialist in minimal access surgery. Laparotomy under the same anaesthetic should now rarely be required.

9.47 Are there any special points about embedding and partial perforation?

If part of a partially translocated device can be grasped within the uterus it might be possible to remove it transcervically. However, this should be done with great gentleness. It is possible for the part of the device which is through the uterine wall to be adherent to bowel or bladder. Removal at hysteroscopy under ultrasound or laparoscopic control is much safer in such cases (*see also Q 9.124* and *Fig. 9.11*, p. 443).

PELVIC INFECTION

9.48 Do IUDs cause pelvic inflammatory disease (PID)?

 The evidence-based answer to this question now is 'no!' (*see Q 9.50*). Although studies have repeatedly shown an increased risk of such infections in IUD-users as compared with controls, the controls are protected (*see Q 9.49*). When they occur, in some studies, attacks appear to be of greater severity than in cases without the associated foreign body.

According to Weström, one severe attack of laparoscopically diagnosed PID of any type carries a 1-in-8 risk of infertility due to tubal occlusion; two attacks, a 1-in-3 risk; and three attacks a 1-in-2 risk. So this infection risk has rightly become the greatest single anxiety about the IUD method, particularly for use by nulliparae, especially since the Dalkon Shield disaster of the 1970s (*see Q 9.62*).

> PID is primarily caused by people, not by devices; and the people are most often MEN, bringing the infection into what the woman believed to be a monogamous relationship.

9.49 What is the actual frequency of PID among IUD-users?

The absolute risk varies enormously according to the background rate of (sexually transmitted) PID in the population studied. The problem is that in most comparative studies the controls have been themselves protected against infection, either by using barrier methods or the combined pill. Progestogen-containing (i.e. mucus-altering) contraception generally about halves the risk of PID (*see Q 5.60*).

Weström [*American Journal of Obstetrics and Gynecology* 1980;138:880–892] studied all women aged 20–29 in the town of Lund, Sweden, and found the incidence of PID per 1000 woman-years to be 52 for IUD-users, compared with 34 for sexually active users of no contraception, 14 for barrier-method-users and 9 for pill-users. This study usefully shows that the lion's share of the sixfold difference at that time (early 1970s) when

IUDs were compared with pills was caused by the protective effect of the latter: fourfold compared with users of nothing.

9.50 As shown by that Weström study, a doubling of the risk of PID through use of the IUD would surely still be important?

Definitely, but even that is a huge exaggeration. Factors like diagnostic bias are operative: PID is more likely to be thought about/diagnosed when pelvic symptoms occur in IUD-users. Several studies have shown low or absent risk in women claiming only one sexual partner – and that's even without good information about what their partner is up to!

More convincingly, in the massive WHO study to be described (*see Q 9.54*) there was not one single case of PID reported among 4301 women fitted with IUDs in China in the 1980s: a country where true (two-sided) monogamy was then a reality, and, at that point, virtually an STI-free zone (not so now). Two other Chinese trials referenced in an excellent review by David Grimes [*The Lancet* 2000;356:1013–1019] and totalling 3300 women, also reported no cases of PID at all. If 7600-plus IUDs can be fitted (anywhere) with not a single attack of PID during follow-up, is not the following slogan fair comment:

> **IUD/IUS slogan 6**
> IUDs, intrinsically, cannot be the cause of the PID that may occur in IUD-users.

What PID really stands for, surely, is 'penis-induced disease' . . . rather than what you see in the Glossary on p. xiii!

9.51 So what factors have been suggested as affecting the rate of PID in IUD-users?

In summary, and in order of clinical importance, the factors are:

1 the woman's risk of acquiring or having acquired a sexually transmitted pathogen
2 the insertion process, combined with point (1) (*see Q 9.54ff*)
3 features of the IUD:
    (a) foreign body effect – unlikely (*see Q 9.61*)
    (b) the cervical tail(s) – very unlikely if they are monofilament (*see Q 9.62*).

9.52 What features of the woman can influence the PID rate?

Age, acting as a marker for the risk of STIs. The risk is highest in young women under 20 and declines in a linear fashion as age increases (*Fig. 9.4*).

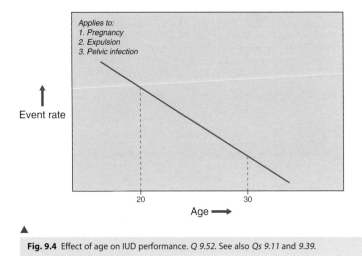

Applies to:
1. Pregnancy
2. Expulsion
3. Pelvic infection

Event rate

20   30

Age ⟶

▲

Fig. 9.4 Effect of age on IUD performance. *Q 9.52*. See also *Qs 9.11* and *9.39*.

In a study at the Margaret Pyke Centre, the incidence of infection was 10 times greater below the age of 20 than it was above 30 – although the 871 women were all nulliparous, had received the same type of IUD (Copper 7), at the same centre and all in the first 10 days of the cycle.

There is no evidence that the uterus becomes more resistant to infection with age and, because the isolation of specific cervical pathogens and rates of PID in non-IUD-users show a decline with age and correlate with sexual lifestyle, this again is indirect evidence that the vast majority of cases of PID in IUD-users are primarily sexually acquired.

It needs to be stressed again that the infection is often transmitted to a woman:

■ who is practising monogamy (serial monogamy, anyway) by her partner who is not
■ at the time of partner change.

Very often, if the right questions are asked, the attack of PID comes after a recent partner change. After the age of 30 it is an observed fact that partner change becomes less frequent.

9.53 So how should we question and counsel women who wish to use the IUD method?

Verbal screening concerning lifestyle of self/partner and recent partner change(s) is of great relevance (*see Qs 1.14, 9.120*) but unlikely to be sufficient: in a study during the mid-1980s by the Margaret Pyke Centre,

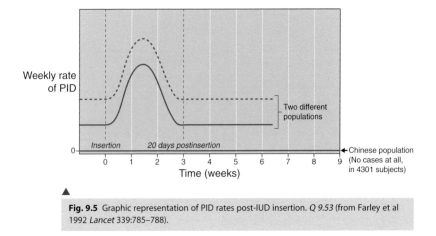

Weekly rate of PID

Two different populations

Insertion   20 days postinsertion

Chinese population (No cases at all, in 4301 subjects)

Time (weeks)

Fig. 9.5 Graphic representation of PID rates post-IUD insertion. *Q 9.53* (from Farley et al 1992 *Lancet* 339:785–788).

the background rate of *Chlamydia* carriage was 2.4% in the general clinic population but higher – 8.2% – in the pre-IUD group who had first been sensitively questioned about their likely exposure!

Thus, in most metropolitan areas of the UK today, I consider it suboptimal to fit copper or progestogen-releasing devices in young women without microbiological screening: the money for pre-insertion *Chlamydia* testing must just be found. This argument is greatly strengthened by the WHO study depicted in *Fig. 9.5* and the discussion that follows.

9.54 **What light is thrown on this PID problem by the thorough database review of international WHO studies published in 1992 [Farley TM et al *The Lancet* 339:785–788]?**

One of 10 types of IUD had been inserted in 13 trials (12 of them RCTs). There were 22 908 IUD-users (almost all parous) from five continents, fitted and followed up to a common protocol from 1975 to about 1990, and there were no less than 51 399 years of follow-up. Of the users, 9% were using the inert Lippes loop, copper IUDs were used by the majority – 17 019 women – and hormone-releasing devices (the Alza progesterone T and the LNG-IUS) were used by the remainder (16%).

The overall rate of PID among the women recruited was low, 1.6/1000 woman-years of use (contrast with *Q 9.49*!), and lower still in the late 1980s – suggesting that later in the trials in all centres there was greater care in user selection, because there was no prescreening or antibiotic prophylaxis. The most important findings were:

■ PID risk was more than six times higher during the first 20 days after insertion than later; the risk was constant and relatively low thereafter for up to 8 years, with no evidence that it was then any higher than the local background rate (see *Fig. 9.5*).

■ PID rates varied by geographical area. They were highest in Africa and nil in China, and were inversely associated with age. This mirrors exactly the background risk of sexually transmitted diseases (STIs).

■ Whether considered individually or grouped by type, the PID rates for copper-bearing, hormonal and inert IUDs were statistically indistinguishable. For all these devices this makes a specific IUD factor in the attacks very improbable, especially as previous studies were readily able to show that one device, the Dalkon Shield, did specifically increase PID risk (*see Q 9.62*).

■ In China, 4301 IUDs were inserted and not a single case of PID was reported either in the critical first 3 weeks or later!

9.55 It looks, then, as though insertion time is the main danger time for IUDs, but why?

The post-insertion infection 'bulge' of *Fig. 9.5* is most unlikely to be because of bad insertion technique (i.e. the doctors introducing new organisms) occurring only among the doctors outside China. Westergaard et al [*Obstetrics and Gynecology* 1982;60:322–325] showed that carrying out a termination of pregnancy in the presence of *Chlamydia* or gonococcal infection of the cervix increased the risk of postabortal infection about threefold.

IUD insertion is another procedure that can temporarily impair (at a cervical level) the mechanisms that protect the upper genital tract from organisms. This was shown by Mishell et al [*American Journal of Obstetrics and Gynecology* 1966;96:119–126]. Although the doctors in all the centres were searching for monogamous women, they might well have been successful in this search only in China. In mainland China, through the 1970s and 1980s (it would not be true now), monogamy was the norm, and it was also two-sided, with a consequential very low incidence of STIs of all kinds.

As there was no systematic prescreening, in the other countries, PID-causing organisms (especially *Chlamydia trachomatis*) are presumed to have been present in a proportion of the women.

In a later study from California [Walsh T et al 1998 *The Lancet* 351:1005–1008] when there *was* effective prescreening (verbal plus microbiological), the post-insertion 'bulge' of PID was – unsurprisingly – not detected even when antibiotics were not given. The screening of clients was so good that few, if any, pathogens would have been in the lower genital tracts of the subjects, and the incidence of PID was minimal (1:1000 in early months of use regardless of antibiotic treatment).

So in the WHO studies without prescreening the process of insertion would enable clinically silent infection to spread from the lower genital tract, where it had been, into the upper genital tract – therefore becoming symptomatic PID. Everywhere except in China. In summary:

■ The greatest risk of PID is in the first 20 days, believed to be caused by pre-existing carriage in the lower genital tract of that woman of sexually transmitted pathogens (STI organisms).

■ PID rates thereafter, like pre-insertion, relate to the background rate of STIs.

■ Insertions should ideally only be through what I lightheartedly call a 'Chinese cervix', minimizing the IUD-related post-insertion 'bulge' of PID (*see Fig. 9.5*).

9.56 So what is a 'Chinese cervix', as you use the term?!

Quite simply, it is a pathogen-free cervix! *Either* because the woman comes from a society/culture where, quite simply, there are no such pathogens (an almost unique feature of the Chinese mainland in the 1970s and most of the 1980s) *or* because she has been so effectively screened by a combination of verbal screening and assessment *and* – except when assessed as personally at very low risk – at least by an accurate *Chlamydia* test.

9.57 In summary, what are the practical implications for arrangements at IUD insertion in a society with a moderate or high prevalence of STIs?

Defining 'moderate prevalence' arbitrarily as over 5% *Chlamydia* carriage, it is my view that:

1   All prospective IUD-users should be questioned closely about their own STI risk, which means a proper sexual history (*see Q 1.14*), including the ticklish issue of how likely it might be that a pathogen might have been transmitted from a sole current partner who is not himself monogamous and then:

2   Ideally this verbal screening, taking the background factor of age under 25 into account, should be supplemented by microbiological screening at least for *Chlamydia*, prior to IUD insertions or reinsertions.

3   Evidence of recent exposure to an STI or a purulent discharge from the cervix indicates more detailed investigation at a genitourinary medicine (GUM) clinic anyway.

4   If *Chlamydia* is detected, an urgent GUM appointment should follow. Unless there is clinical PID (requiring more vigorous treatment), treatment is usually by doxycycline 100 mg bd for 7 days, or azithromycin 1 g stat, *after* other STIs have been looked for. Contact tracing should be arranged and the IUD insertion postponed – maybe indefinitely. There should certainly be a serious reappraisal of the

implications of her (and her partner's) lifestyle for use of this method – most particularly, as usual, if she is nulliparous.

5   If the *Chlamydia* result is negative, this, now highly likely to be a pathogen-free 'Chinese cervix', should be very thoroughly physically cleansed before the device is inserted – following the manufacturer's instructions with minimum trauma.

9.58   What if the (copper) IUD needs to be inserted before the results of the recommended *Chlamydia* screening are known – which is the norm in emergency contraception cases? Could one not eliminate the post-insertion 'hump' of infection shown in *Fig. 9.5* by simply routinely prescribing the appropriate antibiotics?

Because attenders for emergency contraception (EC) are known to be at high risk of *Chlamydia* [FSRH Guidance (April 2006). Emergency contraception. *Journal of Family Planning and Reproductive Health Care* 2006;32:121–128], in my view, full antibiotic treatment (as detailed in *Q 9.57(4)*) should normally be given with 100% follow-up to enable contact tracing if the *Chlamydia* test does return positive.

But some will dispute this because a Cochrane Review [Grimes DA et al 2002 Cochrane Library, Issue 4. Oxford, Update Software] was not able to demonstrate that prophylactic antibiotic use prior to *routine* IUD insertion conferred any benefit, except for a significant reduction in unscheduled return visits to the provider clinic in one Kenyan study. Aside from the fact that evidence is lacking for similar treatment at the time of *emergency* IUD insertion, in my opinion the four main RCTs in the excellent review by Grimes could not detect an advantage. This would be either because, through excellent screening, the women studied were at too low a risk without prophylaxis (Walsh's Californian study, *see Q 9.55*, and probably the study from Turkey) or perhaps because the studies in Kenya and Nigeria gave inadequate treatment (a single 200-mg dose of doxycycline pre-insertion).

Even within the Cochrane Review there is the statement:

> In populations with a high prevalence of sexually transmitted diseases, such as Kenya [Sinei 1990] prophylaxis may offer modest protection against both pelvic inflammatory disease and unscheduled visits to the clinic.

Now, according to the Faculty of SRH guidance mentioned above, EC-requesters in the UK are indeed such a population with respect to *Chlamydia*. Pending more data, therefore, I would withhold a proper course of prophylactic antibiotics from a prospective IUD-user in these particular circumstances only rarely, if verbal screening of the particular individual was very convincing that she was at *low risk*. I would also, for safety, then arrange, in the absence of this preventive treatment, for there to be contact at 7 days, at least by telephone (*see Q. 9.59*).

Note that if the high-risk circumstances of the individual do justify that antibiotic, they would certainly justify also doing a *Chlamydia* test so as to have the option of contact tracing – and to minimize the woman's risk of later (re-)infection by her partner.

9.59 What are the implications of *Fig. 9.5* for follow-up?

One possible policy is that there should be a routine first post-insertion visit after 7 days (additional to the routine 6-week follow-up): designed to pick up any women with post-insertion infection (during the highest-risk time of *Fig. 9.5*).

However, now that effective *Chlamydia* screening by a highly sensitive DNA test is available, it works well in practice in an elective case, or emergency non-antibiotic-treated cases, to give women a handout at the insertion visit, with a list of the symptoms suggestive of PID:

- low abdominal or pelvic pain, especially if any post-insertion symptoms had initially improved
- dyspareunia
- abnormal or offensive vaginal discharge
- a temperature above 38.3°C, especially if preceded by rigors.

In a clinic service they are instructed to telephone the Advice Sister should they be in the slightest doubt. In general practice, a similar handout could be used and it might be advisable for the woman to be asked routinely to 'touch base' by telephoning the Practice Nurse about a week after insertion.

9.60 How do you manage those who report problems?

If examination reveals cervical excitation tenderness and/or adnexal tenderness, then an urgent GUM appointment is indicated. If frank PID is confirmed, sometimes laparoscopically (*see Q 9.65*), metronidazole may need to be added along with a full 2 weeks of doxycycline.

9.61 What features of the device itself might increase risk of PID, and how might they be changed?

As we have seen, PID is primarily a 'self- or partner-inflicted wound'. Because IUDs are foreign bodies they have the potential suggested in early studies such as by Vessey et al 1981 [*British Medical Journal* 282:855–857] to promote the severity of attacks and perhaps facilitate secondary invaders. However, studies summarized in the review by David Grimes in 2000, quoted in Q 9.50, do not support this: more evidence is needed.

If the foreign body effect of IUDs is indeed a factor in worsening (sexually acquired) PID, it cannot – by definition – be eliminated. However it is *theoretically* reducible by:

- elimination of the plastic carrier, as in the GyneFix (*see Q 9.139*)
- release of progestogens into the cervical and uterine fluids, which might hinder transfer of pathogens to the upper genital tract with the LNG-IUS, although whether this truly lowers PID risk is not proven (*see Q 9.144*)
- similar release of antiseptic substances – attempted in small experiments, never taken further.

9.62 What could be the effect of the threads traversing the cervical canal?

The thread of the now defunct Dalkon Shield was multifilament in design and this was shown to act as a 'wick'. This was disastrous and, because a very few Dalkon Shields might still be in situ, they should always be removed on suspicion of their presence.

9.63 So should we go back to using threadless IUDs, like the old Birnberg Bow?

No. The RCTs quoted in *Q 9.50* have shown no difference in PID rates between thread-bearing and thread-free IUDs, and vanishingly low or zero rates of important infections anyway among thread-bearing device users in low-risk populations.

Pending more data, any adverse influence of the threads must be very small in practice, and more than outweighed by their usefulness during IUD follow-up and to simplify device removal.

9.64 How would you summarize practical implications, especially of the WHO studies (*Qs 9.53–9.58*)?

- Monogamous parous women with monogamous partners as in China in the 1980s can use IUDs with absolutely no fear of PID.
- Monogamous young nulliparae can definitely consider the option, but always as a second choice (WHO 2, or sometimes WHO 3, depending on the discussion about sexual lifestyles of self or partner) because they do not have that cushion, of one or more babies already in the cot.
- All potential and current users need to be informed/reminded where the infection really comes from because, as the 1992 WHO authors put it, 'exposure to sexually transmitted disease rather than type of IUD is the major determinant of PID'. Especially at times of partner change, users need to insist on condom use as well as their IUD.

■ Around the crucial time of insertion, the measures described in
Qs 9.53–9.57 need to be implemented.

■ There should be very vigorous treatment and contact-tracing of PID
when it happens.

■ Providers should minimize the number of (potentially dangerous)
reinsertions by choosing devices with the longest possible long-term
efficacy (see Q 9.133).

9.65 How should significant IUD-associated pelvic infection be managed?

Laparoscopy is indicated in severe cases to establish the diagnosis. Ideally,
full bacteriological screening at a GUM clinic should be performed. If such
detailed bacteriology is impossible, often because treatment is urgent, at
least endocervical swabs should be taken first into the appropriate transport
media. The usual first choice of antibiotic would be a tetracycline (preferably
for at least 2 weeks, to treat the most common and possibly most harmful
pathogens, namely *Chlamydia* and *Neisseria gonorrhoeae*), with 5 days of
metronidazole to deal with the frequently associated anaerobes.

9.66 Should the IUD be removed?

Data available do not support a better outcome to treatment of frank PID if
the IUD is removed (see the Grimes reference in Q 9.50) although, if there is
not a good response within 48 h to appropriate antibiotics, most authorities
would remove it. If it is removed, there should be urgent consideration of
postcoital contraception according to the menstrual and coital histories (see
Qs 9.13, 9.14) – not omitting also, as gynaecologists so often do, to arrange
with the woman a new long-term method of birth control.

9.67 Should there be any other action, after IUD-associated PID?

Regrettably, healthcare providers in most cultures still pussyfoot around
this matter, but the sexual contacts of all such women should be traced and
appropriately treated. There are a minimum of three individuals to be
treated, the index case, her partner and his other partner.

Moreover, a very clear warning should be given about the disastrous
effects of recurrent PID (reaching, after three hospitalized attacks, a tubal
occlusion rate of one in two); along with advice about condom use to
avoid another attack, let alone that other risk she may also be running, of
HIV infection. All this is not being judgmental, just good preventive
medicine.

9.68 Is pelvic infection always a contraindication to an IUD?

If currently acutely or chronically present, this is an absolute
contraindication (WHO 4). Moreover, all women reporting deep

dyspareunia or with tenderness of the pelvic organs, whether on palpation or caused by cervical excitation, should not receive an IUD until infection has been excluded.

9.69 What about a history of past pelvic infection?

If this was not severe, more than 6 months ago and there has been no recurrence, and currently the woman is free of any symptoms or signs, then (after full discussion and counselling) IUD insertion is only relatively contraindicated (WHO 3). It would still be preferable that such a woman should have at least one living child.

Rescreening for STIs, especially *Chlamydia*, should be done and there should be serious consideration of tetracycline 'cover' for the insertion.

The woman might need to be advised to use condoms as well, subsequently. She should also be warned to return exceptionally promptly at the first sign of another PID attack.

Past severe or recurrent infection is WHO 2 in a case at risk of endocarditis (*see Q 9.89*).

9.70 What does it mean when a cervical smear report says 'Actinomyces-like organisms (ALOs) are present'? Is it necessarily Actinomyces israelii?

This bacterium is normally a harmless commensal in the mouth and gastrointestinal tract but has the potential to do harm (*see Q 9.72*). In the lower female genital tract it is almost never detected by cytology (or culture) except when a foreign body is present, the most common being an IUD or IUS. But not all reports of ALOs are necessary this particular organism.

There is also an association with bacterial vaginosis (BV) – which itself has been found more common in IUD-users than controls (*see Q 9.174*).

9.71 How often are ALOs found in the cervical smears of IUD-users?

In some studies, the frequency with which ALOs have been reported in routine smears appears to relate in a linear fashion to the duration of use of the device: whether inert, copper or LNG-containing. After 1 year's use in one review, 1–2% of smears were positive, rising to 8–10% after 3 years.

It was initially thought that copper prevented the carriage of these organisms. It is now believed that the main explanation for lower incidence is the shorter average duration of use of copper than inert devices (plus, in the past, more frequent changes, *see Q 9.74*).

9.72 What is the most serious potential significance of the finding of ALOs in the cervical smear?

Frank actinomycosis is an extremely serious and debilitating condition, featuring granulomatous pelvic abscesses. A fatal outcome has been reported in one IUD-user and other women have been known to require pelvic clearance as a lifesaving measure. However, the incidence of this complication is extremely low, even allowing for under-diagnosis among women with severe IUD-related infections. In the context of millions of woman-years of IUD use there have been only a few hundred cases reported in the whole world literature.

In short, it seems clear that actinomycosis represents a very small part of the spectrum of pelvic infection associated with IUDs.

9.73 What action should be taken when a cervical smear from an established user of an IUD or IUS is reported as showing ALOs?

The protocol that follows is only partially evidence-based but, substantially, it is that of the Faculty of Sexual and Reproductive Healthcare as first issued in January 1998 and subsequently reissued. Pending more data:

- The patient should be recalled without delay and questioned carefully about the occurrence of pain, deep dyspareunia, intermenstrual bleeding or excess discharge, and dysuria.
- *She should always be examined.* If, as is the rule, she is completely asymptomatic and examination is normal, proceed directly to Q 9.74.
- If the bimanual examination is not entirely normal, if there is even mild adnexal or uterine tenderness on examination, or cervical excitation tenderness, or any mass is felt,
- an ultrasound scan should be arranged. If this shows adnexal mass(es), immediate referral is indicated.
- If actinomycosis rather than a 'normal' form of PID is suspected, referral should be generally to a gynaecologist rather than a department of GUM – again, especially if there is an adnexal mass.
- In my view, the knowledge that ALOs are present should markedly lower the threshold for IUD removal, whatever other action is taken.
- Investigations might include (preferably after personal discussion with the microbiologist): endocervical swabs, culture of the removed IUD (threads excised) and endometrial biopsies for culture and histology. If the laboratory recommends antibiotic therapy, penicillin or erythromycin are usual choices but in high dose often for several weeks. If other anaerobes such as those causing BV are diagnosed, metronidazole 400 mg bd for 5 days or more may also be advised.
- The patient should be followed up to check for cure, and another method of birth control arranged.

9.74 What action should be taken if ALOs are reported and there are absolutely NO symptoms or signs at all (pelvic infection not suspected)?

If so many long-term IUD-users carry ALOs, and so very few ever develop symptoms, more morbidity (through resulting pregnancies) could be caused by insisting on ceasing the method than by simply monitoring the situation.

All asymptomatic women should first be counselled about the potential (small) risk and taught the symptoms of pelvic actinomycosis. At the Margaret Pyke Centre there is a helpful leaflet describing the two management options:

OPTION A: REMOVAL OR CHANGE OF THE IUD OR IUS

This is a popular course of action, particularly for copper IUDs, because it usually leads to a more reassuring situation for the woman. In 1984 a small study at the Margaret Pyke Centre, and a later study of 100 women in Newcastle upon Tyne, showed that device removal – *without* any antibiotic treatment – was followed by disappearance of the ALOs from the subsequent cervical smears. At the Margaret Pyke Centre this clearance occurred with or without immediate reinsertion.

Although later experience shows that such clearance is not invariable, we find that most women after counselling now elect to try device removal, with replacement or switching to another long-term method. The removed device does not need to be sent for culture.

After one case at the Margaret Pyke Centre developed full-blown actinomycosis – subsequent to being asymptomatic at IUD removal without reinsertion, and being discharged because she did not need contraception postmenopausally – I now recommend follow-up at 3 rather than 6 months in every case. The woman should also be counselled to return at any time should she have any of the symptoms in Q *9.73*.

If at the follow-up visit a bimanual examination and repeat smear show no abnormality, she can simply return to having regular cervical smears on her local screening programme (e.g. every 3 years).

OPTION B: LEAVE THE IUD OR IUS IN SITU, WITH MONITORING BY REGULAR FOLLOW-UP EXAMINATION ARRANGED EVERY 6 MONTHS

The follow-up is for a *bimanual examination* and enquiry (and reminder) about relevant symptoms, i.e. pain, deep dyspareunia, intermenstrual bleeding or excessive discharge, and dysuria.

The woman is additionally advised, with back-up written instructions, that if these should ever occur she must – without fail – return before her next routine visit. She should agree to be contacted at home or through her general practitioner if she defaults from follow-up.

Cervical smears are likely to continue to show the ALOs and are hence only repeated at the frequency of local screening guidelines.

In both cases, if BV is diagnosed (characteristic odour and history with pH more than 4.5) it should be treated with metronidazole 400 mg bd for 5 days.

COMMENT

Option A as compared with Option B has the potential to reduce both a woman's ongoing anxiety about harbouring a potential pathogen 'down below' and our burden of responsibility for long-term follow-up. But each case should be individualized and other factors, such as the cost of a new LNG-IUS when her existing one is suiting well, might also come into the equation.

PAIN AND BLEEDING

9.75 What is the most frequent complaint of users of copper IUDs?

 In practice, the most frequent problem is increased bleeding, frequently accompanied by cramp-like menstrual pain, and the two are often considered together. However, it is a good working slogan that:

> **IUD/IUS slogan 7**
> Pain plus bleeding in an IUD-user has a serious cause until proved otherwise.

Thus, to label these as a 'side-effect' should only be after exclusion of the more important possible causes: pregnancy-related (miscarriage, ectopic) or otherwise (partially expelled, malpositioned or perforated device; or PID) (*see* Qs 9.20, 9.21).

9.76 What types of bleeding pattern are observed by IUD-users?

The loss at the menses might be heavier and/or longer: the latter typically because of light premenstrual bleeding, or spotting, before and after the flow proper. There might also be intermenstrual bleeding or spotting, too light to cause anaemia but often very troublesome to the woman.

9.77 How often do IUD-users discontinue the method because of pain or bleeding?

About 5–20% of users of inert or copper IUDs have the device removed because of bleeding and pain within the first 12 months. Of the remainder, approximately half will admit to annoying bleeding symptoms that they have learnt to live with and some will subsequently discontinue the method for the same reason. (Measurement of the loss has shown that inert devices roughly double the measured volume of flow, whereas the smaller copper ones increase the amount only by about 50%, that is about 20–30 mL on average.) Nevertheless, removal rates were not dramatically improved when copper devices arrived. This is doubtless because none have eliminated the annoyance for some women of prolongation of duration of flow and intermenstrual spotting.

These last two bleeding problems are still features of at least the early months of use of progestogen-releasing devices like the LNG-IUS, even though they positively reduce the measured volume of loss and often eliminate pain. Perseverance is usually rewarded by frank amenorrhoea or infrequent light bleeds (*see Q 9.145*).

9.78 Is copper a haemostatic agent?

Menstrual blood loss measurement studies of my own in the 1970s, comparing Lippes loops with and without copper bands (but otherwise identical), showed clearly that the measured mean volumes were similar. Indeed, the duration of loss in the copper-using group was slightly but significantly increased. Hence it is possible to be definite that the reduced amount of bleeding with copper devices is a function merely of their smaller size and surface area (*see Q 9.9*).

9.79 What is the cause of the increased bleeding as an IUD symptom, with or without pain?

- Various types of malposition can cause both symptoms.
- The fact that the cavity of the uterus is distorted congenitally or by fibroids might be missed, causing pain as the uterus attempts to expel the device. Coincidental polyps are also possible.
- Especially in nulliparae, whose cavities tend to be smaller, the fitting of a device that is too long or too wide (*see Q 9.92*) can similarly cause cramping pain. The stem of a device that is too long projects into the sensitive isthmic part of the uterus and pain might also result from penetration of the myometrium by the side arms.
- Perforation of the cervix by the stem of the device can result from partial expulsion and also cause pain (see *Fig. 9.11* (p. 443) and *Q 9.124*).

In all these cases following bouts of cramping, some at least of the observed intermenstrual bleeding (IMB) can be caused by mechanical trauma to the endometrium. According to some X-ray studies, small-framed devices that float too loosely in a large cavity can also cause some IMB, but without pain.

The LNG-IUS (*see Q 9.143ff*) has the same mechanical limitations as the Nova-T 380, whose shape it shares, yet when properly located improves uterine pain in most women (as well as dramatically reducing quantity of bleeding).

GyneFix (*see Q 9.139*) was expected to eliminate or minimize the problems listed above, through its unique implantable technology. Surprisingly, however, a systematic review [O'Brien PA et al 2002 Cochrane Library, Issue 1. Oxford, Update Software] did not demonstrate improvement in bleeding/pain removal rates as compared with standard framed copper IUDs.

9.80 What is the uterine mechanism for IUD-related bleeding and pain?

Insertion of IUDs leads to a high concentration of plasminogen activators, which increase fibrinolytic activity and hence lead to more blood flow. Linked in some way with these changes are alterations in the prostaglandin responses of the endometrium during menstruation. Prostacyclin activity is increased and this causes vasodilatation and inhibition of platelet function. An increase in other prostaglandins probably explains the increased menstrual cramps, but not why some users are affected so much less than others.

9.81 Are there any drugs that can reduce the menstrual flow and pain in IUD-users?

There is no very effective therapy for the problem of prolonged spotting. However, for the heaviness of flow at the menses, antifibrinolytic agents are certainly effective. Tranexamic acid is available but it is not certain whether the benefits of treatment outweigh its risks, particularly as it is not an analgesic. The pain-relieving PGSIs are therefore normally preferable for initial trial, particularly mefenamic acid (1500 mg), ibuprofen (1200 mg) and naproxen (1500 mg). (Amounts in parentheses are totals for each day, to be taken in divided doses.) These drugs need only be taken from the onset of menstruation for so long as the patient feels the benefit from treatment. Response is very variable (*Fig. 9.6*) but some women report that the flow diminishes rapidly within an hour of taking a tablet.

9.82 Do many women persevere for long with an IUD if they have to take drugs regularly to cope with bleeding and/or pain?

Not as a rule. Few women would be happy to continue for years taking powerful drugs with each menstruation and doctors too would be worried by possible long-term risks. Antiprostaglandin drugs are certainly very useful to reduce the cramps at IUD insertion, and both pain and bleeding over the first few cycles. In practice, however, few women continue to take

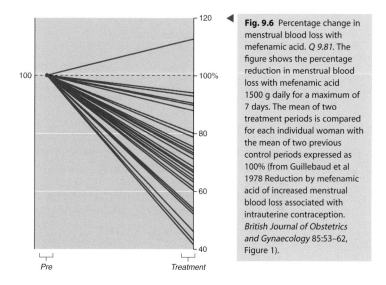

Fig. 9.6 Percentage change in menstrual blood loss with mefenamic acid. *Q 9.81*. The figure shows the percentage reduction in menstrual blood loss with mefenamic acid 1500 g daily for a maximum of 7 days. The mean of two treatment periods is compared for each individual woman with the mean of two previous control periods expressed as 100% (from Guillebaud et al 1978 Reduction by mefenamic acid of increased menstrual blood loss associated with intrauterine contraception. *British Journal of Obstetrics and Gynaecology* 85:53–62, Figure 1).

them (except intermittently for dysmenorrhoea) and the majority either live with their symptoms or eventually give up the IUD method. A better alternative might be to exchange the IUD for an IUS (*see Q 9.143ff*).

SELECTION OF USERS AND OF DEVICES

9.83   How are the absolute contraindications (WHO 4) to IUD or IUS use best classified?

These mostly relate to the adverse side-effects that we have already considered. They can be classified into *temporary* absolute contraindications, which imply some variable delay before possible later insertion, and *permanent* WHO 4 contraindications. In general, absolute contraindications apply to both IUDs and IUSs, but relative contraindications do not always apply to the IUS (*see below*).

9.84   What are the (possibly) temporary absolute contraindications to IUDs and IUSs?

■ Undiagnosed *irregular genital tract bleeding*. This is for fear of wrongly attributing post-insertion bleeding to the IUD when in fact it is due to important uterine pathology, such as carcinoma of the endometrium.
■ Suspicion of *pregnancy*.
■ *Post septic abortion*, current *pelvic infection* or undiagnosed pelvic tenderness/deep dyspareunia or *purulent cervicitis* (*see Q 9.88*).

- Therapy causing *significant immunosuppression*, i.e. more profound than use of low-dose corticosteroids (*see* Q 9.88).
- *Trophoblastic disease* while hCG still elevated, for fear of uterine wall involvement in the disease process. (WHO 1 when hCG undetectable).

9.85 What are the permanent absolute contraindications to IUDs and IUSs?

1 *Markedly distorted uterine cavity*, or cavity sounding to less than 5 cm depth (see *Fig. 9.10* (p. 435) and *Q 9.91*). However, this finding signifies only category WHO 2 (broadly usable) for the GyneFix frameless device (*see* Q 9.139).

2 Known true allergy to a constituent (*see* Q 9.87).

3 *Wilson's disease* (copper devices only). WHO 4 is precautionary, no good data (FSRH Guidance. Intrauterine contraception (2007). www.fsrh.org).

NB: In previous editions it was stated that the WHO 4 category for IUDs or the IUS should include those at highest risk of *bacterial endocarditis,* namely those with a prosthetic heart valve or with the history of a past attack. Current practice has changed. The IUD or IUS is 'broadly usable' (WHO 2), along with appropriate advice as in Q 9.89.

9.86 What are the relative contraindications to copper IUD use?

These often do not apply to the LNG-IUS (*see the note, below*). They vary in their importance: the WHO classification is useful (*see* Q 5.121). WHO 3 means use very cautiously, other contraceptive options being preferable, and WHO 2 signifies broadly usable, benefits outweigh risks. Unless otherwise stated, the factors listed here are WHO 2, meaning in the individual case that the IUD could even be her best choice, in comparison with alternatives. Some are considered in more detail later.

1 *Between 48 h and 4 weeks postpartum*: excess risk of perforation, so is WHO 3.

2 *Known HIV infection*: if controlled by drug therapy this is only WHO 2 (*see* Q 9.88). Eventual interference with the immune system by the virus in AIDS can be expected to increase the risk of severe infection (WHO 3). But the LNG-IUS is an excellent choice in either state because of its added advantages of reducing pain and blood loss (WHO 1) – plus added condom use as routinely advised.

3 Recent *exposure to a high risk of a sexually transmitted disease* (e.g. after rape): ideally, the insertion should be delayed until after full investigation, but in emergency situations, such as for postcoital contraception, a copper IUD is permissible (WHO 3) with full antibiotic cover (after swabs for bacteriology have been taken, *see Qs 10.23 and 10.27*).

4 *Structural heart disease* with bacterial endocarditis risk, however severe. This classification is new, see *Q 9.89*. In my view the new (2008) guidance supports WHO 2, 'broadly usable' but with specific advice (end of *Q 9.89*).

5 *Past history of tubal ectopic pregnancy* in *nulliparae* (*see Q 9.31*): WHO 3 if the most effective banded copper IUDs or the LNG-IUS are used but it would be better still to use an anovulant method. Also, past history of tubal surgery, or other very high ectopic risk, in those still wanting a child would be WHO 3. Even among parous women the risk of recurrence of this dangerous condition implies some caution (WHO 2). WHO itself is less cautious, and calls past ectopic always WHO 1 – on a *population* basis (*see Q 9.29*).

6 With any prosthesis that can be prejudiced by blood-borne infection (e.g. *hip replacement*), IUDs are certainly usable, appearing in category WHO 2 solely to flag up consideration of possible antibiotic cover for the insertion.

7 Past history of definite pelvic infection (*see Q 9.69*).

8 Lifestyle with frequent partner change, risking STIs.

9 *Suspected subfertility already*: WHO 2 for any cause or WHO 3 if the questionable fertility relates to a tubal cause.

10 *Nulliparity and young age*, especially less than 20: the reason this is WHO 2 – and in some young women after a good sexual history it might be WHO 3 – is concern about increased risk of infection and also not having the 'cushion' of having least one child. But as we saw above, neither the IUD nor LNG-IUS themselves *cause* PID and so are very usable in selected cases. Summation, as usual, with other factors in this list can make the caution stronger (up to WHO 4). Expulsion is also more common in nulliparae, regardless of device design.

11 *Diabetes*: WHO 2 allegedly for infection risk but the IUD is preferable to several of the hormonal methods for diabetics; and the LNG-IUS can be an excellent choice (*see Q 9.90*). (WHO says always WHO 1.)

12 *Fibroids or congenital abnormality without too marked distortion* of the uterine cavity (*see Q 9.91*): WHO 2 for framed IUDs or IUSs; WHO 1 for the GyneFix.

13 *Severely scarred uterus*, e.g. after myomectomy: WHO 3.

14 *Severe cervical stenosis*: pretreatment with estrogen can help (*see Q 9.34(3)*).

15 *Heavy periods*, with or without anaemia, before insertion for any reason, including anticoagulation. This is an indication for the LNG-IUS: WHO 1.

16 *Primary dysmenorrhoea*: but the LNG-IUS (which will benefit most cases of dysmenorrhoea, *see Q 9.144*, provided the uterus tolerates its frame) can be tried.

17 *Endometriosis*: there is no proven link but part of the mechanism of endometriosis might be retrograde menstruation. Hence, prudence dictates it might be preferable not to increase this with a copper IUD. However, here again the progestogen-releasing LNG-IUS is a good option: WHO 1.

18 *Penicillamine treatment*, whether for Wilson's disease (WHO 4 for copper IUDs anyway) or rheumatoid arthritis: there are one or two anecdotes of in situ pregnancy occurring in penicillamine-treated users of copper IUDs – possibly due to interference with the contraceptive action of the copper. This is unproven; inert or progestogen-releasing IUDs would not be affected.

19 *After endometrial ablation/resection* (*see Qs 11.53 and 11.54* for more about this). LNG-IUS can be used in selected cases. Finally:

20 Past perforation of the uterus is only WHO 2 (*see Q 9.42*).

> The LNG-IUS (*see Q 9.143ff*) is actually indicated for (2), (15), (16) and (17) above, and poses no added problem for (18).

9.87 Can copper IUDs cause local or systemic allergic reactions?

Definite cases have been reported, although they are rare. For instance, one case reported in 1976 presented with urticaria, joint pains and angioneurotic oedema, and positive scratch tests showed a true copper allergy. I had one clear case of marked reversible uterine pain and tenderness plus vaginal discharge, with no evidence of infection, resolving immediately after removal of the device. Referral to a dermatologist for specific allergy tests might be indicated, although most contact allergies to metal bangles or rings are not due to copper.

9.88 Is there evidence that antibiotics, antiprostaglandin or immunosuppressive drugs might impair the efficacy of IUDs?

As there is no evidence that the inflammatory reaction in the uterus and tubes of IUD-users is normally caused by any infective process, the few reports of pregnancy occurring during antibiotic use can be dismissed as coincidences. One study comparing pregnancy rates in IUD-users with and without rheumatoid arthritis has shown no evidence that interference with endometrial prostaglandin metabolism by PGSIs can impair IUD efficacy, although this had been suggested in a study from France.

There are reports that immunosuppressed transplant patients are more likely to become pregnant if they use IUDs. Probably more important is the risk of severe and silent infection. Hence, other methods of birth control should be advised if such drugs must be used (not including corticosteroids, except for high-dose regimens).

9.89 What are the implications for IUD-users of significant anatomical lesions of the heart?

The long-standing concern here related to a possible increased risk of life-threatening bacterial endocarditis, due to bacteraemia occurring during the insertion. Those at highest risk have a prosthetic valve or a past history of the disease. But in March 2008 NICE (www.nice.org.uk) issued new clinical guidelines, which have introduced a significant change to clinical practice since the last edition. Antibiotic prophylaxis is NO LONGER recommended when clients at even the highest level of risk are undergoing invasive procedures such as IUD/IUS insertion (or difficult removal). Whilst the latter remains in my view WHO 2 since it can, sometimes, cause bacteraemia, there is no clear association between recent interventional procedures and subsequent infective endocarditis: including in dentistry, where bacteraemia with relevant organisms is frequent. To put this into context, the evidence considered by the Guideline Development Group showed that simple toothbrushing can cause repetitive bacteraemia episodes which, cumulatively, pose almost certainly a greater risk for infective endocarditis than any single interventional procedure. Antibiotic prophylaxis for the latter is not cost effective and may lead to higher mortality from adverse effects, especially fatal anaphylactic reactions, than not using preventive antibiotics.

All patients at risk of endocarditis given an IUD/IUS should be advised:

- how to recognize symptoms of infective endocarditis and instructed to seek expert advice if they occur subsequent to the insertion, and
- to persevere with good oral hygiene (daily tooth-cleaning and flossing).

Finally, any relevant infection (specifically pelvic inflammatory disease) should be promptly investigated and treated in all users of intrauterine contraception who have this endocarditis risk.

9.90 What are the implications of diabetes for a potential IUD-user?

It was suggested in a study from Edinburgh that diabetes rendered both inert and copper IUDs less effective. However, other workers, notably in Scandinavian countries, have completely failed to show this association.

More relevant is the fear that diabetes might make any pelvic infection more severe than it otherwise would be. However, the IUD, or perhaps even better the LNG-IUS, remains a valid option, particularly for diabetics at low risk of STIs. WHO is probably right to call this WHO 1.

9.91 Can an IUD or the LNG-IUS be used by a woman with uterine fibroids?

The answer is 'yes', provided the cavity of the uterus is not distorted by any submucous fibroid and (as will normally follow) she does not suffer from menorrhagia. After careful bimanual examination, and the usual discussion about future fertility, etc., provisional arrangements can be made for the device to be inserted. The woman should be warned that plans might have to be changed if, early in the insertion procedure, the uterine sound detects an obvious submucous fibroid (as in *Fig. 9.10*, p. 435).

Where the facilities exist, a pre-insertion ultrasound scan is crucial, requesting specifically that the uterine cavity be checked for distortion by submucous fibroids. If there is distortion, a GyneFix can still be tried or, in the absence of marked cavity intrusion, the LNG-IUS, to control heavy periods – with warning about increased risk of expulsion and of malposition (this is where an implantable version of the latter would be so useful).

CHOICE OF DEVICE

9.92 How can one select the best IUD for each woman?

Feet come in different sizes and shapes, and shoes therefore come in many different fittings. Even without recognized distortions of the uterine cavity (see *Fig. 9.10*, p. 435), the sizes and shapes of uteri similarly vary. There is no fixed relationship between total uterine length as measured with a standard uterine sound, and uterine cavity length, which can comprise as little as one-third of the total (*Fig. 9.7*). Maximum fundal width also varies between individuals, and is less in vivo than when measured on hysterectomy specimens. The living uterus is a muscular organ, which contracts and relaxes and whose tonus also varies with the menstrual cycle (*Fig. 9.8*). Yet traditional framed IUDs came in constant shapes and in sizes that are sometimes too large for the cavity in which they are to be placed.

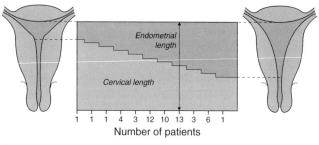

▲

Fig. 9.7 Measured endometrial and cervical lengths. *Q 9.92*. Eleven different combinations were noted in a series of 55 patients, all with the same total uterine axial dimension of 7 cm (from Hasson 1982 Uterine geometry and IUCD design. *British Journal of Obstetrics and Gynaecology* Supplement 4:3, Figure 3).

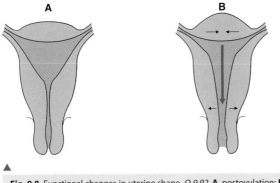

Fig. 9.8 Functional changes in uterine shape. *Q 9.92*. **A**, postovulation; **B**, at menstruation (from Hasson 1982 Uterine geometry and IUCD design. *British Journal of Obstetrics and Gynaecology* Supplement 4:3, Figure 2).

The manufacturers have usefully now produced several smaller IUDs, notably the banded Mini TT 380 Slimline. The size of this is reduced to 23 mm wide × 30 mm long and it is 'suitable for minimum uterine length of 5 cm' on sounding. Unhelpfully, the inserter tube is no thinner than for the larger TT 380 Slimline which is 33 mm wide × 37 mm long.

In theory, the best approach for smaller or distorted cavities must be the implantable (frameless) technology of GyneFix. Experience with this on the ground in the UK has been disappointing, however (*see Qs 9.140, 9.141*). Hopefully, further development, especially of the inserter mechanism, will deal with the problems and additionally lead to a viable hormone-releasing product.

9.93 Given the range of IUDs available in the UK, what is your normal first choice for a parous woman?

The main framed devices available are shown in *Fig. 9.9* (see also *Figs 9.12 and 9.13*).

In the UK the T-Safe Cu 380A and its clones named in *Fig. 9.9* – a successful series of banded devices – are now the 'gold standard' for copper IUDs, with one of the lowest cumulative pregnancy rates so far reported (*see Q 1.10*) and a UK-approved intrauterine lifespan of 10 years (indeed the evidence-base supports use for at least 12 years; Dennis J et al 2002 *Journal of Family Planning and Reproductive Healthcare* 28:61–68) – meaning a bargain price of about £1 per year. None of the other framed IUDs available perform better, nor can they be left in situ for so long, which is a major advantage, given the risks at every insertion/reinsertion. See IUD slogan 1 at *Q 9.21*.

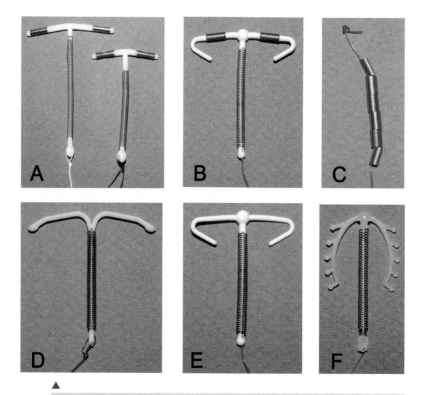

▲

Fig. 9.9 Copper IUDs. **A**: T-Safe Cu 380A QL (Quick-Load) (FP Sales) or TT 380 Slimline (Durbin) and related Mini TT 380 Slimline with shorter stem and narrower 'armspan' (Durbin); **B**: Flexi-T 380 (FP Sales); **C**: GyneFix (Durbin, FP Sales); **D**: Nova-T 380 (Schering); also UT 380 Short (Durbin) with short stem; **E**: Flexi-T 300 (FP Sales) with short stem; **F**: Multiload Cu375 (Organon) or Load 375 (Durbin). *Q 9.93*. Images reproduced by kind permission of Dr Anne MacGregor.

9.94 **Is the new Nova-T 380 with 380 mm² of copper wire improved as compared with the old Nova-T 200?**

Yes. The Nova-T 380 is certainly more acceptable for use (at least to 5 years) than its predecessor. In the UK Family Planning Network study of 574 users, its cumulative failure rate to 5 years was good, 2 per 100 women. But in the only RCT so far reported [Haugan T et al 2007 *Contraception* 75:171–176] among 470 volunteers its cumulative failure rate per 100 women at 3 years was 3.6, compared with 1.7 among 487 users of a clone of the banded T-Safe Cu 380A. The main difference occurred in the first year of use.

More important than its probable lower effectiveness, it suffers from not being evidence-based for use beyond 5 years, which is the chief advantage of its banded rivals (*see Qs 9.21, 9.93*). But its small inserting diameter of 3.7 mm when loaded makes it easy to insert in nulliparae. This makes it or its short-stemmed version (UT 380 Short, see legend to *Fig. 9.9*) a reasonable choice for emergency contraception when required by a nulliparous woman, above all if the plan is for it to be removed in the next cycle when the woman is established on a more appropriate method (*see Q 9.97*).

9.95 What do we know about the Flexi-T 300 and the Flexi-T + 380 IUDs?

In an RCT referenced in the Dennis article (*see Q 9.93*), among 300 users the former (shown at E in *Fig. 9.9*) had a failure rate of 2.5 per 100 to 3 years, which was higher (but not statistically so) than experienced by 300 users of the banded Cu T 380A comparator. It also had a significantly higher expulsion rate. Like the Nova-T 380 it has a narrow inserter tube and is exceptionally easy to insert by a direct push technique, making it another option for emergency contraception.

But for all likely long-term users I still rate as first choices, if they can be fitted successfully, the T-Safe Cu 380A or its smaller version bearing the same amount of copper, the Mini TT 380 Slimline. The Flexi-T + 380 IUD (B in *Fig. 9.9*) is banded and being 28 mm wide × 32 mm long it is 5 mm wider and a couple of millimetres longer than the 300 version, though inserted by a similar direct push technique. Its main problem is that there seem to be no efficacy data available.

9.96 When would you recommend use of Multiload IUDs?

These are no longer stocked in the services to which I am affiliated. Multiload IUDs tend to cause greater cervical discomfort (at removal as well as insertion) and are not well enclosed in a sterile tube while traversing the endocervical canal. Only the more effective 375 version should now be used. It remains licensed only to 5 years and its efficacy is lower than the banded Cu T 380A comparator in most studies. Even its expulsion rate does not (as used to be taught) show any comparative advantage.

9.97 Which IUD do you select for the nulliparous woman?

- ■ If the method is used, after discussion of all the young woman's options, the preferred choice for long-term use among marketed IUDs by a nullipara remains a banded product, if it can be comfortably fitted: either the Mini TT 380 Slimline or possibly (*see Q 9.95*) the Flexi-T + 380 (B in *Fig. 9.9*).
- ■ If available, the GyneFix (*see Q 9.139ff*), with its minute physical size (*see Q 9.61*), narrower inserter and low expulsion rate, is also an excellent

choice, above all for the tiny or distorted uterus. The special insertion skills it requires, the risk of unnoticed expulsion and its higher price are the main obstacles.

■ If the internal os is very tight, either the Nova-T 380 or the UT 380 Short (see D in *Fig. 9.9* and legend), or perhaps the Flexi-T 300, may have to be used – all are unbanded.

■ The LNG-IUS (*see Q 9.148ff*) still has the problems for the present (*see Q 9.145*) of being on a frame rather than implanted and inserted through a relatively wide tube. However, it can be a godsend if the young woman has painful periods, and some data suggest it would reduce (not eliminate) the risk of PID.

9.98 Which device do you choose for women who have expelled a previous IUD?

■ First, I would evaluate the possibility of a distorted uterus (congenitally or by fibroids), and, if in doubt, do a pelvic ultrasound scan. The earlier insertion might also have been done during a heavy day of the woman's period (*see Qs 9.15, 9.16*).

■ The GyneFix has, in one series, the lowest known expulsion rate: but only if it is inserted by a healthcare provider with the required skill and experience (*see Q 9.139*). But

■ All the variants of the T-Safe Cu 380A IUDs (A in *Fig 9.9*) come next for expulsion risk and would normally be tried next, or again.

■ Because the commonest reason for expulsion is less-than-ideal placement of the first IUD, it may be entirely appropriate for an experienced practitioner to use the same type as just expelled – indeed, this may not be avoidable if the woman needs a LNG-IUS on specific gynaecological grounds.

INSERTION TIMING AND PROCEDURE

9.99 What is the importance of correct insertion?

This cannot be overstressed. A good 'revision test' is to check for yourself in *Qs 9.20 and 9.21* how true it is as in 'IUD/IUS slogan 1' that poor insertion technique is capable of producing every one of the eight IUD problems listed.

9.100 When should one perform so-called interval insertions?

COPPER IUDS, WHETHER FRAMED OR FRAMELESS

See Qs 9.15–9.17 for discussion of the optimum time in menstruating women, which is any time from around the end of the main menstrual flow through to day 12 of a 28-day cycle, normally. But this can be extended for copper IUDs to day 19 (adjusted for cycle length) even if contraception has been effectively non-existent up to that day, using it as a postcoital (anti-implantation) method. Thereafter, insertion could be even later if you are confident that there cannot already be an implanted pregnancy from intercourse earlier in the cycle, or up to 5 days after a single act of unprotected intercourse late in the cycle (*see Qs 10.14, 10.33*).

THE LNG-IUS

See Q 9.143. In brief, the speed with which this extremely effective method operates is not great enough within the first cycle for it to act as a postcoital method. Conception in the cycle of insertion would be of special concern because of the extremely high endometrial concentration of LNG hormone. Therefore, in cycling women it is recommended that insertion is performed within the first 7 days. If any later, there must be 'believable and really effective' contraception up to the day of insertion and condom use thereafter at least for the next 7 days.

> Ensure that, *as a routine,* all who plan to have an LNG-IUS are started on a more effective method than condoms (e.g. the combined pill), so the insertion can be performed without that conception anxiety, on any mutually convenient date.

Note that the above is a similar policy to what was recommended for Implanon (*see Q 8.68*).

9.101 When should IUDs be inserted following a full-term delivery?

POSTPARTUM

Normal policy in the UK is for IUD insertion to be delayed until the postnatal visit, i.e. at about 6 weeks. This is fine for lactating women, but if she is not breastfeeding, the woman will need to use another method of birth control from the fourth week (*see Q 5.50*). Hence, insertion during that fourth week by an experienced clinician may sometimes be contraceptively preferable, depending on the amount of lochia and satisfactory uterine involution (*see Q 11.22*).

POST DELIVERY

Insertion directly after delivery of the placenta, with careful fundal placement, manually or using a sponge-holder or ring forceps, has been shown to have higher (but in some circumstances acceptable) subsequent expulsion rates. Insertion slightly later is also a possibility, up to 48 hours.

9.102 What is the optimum insertion time after lower segment caesarean section?

A T-Safe Cu 380A or other IUD or IUS can be sutured to the fundus with chromic catgut, by way of the lower segment incision. However, normal practice is to defer insertion at least to 6 weeks (some would say 8 weeks) to be sure of complete healing of the lower segment scar. As, after involution, this potential weakness finishes up very low – at the level of the internal os – there would in fact be no objection to the insertion by an experienced, careful clinician at the same time as for other women (i.e. at about 6 weeks).

Puerperal infection (with or without operative delivery) would indicate postponement – if indeed an IUD insertion were ever to be appropriate.

9.103 When should IUDs be inserted following any kind of abortion?

Careful studies have shown that immediate insertion at the time of evacuation of the uterus – whether for legal induced abortion or following an incomplete miscarriage – can be good practice in selected cases. Surprisingly to many, no statistical differences with respect to subsequent infection were found in RCTs that compared outcomes in women receiving versus not receiving a framed copper IUD at the time of uterine evacuation in the same service [systematic review by Grimes, 2002].

The expulsion rate in the above studies was higher than for interval insertions, but this can be dealt with by follow-up and replacement of the IUD as necessary.

The above studies were performed by experts; there is the fear that in less experienced hands a fragment of products of conception might be retained and the insertion of a foreign body might then both facilitate infection and render such infection more severe. But insertion of IUDs or IUSs at the time of the evacuation could be good practice almost routinely in parous women, and fairly often in nulliparae, if only there were:

■ preliminary full counselling
■ an ultrasound scan machine in the theatre, as is increasingly the case, to ensure no retained products
■ microbiological screening (for *Chlamydia* anyway)
■ antibiotic chemoprophylaxis (*see* Q 9.58).

9.104 Do you have any practical tips for IUD/IUS insertion in an older perimenopausal woman whose cervix might be tight despite previous parity – due to hypoestrogenism?

This is a very real problem that we faced at the Margaret Pyke Centre during our (highly successful) studies of the LNG-IUS as the progestogen component of HRT. The solution, which can dramatically improve (soften) the cervix, is to give a good dose of standard HRT estrogen for 1 month before the planned insertion, systemically or to the vagina – followed by local anaesthesia and dilatation on the day.

9.105 What are the minimum practical requirements for insertion of IUDs or the LNG-IUS?

■ A firm couch at a convenient height.

■ A good adjustable light.

■ Sterile equipment:
- bivalve speculum
- Stiles or Allis holding forceps, preferably not a toothed tenaculum, to reduce cervical pain (*and see Q 9.109 re LA to the cervix*)
- sponge forceps
- uterine sound
- galley pot plus swabs for sterilizing solution
- scissors
- gloves (if they are not sterile and a no-touch technique is planned, meaning no manual contact with any part of an instrument entering the uterus, great care must be taken to maintain a 'sterile field' over one side of the trolley: ensuring the handle ends that have been touched are systematically placed to the opposite side)
- Spencer–Wells forceps.

■ In reserve:
- local anaesthetic, needles and syringes
- small cervical dilators up to 6-mm diameter
- an emergency tray (*see Q 9.119*), and an oxygen cylinder and mask.

■ *An assistant in the room*: as a chaperone, to aid sterile technique, for added reassurance – and to help in a rare crisis (*see Q 9.115ff*).

9.106 What are the characteristics and qualities of a good IUD doctor/nurse, regardless of devices and services?

■ First and foremost, the clinician (doctor or nurse) should be really well trained, which means excellent bimanual and speculum technique for a start, followed in the UK by the theoretical and practical training now organized by the Faculty of SRH. This is in two stages for doctors, but special arrangements (though similar in their essentials) can be made for nurse practitioners who have the backing of their local service: the basic diploma is followed by a special advanced course leading to the Letter of Competence in intrauterine contraception techniques (including cervical local anaesthesia and the management of 'lost threads'). This brief apprenticeship training with a good instructing doctor beats any amount of book-learning.

- Before attempting insertion in any patient, some initial practice with the same devices using a small plastic model and working through the manufacturer's instruction sheet is, in my view, essential. Such a 'dry run' should also never be omitted whenever a new device (e.g. GyneFix) or new inserter (e.g. recently for the T-Safe Cu 380A and LNG-IUS) arrives on the contraceptive scene.
- Initial competence with any device should be maintained by continuing experience, and this cannot be by inserting only one device every 3 or 4 months (12 IUDs or IUSs per year is the Faculty's accepted minimum).
- During both examination and insertion, gentleness as well as competence should be the rule in all manoeuvres, especially when the sound or loaded inserter enter the uterine cavity (such gentleness is not the same as hesitancy or being excessively slow).
- Last but not least, the clinician should be a good communicator, able to use plenty of that 'aural Valium' whose route of administration is the ears – also known as 'vocal local'!

9.107 How does the insertion process begin?

(Obviously – except for EC cases – it should actually begin at an earlier visit: with counselling and assessment both by history and (usually) examination, well ahead of the insertion. These aspects are considered later at Q 9.120).

- First, on the day, make yourself known to the woman if you as the practitioner were not involved in the earlier counselling. Even a brief initial conversation helps, followed by a matter-of-fact and informative commentary throughout the insertion procedure.
- Check that she was advised to take a PGSI as premedication (*see* Q 9.108) and, if so, when she took it.
- Discuss sensitively the results of any screening for STIs, primarily *Chlamydia*. Make a decision about whether she is to receive antibiotic cover (*see* Qs 9.57, 9.58).
- Discuss the use of local anaesthesia, at least at the 12 o'clock position on the cervix (*see* Q 9.108).
- Above all, make it explicit that *she is in control and that you are there for her, under her authority*. During the procedure give warning of any actions that might cause discomfort, e.g. the needle for paracervical block or the application of the Allis or Stiles forceps.

9.108 What are the indications for pre-insertion analgesia or local anaesthesia?

Analgesia

Researchers into pain relief have noted over many years that, as a very general rule, analgesics work more effectively and at lower dose when given in advance to *pre-empt* a pain than when trying to get rid of it once it is present. Back in the early 1980s in an RCT at the Margaret Pyke Centre [Guillebaud J, Bounds W 1983 *Research and Clinical Forums* 5:69–74] we showed, using visual analogue scales, that the scores for the cramping pain following insertion were statistically lower after premedication with a PGSI (we used mefenamic acid 500 mg about 45 min before the actual procedure). But scores for the more immediate somatic pains such as that from the holding forceps (see below) were NOT reduced.

At the Margaret Pyke Centre it therefore became the norm – followed very widely now elsewhere – that all women were offered premedication with a PGSI, normally mefenamic acid 500 mg, 30–45 min before the expected time of the procedure (checking first for contraindications). Later and in other services we simply suggested the woman swallow 400 mg of her own ibuprofen at the point of leaving home for her appointment.

A small subgroup who are unusually anxious benefit, additionally, from a short-acting benzodiazepine.

Local anaesthesia (LA)

Most women – but definitely not all – if questioned after an uncomplicated IUD insertion without LA tend to have the view that an LA needle would have caused more discomfort than it would have stopped. However, there is a group so questioned who clearly suffered and who are very clear that the pain began the instant the tenaculum (holding forceps, of whatever design) was applied. This pain varies immensely and completely unpredictably between women (sometimes marked in a relaxed parous woman, yet hardly noticed by an anxious one). When severe it seems to make the rest of the insertion process more painful than would be expected.

An initial 1-mL dose of 1% plain lidocaine to the anterior lip of the cervix at the 12 o'clock position 1 min ahead of the tenaculum completely abolishes this pain. In a brief survey of mine, women who had previously suffered in this way said that the pain from the needle was absolutely negligible by comparison.

Personally, I therefore always *offer* LA to *all* women, regardless of their parity, even if it will only be this tiny injection at the 12 o'clock position.

A smaller subgroup, often nulliparous or perimenopausal, or where dilatation to Hegar 5 or, rarely, 6 is likely, or for intrauterine manipulation (e.g. for 'lost threads'): these will benefit from a good *paracervical block* in addition. I use about 10 mL in all of 1% plain lidocaine or equivalent. This is injected through the finest possible needle (e.g. a dental needle) 1–2 mL first at 12 o'clock intracervically, and the rest – either through the cervical canal or laterally into the cervix itself – is delivered close to the internal cervical os at about 3 o'clock and 9 o'clock. NB: *wait* for 3 min for this to act. After training, this is neither a difficult nor significantly time-consuming addition to the procedure.

> **Practical tip**
> Note that there are two distinct pains to be treated:
> 1 Premedication with a PGSI (e.g. ibuprofen 400 mg) treats the (delayed) fundal cramps, while:
> 2 LA (by gel, or injection at 12 o'clock – or, less often, a full cervical block) is for the more immediate, somatic, mainly cervical component.

9.109 How important is the initial, personally performed, bimanual examination (BME)?

This is crucial: so much so, I teach that the practitioner who has forgotten and started doing an insertion should cease forthwith and unsterilize, even though it means scrubbing up again after the BME!

It has two main purposes:

■ First, to ensure that there is no uterine or adnexal tenderness, especially on moving the cervix. (Check verbally that there is also no dyspareunia.) Positive findings mean that the insertion should be postponed.

■ The second essential purpose is to identify the size, shape, mobility, and direction and position of the fundus.

9.110 Which is the best position for the patient to adopt during the insertion?

Most insertions in the UK are performed with the patient in the dorsal position, but lithotomy or its near-equivalent working from the *end* of the couch is preferable for GyneFix insertions.

Sometimes access is radically improved by using the left lateral position, which after all is equivalent to lithotomy rotated through 90°. This is of particular value if the cervical canal is very flexed and the cervix points directly either anterior or posterior. The left lateral does lead to loss of eye contact with the woman, though, and this must be replaced by better-than-average verbal communication.

9.111 Do you find 'Instillagel' into the cervix is a helpful alternative to full paracervical block?

Frankly, in my experience, the answer is 'no' – I no longer use or recommend it. A pity, as it would be so good to have a 'non-needle' option. The technique uses 2% lidocaine antiseptic gel and just sufficient of this 'Instillagel' is injected via a special Instillaquill to fill the cervical canal up to the internal os. If more than 1.5–2 mL is used, it causes uterine pain – and might theoretically push cervical pathogens into the uterus.

There must then be a minimum wait for it to act. A significant ($p < 0.05$) benefit was shown in a small trial of this in 1996 in Leeds after waiting only 1 min before passing the sound. To me it is counterintuitive that it could ever work so fast; after all, EMLA local anaesthetic cream for skin is recommended for application a minimum of 1 h ahead. I wonder if the study was an example of a type 1 error (positive result by chance). Could any apparent benefit be through it being a bit of lubricant?

9.112 Should tissue forceps be applied to the cervix, and should the uterus be sounded?

Normally yes: Stiles or Allis forceps cause variable discomfort, reduced to nil if a little local anaesthetic is injected as I recommend routinely (*see Qs 9.107, 9.108*) into the anterior lip of the cervix. X-ray studies have proved that gentle traction straightens the canal and very much assists in passing the sound. The latter is also essential to:

- confirm the direction and patency of the cervical canal
- estimate the length of the uterine cavity (*see Q 9.92*)
- exclude obvious intrusion of any submucous fibroid or uterine septum (*Fig. 9.10*). I teach that this should be done in all insertions by gently rotating the handle of the sound through a small arc.

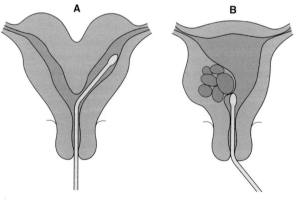

▲

Fig. 9.10 Uterine cavity distorted – congenitally or by fibroids. *Q 9.112. Note:* in **A** it is easy to obtain a normal sounding depth despite a septate uterus. Careful sounding will detect the abnormality, however, and will also identify a submucous fibroid, as in **B**. Such findings need to be confirmed by ultrasound. See also *Q 9.85*.

The sound should be passed with minimal force, rested between the finger and thumb like a loosely held pencil. Note that the anatomy of the cervical canal is variable. Be prepared to repeat the bimanual examination or to withdraw and reinsert the sound if it does not pass readily, or move on to using dilators (Hegar 3–6 should be available).

9.113 What about antisepsis?

This is much less important during the insertion than is prescreening for specific pathogens and, as appropriate, antibiotic cover (*see* Qs 9.57, 9.58). Remember that the flora of the endocervical canal is almost identical to that of the vagina.

All the same, even in the presence of a negative *Chlamydia* test and with no pelvic tenderness on examination, the cervix should still be inspected carefully at the time of the insertion. A purulent discharge could signify the need to postpone the insertion and arrange GUM referral to search for other pathogens.

Otherwise, the cervix should be cleansed thoroughly with a gauze swab usually dipped in aqueous antiseptic, though this has no proven benefit, concentrating on mechanical removal of any mucus at the external os.

9.114 What other practical points should be considered?

- Only at the last minute, and after satisfactory sounding, should the device be loaded into its inserter, for fear that it should lose its 'memory'.
- Some devices (e.g. Flexi-T 380) are primarily 'pushed' into the uterus; most are inserted by a 'pull' technique in which the plunger is kept stationary and the inserter tube pulled back over it.
- We all have a sensible paranoia about perforation but this leads to a tendency for the T-Safe Cu 380A or the LNG-IUS (or Nova-T 380) to be inserted rather low, risking expulsion and even implantation above the device. I teach that after the side arms of the above-mentioned devices have been released, you have an object that is most unlikely to perforate. Therefore, at that point in the insertion sequence for any of these devices, after the arms have just been released from the top of the inserter tube, the latter should be gently advanced towards the fundus. This might mean allowing the cervical stop to be pushed (caudally) by the external os, until the very top of the cavity is reached – always looking at the woman's face so as to be sufficiently gentle throughout. It has surprised me how often I have found that my initial estimate of the fundal depth was a centimetre or more less than the measurement from tip of tube to stop after this has been done.
- Take care that the device finishes in the right plane, by observing the marker wings on the inserter, as well as in the correct high fundal

position. If in doubt, the device should be removed and a new one inserted.

GyneFix has a very specific technique (changed, not entirely for the better in some people's view, when a new inserter was marketed in 2001) that must be learned with the help of the manufacturer's video, polystyrene models and then supervised insertions.

9.115 What about the prevention of the rare IUD insertion 'crises'?

- First, so far as possible, they should be prevented by: the presence of an assistant; a calm and relaxed atmosphere; matter-of-fact chat which provides 'vocal local' – all combined with obvious competence and teamwork.
- During the insertion, gentleness and accuracy while passing both sound and loaded inserter along the cervical canal reduce the incidence of vasovagal reactions.
- Above all, starting at an earlier stage:
  - good counselling and selection of cases, combined with
  - premedication as the norm (*see* Q 9.108)
  - consideration of a benzodiazepine (rarely)
  - usually a small injection of local anaesthetic before attaching the tenaculum
  - consideration of paracervical block if dilatation above Hegar 5 is required during the insertion.

These measures all help but cannot prevent every case. . . .

9.116 What if a vasovagal attack follows despite every precaution?

The patient goes white, may sweat with a slow pulse and could faint. Occasionally there is no warning – be alert!

1. The first thing to do is to abandon the procedure, stop any cervical stimulation and remove a partially inserted device (but, unless symptoms persist, not one that is considered to be well located).
2. The woman's head should be lowered or her feet elevated, and she should be moved into the recovery position.
3. Oxygen (which should be available) can be administered by mask. An airway should be used if the subject loses consciousness. All this takes a bit of time and occupies anxious bystanders, which is excellent because the majority of attacks are self-limiting.
4. At this point, 500 mg of mefenamic acid should be taken, if a PGSI was not already used as a premedicant. If it was, one or two tablets of a non-PGSI analgesic such as co-dydramol may be given.

9.117 What should be done if the woman continues to suffer severe dysmenorrhoeic pains?

If the woman continues in severe pain with pallor for 30 min after the insertion, in my view even a fully inserted device should be removed. The chances of long-term successful use of the IUD/IUS in this situation are too low. In an occasional case one might also be avoiding the later problems of a perforation.

If ultrasound scanning were routinely done before the removal I believe most of these cases would be explained by malposition, or because of an unexpectedly small or distorted uterine cavity.

If the woman wishes, after (usually) a pelvic scan to exclude congenital or acquired problems affecting the fundal cavity, a subsequent attempt with local anaesthesia, an expert practitioner and possibly now using the GyneFix (*see Q 9.142*) is often successful.

9.118 What unusual complications of IUD insertion can occur?

PERSISTENT BRADYCARDIA

If the pulse is persistently less than 40 beats/min, the slow intravenous injection of atropine 0.3 mg (repeated, if felt essential, to a maximum of 0.6 mg) might help, along with oxygen.

If the pulse is absent and the patient completely unresponsive, any competent doctor or nurse ought to be prepared to diagnose *cardiac arrest*, insert an airway and initiate cardiopulmonary resuscitation, Fortunately, this is more than most clinicians will ever be called upon to do in a lifetime of inserting IUDs. Beware of vomiting and the risk of inhalation of fluid when consciousness returns – hence use the recovery position.

ASTHMATIC ATTACK, LARYNGEAL OEDEMA OR OTHER SEVERE ALLERGIC REACTION

Treat urgently with 0.5 mg (contained in 0.5 mL) adrenaline 1:1000, intramuscularly and repeatable, according to the response, to a total of 1 mg.

GRAND MAL ATTACK

This can occur even in the absence of any history of epilepsy or the subsequent development thereof. Known epileptics should take their usual medication for the day concerned.

Any attack is usually self-limiting. Diazepam emulsion 10 mg should be available, ready for intravenous use or as rectal tubes (e.g. Stesolid, often a good route for this situation). One 10-mg dose is administered, repeatable once if there is no response after 5 min. Epilepsy needs to be distinguished from:

ALKALOSIS DUE TO OVERBREATHING

This causes paraesthesia and carpopedal spasms. Treatment is by reassurance and instruction in (supervised) breathing in and out of a plastic bag.

9.119 In summary, what should be available in the emergency tray?

- A well-fitting facemask and separate airways. Nearby, oxygen cylinder.
- Diazepam emulsion 10 mg either for rectal (Stesolid tubes) or intravenous injection.
- Atropine 0.6 mg for intravenous injection.
- Adrenaline 1 mL of 1:1000 for intramuscular injection.
- Mefenamic acid oral tablets – dose 500 mg.
- Dihydrocodeine 30 mg or as co-dydramol tablets – containing 10 mg with paracetamol 500 mg.
- Benzodiazepine tablets (temazepam 20 mg) for premedication.
- Syringes, needles, etc. as appropriate.

This is all that is required, and most will never be used.

PATIENT INFORMATION AND FOLLOW-UP ARRANGEMENTS

9.120 What main points should be made in advance when counselling any prospective IUD-user?

As usual, a balance has to be struck between creating unnecessary fears that might impair the woman's acceptance and satisfaction with the method, and the need to help her reach an informed and valid decision based on the likely benefits and risks for herself. During counselling, often rightly delegated to the family planning-trained nurse:

- Mention first the many advantages of the method (*see* Q 9.18). Let her see and ideally handle the device she is to receive.
- The possibility of failure, including after unrecognized expulsion, should be mentioned. Although expulsion ought to be particularly rare with GyneFix, the item itself is so small that it might well not be seen: learning to feel the threads is therefore even more important with this IUD than others.
- Attention should be drawn to pelvic infection and ectopic pregnancy. Explain how both are linked with sexual transmission of infections. Take a full sexual history (*see* Qs 1.13, 1.14), including a careful history of

past PID or any treatments at a GUM clinic. Embarrassment should not stop good plain medicine, which is to go on to say something like: 'You know better than I can possibly know what your likely risk of (sexually transmitted) infection might be. This depends both on you and also your partner: have you ever wondered if he has other partner(s)?' Stress also the importance in the future of using condoms in all situations of risk, especially at partner change – and of returning promptly to the clinic should relevant symptoms occur.

At the end of this discussion, make sure and record that she consents to any (*Chlamydia*) screening. Much aggravation has sometimes been caused by the result of a not-agreed-to test when it (unexpectedly) brought to light a partner's infidelity. . . . Record also her verbal consent for the IUD insertion itself.

■ **Examination.** Arrange at least a *Chlamydia* screen if at all possible, and usually antibiotic cover when no result is available (e.g. if the insertion is for EC, see the earlier discussion in *Qs 9.57 and 9.58*).

A bimanual examination will be done later, just before the insertion, but may also be indicated by symptoms at the counselling visit and is essential in older women. Its purpose is to pick up often unexpected pelvic masses, commonly fibroids, which would indicate pelvic ultrasound scanning to check that the fundal cavity is not obstructed.

■ In my view, it should also be pointed out that some discomfort is common during insertion, helped by the use of premedication – with added local anaesthetic as she prefers (*see Q 9.108*), given that it is only fully effective by needle!

■ Problems like perforation are rare but should be mentioned with the aid of the leaflet (see bulleted point below). Honest and accurate answers should be given to all questions (*see Q 5.106*).

■ Finally, counselling should be backed up by a user-friendly leaflet, such as the IUD or IUS ones from the fpa: 'To be read now before the insertion, but also for you to keep for future reference'.

9.121 What instructions should be given to the woman after IUD insertion?

■ She can be reminded that the method is effective immediately.

■ She should also be reminded that if she is ever in future in a very new or not mutually faithful relationship, she should use a condom as well, thereby reducing both the risk of failure and of infection.

■ She should be carefully taught palpation of her cervical threads and advised that this check should be done by self or partner post menstruation, in each cycle, before the device is relied on. (LNG-IUS users with oligo- or amenorrhoea (*see Q 9.143ff*), should do this regularly, perhaps on the first day of each month). *Q 9.171* offers some practical points about cervical palpation. If she becomes unable to feel the threads, or palpates the hard end of the device, she should be told to take additional contraceptive precautions and arrange an early examination.

■ As sperm can be bio-vectors of STI pathogens and the process of IUD/ IUS insertion interferes with protective mechanisms at the cervix (*see Qs 9.54, 9.55*) it is my personal policy to recommend abstinence for the next 3 days only.

■ Tampon use is also discouraged for 3 days, hopefully allowing enough time for the cervical barrier to be reconstituted.

■ *Important*: before leaving after the insertion, she should be given instructions, preferably backed by a handout, concerning the new symptoms (arising after those from the insertion have subsided) that should lead her to telephone the clinic/surgery immediately, during the critical next 3 weeks (*see Q 9.59*).

■ If she has neither had prescreening with a known negative *Chlamydia* result nor is being given antibiotic prophylaxis, then it is best to arrange a follow-up visit at about 1 week (*see Qs 9.52, 9.122*).

9.122 When and for what purpose should the first follow-up visit take place?

About 6 weeks after the insertion is the usual timing, on a date planned to be after the first expected menses, so as to exclude partial or complete expulsion.

However, the important data discussed in *Qs 9.54–9.59* suggest that making an earlier visit routinely at about 1 week would be ideal, if steps have not been taken to ensure a pathogen-free cervical canal! The woman should be advised (*see Q 9.50*) to telephone for advice and if in doubt attend as an emergency for examination, if in the crucial first 20 days post insertion she has pain or other symptoms that might be PID-related.

At the routine 6-week visit, which remains important to 'round off' the insertion process:

■ The woman should be asked:
  – about all relevant symptoms (*see Q 9.59*) and
  – whether she can feel her threads, being re-taught as indicated.

■ She should also have a speculum examination during which the threads should be seen. As a general rule, in my view, but especially if the threads have apparently lengthened, the lower cervical canal should be sounded. This can be done most simply by using the omnipresent throat swab or even a Cytobrush (not advanced higher than the internal os). In this way *partial expulsion* of a framed IUD can be detected and the device replaced before an avoidable intrauterine pregnancy occurs.

■ A bimanual examination should also be performed in every case, to detect tenderness and any adnexal or uterine enlargement.

9.123 How frequently should subsequent visits take place?

After the first one or maximum two follow-ups in the first 6 weeks, for women without symptoms UKSPR follows WHO in recommending *no routine follow-up appointments*.

■ More important than any routine pelvic examination is an 'open house' policy and an IUD programme that makes it really easy for a user to obtain medical advice and help at once should a new problem occur, notably an attack of pelvic infection or an ectopic pregnancy or 'lost threads'. She should therefore be fully taught, with a leaflet, about all the symptoms that require prompt action and know where to obtain telephone advice.

■ Iron deficiency anaemia is very easy to miss in long-term users with heavy bleeding. This should be excluded or treated if present.

9.124 Are IUDs always easy to remove by simple traction on the thread(s)?

Not if the threads are absent in the first place (*see Q 9.36*) or 'lost' (*see Q 9.34*). But even without this problem the device might be malpositioned or embedded, or there might be a type of partial cervical perforation (*Fig. 9.11*). In such cases it is sometimes possible, under local anaesthesia, to grasp the device and push it in a cranial direction to disimpact it first. Excessive traction at removal must always be avoided, especially under general anaesthesia, for the reason noted in *Q 9.47*.

GyneFix is removed by simple firm traction and is more comfortable done positively, not tentatively. A study at the Margaret Pyke Centre in 2003 found the GyneFix to require an unusually strong pull of 6 Newtons, compared with a mean of 2.2 Newtons for the comparator banded device (almost identical to the T-Safe Cu 380A). There was no significant difference in the pain reported on visual analogue scales and with both devices the women anticipated more pain than they actually experienced. This result is worth using, to reassure women prospectively.

9.125 Do you have any tips for removal of IUDs that are a bit stuck after the menopause? Must they always be removed at all?

This is mainly a problem when removing inert IUDs or Multiload 1 year after the last period. One solution is to prescribe natural estrogen, e.g. one complete cycle of Premarin 1.25 mg daily beforehand; this will soften the

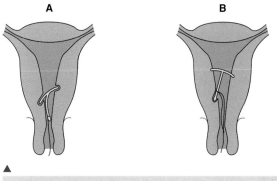

Fig. 9.11 Two varieties of partial cervical perforation. *Q 9.124*. Both of these could cause difficulty in removal. Each is best treated (under appropriate anaesthesia) by grasping the end of the device and pushing in a cranial direction before traction.

cervical canal. Mefenamic acid 500 mg as a premedicant also helps, as for other uterine manipulations (*see Q 9.34(3)*).

It is actually a matter of debate whether devices that are very 'stuck' (with or without avulsion of the threads) do have to be removed after the menopause – or an LNG-IUS that is found to be embedded, having been inserted at endometrial ablation. The postulated risk of a pyometrium is small and can be dealt with in the individual case. I would, personally, not now feel the risks of a general anaesthetic were justified for any difficult removal of IUDs postmenopausally, and would simply warn the woman to seek advice at any time later if she were to develop an offensive discharge.

An exception would be the presence of ALOs on a cervical smear in a perimenopausal woman (see the case reported in *Q 9.74*), where the device certainly must be removed and at least one follow-up visit at 3 months arranged.

9.126 Are IUDs a genuine cause of male dyspareunia?

Certainly, above all if a framed device is partially expelled so that its end just protrudes from the external cervical os! More commonly, some men notice the threads of the device.

If this problem is not resolved by slightly altering positions of intercourse, the threads should be trimmed – but not to within a few millimetres of the os, as this can actually worsen the situation. Rather, if necessary, they should be shortened to lie wholly within the cervical canal. Ensure that this is noted in the records and that the woman will report the fact to any future doctor. Long-handled Spencer–Wells forceps should easily retrieve the threads when removal is required.

9.127 Is short-wave diathermy treatment contraindicated in IUD-users?

This treatment is now rarely given to patients with chronic pelvic pain, in whom removal of the device would normally first be tried. However, if there is an IUD present there is certainly a theoretical possibility that the copper wire might heat up. Experiments with devices in recently excised hysterectomy specimens have shown no obvious damage or charring to the endometrium, and the devices have merely become pleasantly warm. So this treatment is relatively contraindicated (WHO 2).

9.128 Are modern methods of imaging dangerous for the IUD-wearer, specifically nuclear magnetic resonance imaging (MRI)?

Ultrasound is harmless, X-rays have no added risk, and (provided, as all modern IUDs are, the device is non-ferrous) on strong theoretical grounds backed by some data, MRI should cause no problems. In vitro studies on a copper T 380A IUD placed within the magnetic field found no significant temperature changes, no static deflection, and no turning motion of the device with different gradient pulses of MRI. The authors concluded that the IUD has no magnetic or magnetizable components, and that screening women for the presence of an IUD or removal of the device prior to an MRI scan is unjustified [Penney G et al 2006 For women with an intrauterine device in situ who undergo magnetic resonance imaging, is there a risk of displacement of the device? *Family Planning Masterclass*. RCOG Press: London, pp. 171–172 and at http://www.fsrh.org/admin/uploads/No624.pdf].

However, with steel devices (e.g. the historical M-device and the outdated Chinese coiled ring IUDs which are still present in the uteri of some visitors to the UK) there would truly be a potential hazard of internal trauma, due to movement of the ferrous metal caused by the powerful magnetic field.

9.129 Are IUDs containing copper affected by any vaginal preparations?

No – there is no clear evidence that material from the vagina reaches the copper or affects the biochemical processes that cause the contraceptive effect (*see* Q 9.5).

DURATION OF USE – AND REVERSIBILITY

9.130 Do the white deposits on copper IUDs removed after varying durations within the uterus cause an increased risk of failure or have any other clinical significance?

These deposits have been studied intensively. They contain organic material along with calcium, sulphur and phosphorus and other inorganic elements.

They are not now thought to be linked with IUD failure. Many women's devices never develop this deposit. When present, if the IUD is copper-bearing it seems that sufficient copper can pass through the deposit to continue the contraceptive effect. It is not an important factor in the rate of copper elution (*see* Q 9.132).

The explanation for failure of modern IUDs that are so effective when correctly located is, nearly always, less-than-ideal placement within the uterine cavity (*see* Qs 9.11, 9.12).

9.131 How often should inert IUDs be replaced?

In the few women who still retain these, and with the exception of the Dalkon Shield, they should never be routinely replaced without a special reason. One possible reason would be ALOs on a cervical smear (*see* Qs 9.70–9.74).

9.132 How often should copper IUDs be replaced?

All the marketed devices have an officially approved duration of 5 or 10 years. The reason for any limit is anxiety that the amount of copper available for release from the device might decline to a level at which the pregnancy rate would increase. Yet the recommended banded copper IUDs have shown no increase, and indeed a *decline*, in the annual conception risk even when fitted under age 40, for as long as they have been studied (namely, over 12 years).

At present the Mini TT 380 Slimline is only licensed for 5 years' use, yet it contains exactly the same surface area of copper as its larger relatives (the T-Safe Cu 380A and all its clones, see legend to *Fig. 9.9*). Therefore 10 years' use should be advised on a 'named-patient' basis (see *Appendix A*) until this changes – as it surely will.

9.133 What are the benefits of long-term use of IUDs?

See slogan 2 at Q 9.21! Long-term studies (especially by WHO and the Population Council) have repeatedly shown a steady reduction with increasing duration of use in:

- pregnancy rates (not with the Nova-T 200, however)
- expulsion rates
- infection rates (overall)
- bleeding/pain removal rates.

Exceptions that show a positive link with duration of use are carriage of ALOs (*see* Qs 9.70–9.74) and ectopic pregnancy – but the latter association is probably confounded by increasing age (*see* Q 9.21).

9.134 What are the explanations for the apparent improvement with duration of use of IUDs in the risks of pregnancy, expulsion, infection and removal for bleeding or pain?

It is too simple to interpret this as a genuine improvement due to the device 'bedding down'. The main point is that the long-term population of IUD-users is highly selected and in all studies is a reduced proportion of those who originally had devices inserted. They are the 'survivors', so to speak. Their success in long-term use has less to do with the passage of time, as such, than with selection for features of the individual women themselves as compared with others earlier in the study:

■ They are likely to have been well fitted with an IUD, which was well matched to the particular shape and size of their uterus.
■ They are obviously well distanced in time from insertion-related expulsion, infection and bleeding/pain.
■ Much the most important factor: women with any side-effects or complications severe enough to have their device removed are, by definition, no longer in the study. For example, the most fertile become pregnant within the first year and have their devices removed, hence the reported pregnancy rates in later years are based on observation of a subgroup of the relatively infertile. Similarly, those whose partners are less likely to transmit an STI to them are over-represented among long-term users.
■ They are also a little older, which helps most problems (*see Qs 9.21, 9.52*).

9.135 What therefore is the view of the UK fpa and the Faculty of SRH regarding long-term use of copper IUDs?

A statement published in *The Lancet* on 2 June 1990 established the principle, which is that even when fitted under 40 (*see Q 9.136*) copper IUDs are usable beyond the strict licensed limits if the evidence supports this. There are examples in *Q 9.132* above: the Mini TT 380 Slimline may be used for longer than the licensed 5 years, indeed the data support both it and its larger but otherwise similarly banded relatives, bearing the same amount of copper, all being used to 12 years provided the criteria in *Appendix A* p. 553 are followed.

Basically, 'if it ain't broke, don't fix it'. But there is one thing specifically to record in the Notes, that no promise was made that the device could not possible fail during the extended use; only that the failure rate is believed to be no higher than it was during the preceding years of successful use.

9.136 What about copper devices that were fitted above age 40?

Since a *Lancet* letter in 1990 that supplemented the statement mentioned above, it has been unchallenged and accepted UK practice that:

> **IUD/IUS slogan 8**
> Any copper device (even one of the copper-wire-only type) which was fitted above age 40 may remain in situ until the menopause . . . (or, for full contraceptive safety, until 1 year after that last period, *see Q 11.34*).

This is good practice because, with diminishing fertility, IUDs almost never fail above age 40. Even when the copper wire has all gone, the plastic frame seems to be sufficiently effective, like an inert IUD would be in these late reproductive years. Moreover, with widespread use of copper bands rather than just wire, there is every reason to expect the contraceptive effects of the copper to continue, right through till 1 year after the menopause.

That *Lancet* statement, like later reports by WHO and others, points out that less frequent replacement minimizes inconvenience, pain, upset and often costs for the woman: as well as bringing major health advantages in reducing all the (re-)insertion-related risks – as already listed at *Q 9.21* and summed up in IUD/IUS slogan 1.

Nevertheless, this policy for long-term use of all IUDs that were fitted above age 40 will often mean well beyond the licensed duration. So the criteria for 'named-patient' usage must be observed (see *Appendix A*, p. 553).

For the policy on possible extended use of the LNG-IUS, *see Q 9.150*.

9.137 How reversible is intrauterine contraception? Do IUDs cause infertility?

The conclusion of the section on this subject in the systematic review of 22 studies by Grimes in 2000 [*The Lancet* 356:1013–1019], including large case–control studies, cohort studies and one RCT, states that 'fair evidence indicates no important effect of IUD use on infertility'.

Subsequent to that review, Doll et al 2001 [*British Journal of Obstetrics and Gynaecology* 108:304–314] concluded from the Oxford/FPA cohort study that 'long term intrauterine device use in *nulliparous women* appears to be associated with an increased risk of fertility impairment'. Later correspondence by Grimes and Guillebaud in 2001 [*The Lancet* 358:6–7, 1460] highlighted several non-causal explanations for the association. In particular, long-term use over the period of the study necessitated frequent IUD replacements, but there was no prescreening of the cervix (*see Qs 9.52–9.58*): so that every reinsertion in the presence of undiagnosed cervical pathogens would equate in the study to an added risk that some long-term users would get tubal factor infertility.

Clearly, the women whose fertility might be impaired by IUD use are more likely to be those who drop out because of medical complications, which could include pelvic infection. However, in two cohort studies (from New Zealand and Norway), there were similar and good conception rates among those who had their IUD removed because of problems and those who discontinued the method in order to conceive. Two large American case–control studies reported in 1985 (references in Grimes 2000, see above) that past IUD use was significantly more common in primary tubal infertility cases than in controls. But most importantly, in one of them – the Cramer study – women who reported only one partner had no significant increase in tubal infertility, regardless of their choice of contraceptive.

For the vast majority of acceptors the IUD is a fully reversible method of contraception. Among those few who do suffer tubal infertility due to PID or ectopic pregnancy, the prime responsibility cannot lie at the door of the IUD itself (*see Q 9.50*). The frequency of this unwanted outcome can be minimized by careful selection of appropriate users by verbal screening (*see Qs 9.83–9.86*), careful IUD insertion (*see Qs 9.99–9.114*) with microbiological screening and consideration of antibiotic cover, and the best possible follow-up (*see Q 9.120ff*), with optimal management of any complications, of fully informed users.

9.138 Are there any special considerations if a woman wants to conceive after using a copper IUD, or the LNG-IUS?

It is usually advised that she uses condoms from the day of removal until the very next spontaneous period, to clear the endometrium of copper or levonorgestrel prior to any possible implantation. This seems 'common sense' to some, although there are no data to support or refute such a policy: and certainly there need be no undue concern if conception is immediate. *See Q 9.23* for the implications of in situ failure of copper IUDs, and *Q 9.145* for the LNG-IUS.

Given the increased likelihood that IUD users might have BV, and the data that this might possibly increase the risk of amnionitis and premature rupture of the membranes, it might be worth at least considering excluding that diagnosis (and treating as appropriate) before IUDs are removed electively to conceive.

GYNEFIX

9.139 What is GyneFix (*Fig. 9.12*), and how is it inserted?

This unique frameless device is the result of some good lateral thinking by Dirk Wildemeersch of Belgium. It is simply a single monofilament

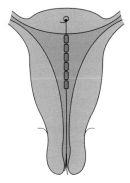

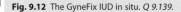
Fig. 9.12 The GyneFix IUD in situ. *Q 9.139.*

polypropylene thread, which dangles in the uterine fundus, bearing six copper bands similar to those on the copper T-380 (*Fig. 9.12*). A small anchoring loop and knot at the fundal end are inserted a measured distance of 9–10 mm into the myometrium by a special stylet, passed through the inserter tube, which is first pressed firmly against the fundus.

Special training is vital for safe insertion of this IUD and is available through the Faculty of SRH.

GyneFix is licensed for 5 years, although this duration can now be extended to 10 years on a 'named-patient' basis (see *Appendix A*), as a result of new data. There was just one failure among 274 users in two ongoing long-term studies (one in China and one run by WHO) between the fifth and ninth years [Wildemeersch, personal communication, 2003].

9.140 How does GyneFix compare with the gold standard, the T-Safe Cu 380A?

The results from the pre-marketing trials in Belgium were very promising, but in UK practice it has failed to live up to expectations and is now very little used. The expected very low expulsion rate (only 0.4% in the first year when inserted by the experts, the initial research team) was not confirmed. Perforations occurred, posing intra-abdominal retrieval problems. The final problem was the introduction of a new inserting system for the device, which many practitioners found rather ineffective for achieving proper implantation of the knot.

With regard to efficacy once implanted, the overall efficacy in a population will depend on how many unrecognized expulsions occur, since there is evidence that they are more easily overlooked when they happen, leaving the woman exposed.

No difference from the 'gold standard' in the rate of bleeding/pain problems or pelvic infection has yet been established by trials or systematic review.

9.141 What are the possible or known problems with GyneFix?

Perforation is always possible with IUDs and this one has a sharp stylet within a quite narrow firm tube. The rate with the new (2001) inserter mechanism is unknown but unlikely to be lower than the 1:1000 rate usually quoted for framed IUDs – and it could easily be much higher in the hands of inadequately trained or inexperienced personnel.

If perforation occurs, the small size of the device can make it very difficult to retrieve laparoscopically. Being frameless, if retrieval fails, it might be judged safer to leave it in the abdominal cavity indefinitely, rather than proceeding to laparotomy.

Expulsion rates were high in the UK experience – see above.

There was no evidence in one preliminary study of either implantation endometriosis or of more than an extremely localized inflammatory reaction at the site of the anchoring knot.

9.142 So what are the criteria/indications for use of GyneFix?

GyneFix costs more than twice as much as the gold standard T-Safe Cu 380A, which is also currently licensed for longer, and so far no head-to-head comparison has confirmed the claimed better performance. The new inserter seems a retrograde step.

For the time being, depending on availability – crucially of an 'expert' to do the implanting – I recommend it for second-line use as follows:

- Small uterine cavities sounding to less than 5.5 cm.
- Distorted uterine cavity on ultrasound scan (assuming an IUD is deemed an appropriate method at all). This includes distortion by fibroids or congenitally – in a bicornuate uterus there would be the option of inserting one GyneFix thread device into each uterine horn.
- Previous expulsion of any framed device.
- History of needing to remove another device within hours of insertion due to excessive cramping pain, where that is attributed to the frame of the previous IUD.
- For selected nulliparae with light or normal periods, upon request, particularly postcoitally.

THE LEVONORGESTREL-RELEASING INTRAUTERINE SYSTEM (LNG-IUS)

9.143 What is the levonorgestrel IUS/LNG-IUS/Mirena – also known as LevoNova?

This Nova-T-shaped device is shown in *Fig. 9.13*. It releases 20 mg/24 h of levonorgestrel (LNG) from its polydimethylsiloxane reservoir through a rate-limiting membrane, over at least 5 years.

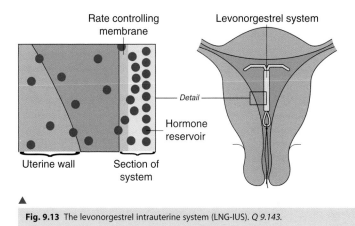

Rate controlling membrane

Levonorgestrel system

Detail

Hormone reservoir

Uterine wall

Section of system

▲

Fig. 9.13 The levonorgestrel intrauterine system (LNG-IUS). *Q 9.143.*

Its main contraceptive effects are local, by endometrial suppression and changes to the cervical mucus and utero-tubal fluid, which impair sperm migration. The blood levels of LNG are about one-quarter of the peak levels in users of the POP, and so ovarian function is altered less. Most women continue to ovulate and in the remainder sufficient estrogen is produced from the ovary even if they become amenorrhoeic as many do: this is primarily a local end-organ effect.

In 2005 there were an estimated 4 million users of this product worldwide.

9.144 What are the advantages of and indications for the LNG-IUS?

■ It has unsurpassed efficacy: a Pearl failure rate of only about 0.2 per 100 woman-years, and in the RCT by Sivin et al 1994 [*Fertility and Sterility* 61:70–77] a cumulative rate of only 1.1 per 100 women at 7 years. This was not different statistically from the 7-year rate of 1.4 for the T-Safe Cu 380A, making them both entirely comparable to female sterilization: whose overall failure rate with a mix of methods in the American CREST study (*see Q 11.50*) was actually 1.4 per 100 women at 7 years!

■ Return of fertility is rapid and appears to be complete.

■ It is highly convenient and has few adverse side-effects.

■ It is, in short, a contraceptive in which the 'default state' is one of contraception, unlike pills and condoms, where the default state is the reverse – conception!

The above advantages are, of course, shared with the T-Safe Cu 380A, which is the best current copper IUD. However, that is where the similarity ends. It fundamentally rewrites the textbooks about IUDs, so that it really deserves a different category of its own (hence the usage 'IUS' for intrauterine system, not IUD).

■ The user of this device can expect a dramatic reduction in amount (more than 90% in numerous studies now) and, after the first few months (discussed below), in duration of blood loss. It is licensed for the first-line treatment of menorrhagia even when there is no need for contraception.

■ Dysmenorrhoea is also generally improved. The LNG-IUS is now the contraceptive method of choice for many women with painful menses even if they are *not* heavy.

■ *Endometriosis*: gynaecologists now recognize the LNG-IUS as often ideal for long-term maintenance therapy, after initial diagnosis and treatment.

■ *Hormone-replacement therapy (HRT)*: by providing progestogenic protection of the uterus during estrogen replacement by any chosen route, the LNG-IUS uniquely, before final ovarian failure, offers 'forgettable, contraceptive, no-period and no PMS-producing HRT'. For this increasingly popular indication, the LNG-IUS is currently licensed only for 4 years before it must be replaced.

■ Although not yet proven in an RCT, the LNG-IUS might reduce the frequency of clinical PID, particularly in the youngest age groups who are most at risk [Andersson K et al 1994 *Contraception* 49:56–72]. This makes it possible to offer the device to some young women requesting a default state contraceptive who would not be good candidates for conventional copper IUDs.

■ The data on file and published for this device show a definite reduction in the risk of extra- as well as intrauterine pregnancy, which can be attributed to its greater efficacy by mechanisms that reduce the risk of pregnancy in any site.

■ It is a good choice for women on enzyme-inducing drugs (*see* Q 9.147), such as epileptics (even if nulliparous), for whom finding effective reversible contraception is essential and yet often fraught with problems.

■ The LNG-IUS is, in sum, a highly convenient and 'forgettable' contraceptive – with added gynaecological value. It is also highly cost-effective (*see* Q 9.149).

9.145 What are the disadvantages of the LNG-IUS?

■ It has the same small risks of expulsion and of perforation and malpositioning as the Nova-T 380, because it uses the same design. It has, in short, all the disadvantages of a frame, which are minimized with GyneFix – and at last the hybrid LNG-releasing IUS that I have been hoping for (using the same anchoring technique as GyneFix) is being trialled: provisionally called FibroPlant-LNG.

■ A more important problem is the high incidence in the first post-insertion months of uterine bleeding/spotting, which, although small in quantity, can be very frequent or continuous and can cause considerable inconvenience. This usually settles to a very acceptable light monthly loss, but it can take 3–6 months to do so.

■ Later in the use of the method, amenorrhoea is very commonly reported.

■ For both of these last effects, particularly the first, 'forewarned is forearmed': implying good counselling in advance of the fitting of the LNG-IUS. In my experience, women can accept the early weeks of frequent light bleeding as a worthwhile price to pay for all the other advantages of the method, if they are well informed in advance and coached and encouraged as appropriate while it is occurring. The amenorrhoea can even be explained and interpreted to a woman as a positive advantage of the method, rather than an adverse side-effect.

■ Women should also be advised that although this method is mainly local in its action, it is not exclusively so: it is a hormonal method. Therefore there is a small incidence of steroidal side-effects, such as bloatedness, breast tenderness, acne and depression. Blood levels are higher in the first 3 months, so women can be informed that, like the annoying bleeding, such symptoms usually resolve during that time.

■ Weight gain did occur, a mean 2.4 kg at the end of 5 years, in the multicentre RCT by Andersson (referenced above). However, the increase was virtually identical (mean 2.5 kg) in 937 copper Nova-T 200 users to that in the 1821 LNG-IUS users. As no one alleges that copper causes weight gain, it seems unlikely that the small dose of systemic LNG was to blame either.

■ Functional ovarian cysts are also more common but are usually asymptomatic, and, if not, should be monitored because most resolve.

■ In the extremely rare event of in situ failure of the LNG-IUS, if the system were not removed well before organogenesis, there is real uncertainty that the fetus might be harmed by the high local concentration of levonorgestrel. Because so few in situ failures have gone to term, there are no outcome data on this. Women must be so informed – so as to have full ownership of any decision about continuing with this unintended pregnancy (in which case the LNG-IUS should be removed at the earliest opportunity). *See also Q 9.148* below for the implications for the insertion cycle.

9.146 What are the contraindications to the LNG-IUS?

Many of the contraindications to this method are shared with copper IUDs (*see Qs 9.83–9.86*, above). The additional few that are unique to the LNG-

IUS, linked with the tiny amount of its LNG hormone that might have systemic effects, are listed below. The manufacturer tends to be more cautious in calling them all WHO 4.

UNIQUE CONTRAINDICATIONS (MAINLY WHO 3) FOR THE LNG-IUS

■ Current liver tumour or severe active hepatocellular disease.

■ Current severe active arterial or venous thrombotic disease (the former is WHO 2 according to UKMEC).

■ Current breast cancer – this is WHO 4 according to UKMEC, but with the LNG-IUS becoming usable on a WHO 3 basis after 5 years' remission (like all the other progestogen-only methods).

 In my view this deprives these women for many years of what might be an ideal contraceptive choice, since:

– the LNG-IUS gives the lowest systemic hormone dose of the hormonal methods

– Backman et al [Obstetrics and Gynecology 2005;106:813–817] could show no difference in incidence of breast cancer between 17 360 users in Finland and the general Finnish female population

– given also the suggestive data that it may protect against tamoxifen-induced pre-cancer changes in the endometrium, in selected cases this WHO 3 status which means usability (if the woman is keen) of the LNG-IUS might be agreed considerably sooner than 5 years: after consultation with the oncologist.

■ Hypersensitivity to levonorgestrel or other constituent (WHO 4).

■ In addition, *the LNG-IUS should not be used as a postcoital intrauterine contraceptive* (failures have been reported); this is because, acting by a hormone, it appears not to act as quickly as the intrauterine copper ion does.

9.147 What about relative contraindications to the LNG-IUS?

If you look through those listed in *Q 9.86* for IUDs, most are irrelevant, or in the very usable category WHO 2, and some such as bleeding and pain are indications!

 If there is structural heart disease and this IUS is chosen, there should of course be full antibiotic cover for the insertion, as more fully discussed in *Q 9.89*. Insertion is the only risky time, though, after which the method is WHO 2.

 Although enzyme-inducing drugs have the potential to weaken the contraceptive effect of a hormonal method, the contraceptive effect of the very high local concentration of levonorgestrel should not be lowered by any effect at the liver. And the Margaret Pyke Centre has now published a small collected series of over 50 such users with only one apparent failure, suggesting that the LNG-IUS does retain, at the least, very useful efficacy for these women (*see Q 9.144*).

The LNG-IUS may be used during breastfeeding (like the POP, *see Qs 7.53–7.57*).

9.148 Are there any special points about insertion of the LNG-IUS?

There are indeed!

It should be inserted no later than day 7 of the normal cycle, because it does not operate as an effective anovulant or postcoital contraceptive *and* because additionally it is potentially disastrous to conceive in the first cycle (*see Q 9.145*). Later insertion is advisable only if there has been believable abstinence or excellent contraception up to that time (usually best to not include condoms in that category!) with continued contraception thereafter (condoms OK), for a minimum of 7 days.

> **Helpful tip**
> Ensure that, *as a routine*, all who plan to have this LNG-IUS are started on a more effective method than condoms after counselling (e.g. combined pill or perhaps Cerazette), so that the insertion can be performed later without the above anxiety and on any mutually convenient date.

The technique of insertion involves a dedicated inserter-system with a tube which is 4.8 mm in diameter. This means that effective local anaesthesia (discussed above) and dilatation to at least Hegar 5 are not infrequently required – although rarely in multiparae, who remain, as for copper IUDs, the primary target population.

> **Two helpful tips (although, as always, no book can substitute for proper practical training):**
> ■ Not only when loading the inserter but also later, when easing the loaded inserter through the internal cervical os, ensure with a finger that the green slider stays in the extreme forward position, nearest the woman. (Otherwise the external tube can slide back through friction so that the side arms of the IUS are prematurely released in the cervical canal.)
> ■ I see as a crucial step that, once the side arms are out, within the uterus, the healthcare professional doing the insertion gently eases the IUS device to the very top of the fundus (as also described for banded copper IUDs, *see Q 9.114 bullet 3*).

9.149 Which women might particularly consider a LNG-IUS?

If it were not for (frequently overestimated) up-front cost considerations, its duration of use only for 5 years and the initial post-insertion bleeding and hormone problems, this method should be reasonably selected not only by almost any IUD-acceptor but also by most women considering sterilization, not to mention all those being advised hysterectomy or uterine ablation for dysfunctional bleeding.

That this is not so tells us more about doctors and other healthcare professionals not sharing all the options – as a human right for women, I would say – and about irrelevant 'baggage' from the past about IUDs and infection (linked with the infamous Dalkon Shield), than it does about any defects of the method.

Women are not going to know about the LNG-IUS unless we tell them: the media doesn't, paradoxically because adverse side-effects are so few and in general in the category 'nuisance' rather than hazardous. Thus there has been no 'Mirena IUS scare' in the media to make people aware of it. Truly, much as we hate 'pill scares', it is also true that there is no such thing as bad publicity!

With regard to the myth about price, NICE in their report (http://guidance.nice.org.uk/CG30/guidance/pdf/English) have clearly established that, when all factors, including continuation rates and the costs of unplanned pregnancies, are taken into consideration, the LNG-IUS (like all the LARCs, in fact) is more cost-effective than the COC by 1 year of use!

The LNG-IUS fulfils many of the standard criteria for an 'ideal' contraceptive:

1 100% reversible, ideally by self
2 100% effective (with the 'default state' as contraception, fully 'forgettable')
3 100% convenient (and non-coitally-related)
4 100% free of adverse side-effects (neither risk nor nuisance)
5 100% protective against STIs
6 Possessed of other non-contraceptive benefits
7 Maintenance-free (needing no ongoing medical intervention).

■ It approaches 100% for reversibility, effectiveness and even, after some delay, convenience. This is because, after the initial months of frequent uterine bleedings and spotting, the usual outcomes of either intermittent light menses or amenorrhoea are very acceptable to most women who are properly counselled. Indeed, in a post-marketing study by Backman et al 2000 [*British Journal of Obstetrics and Gynaecology* 107:335–339] of 17 360 users in Finland, the continuation rates to 3 and 5 years were amazingly high (81% and 65%, respectively) and 'the risk of premature removal was markedly lower among women who had occasional or total absence of menstruation'. Thereby demolishing the myth that women necessarily want to be regularly seeing periods!

■ Adverse side-effects are amazingly few and rarely dangerous.

■ Evidence continues to accumulate, instead, of its 'added value' through non-contraceptive benefits, including a useful reduction in symptoms of the premenstrual syndrome in about half of those receiving it.

■ Although it might be chosen by some young women with heavy menses or unable to accept alternatives, it is particularly suitable for women with heavy *or just painful* periods, or with contraindications to other options.

■ The LNG-IUS can often provide an excellent solution for the contraceptive dilemmas of many women suffering from a range of interacting medical disorders or risk factors, e.g. severe diabetes, SLE (*see Qs 5.136–5.139*) and epilepsy (*see Q 9.147*).

There is then the possible option, in the older reproductive years, of providing the progestogen component of a most useful form of 'contraceptive and no-period HRT' – to follow, if they are later prescribed estrogen by any chosen route.

9.150 Can the LNG-IUS (Mirena) be left in situ at the user's request beyond its licensed 5 years?

A qualified 'yes' to this question. The three answers depend on the context:

1 **LNG-IUS for *contraception*:** effective use is evidence-based, but unlicensed, for up to 7 years. Sivin's study (referenced in *Q 9.144*) in which 174 users continued to the end of the seventh year, and another study from Brazil, provide data that it is effective as a contraceptive for at least 7 years. Therefore:

 ■ For all women under age 35, because of their greater fertility, replacement after the usual 5 years would be advisable.

 ■ But the *older* woman whose LNG-IUS was fitted above the age of 35 might continue for 7 years, at her fully empowered request (but always on a 'named-patient' basis – *Appendix A*, p. 553).

 ■ Furthermore, NICE has stated that any woman who had her LNG-IUS inserted above the age of 45 and who has complete amenorrhoea may continue to use the same LNG-IUS 'until contraception is no longer needed' (*see Q 11.42*).

2 **LNG-IUS as *part of HRT*:** current practice (and the licence) for safe endometrial protection against cancer is always to change at 4 years.

3 **LNG-IUS not being used for either** *contraception or HRT*: it could be left in situ for as long as it continues to work, in the control of heavy and/or painful uterine bleeding, and then removed in the mid-50s.

CONCLUSIONS

9.151 What are your ten resolutions for the conscientious clinician providing intrauterine methods?

1 Remembering that one of the main times of action of IUDs is the last 9 days of the cycle, I will follow the 7-day rule for elective IUD removal (*see Q 9.14*), to avoid 'iatrogenic pregnancies'. I will also be prepared to proceed with IUD insertion up to 'day 19' – adjusted for shortest cycle length – in selected cases (*see Qs 9.15, 10.14*).

2 As the main IUD concerns and contraindications relate to threats to fertility, I will always make this the main point when counselling the nulliparous – but explain that the IUD itself is innocent!

3 As the rates of in situ pregnancy, expulsion and pelvic infection are inversely related to age, I will always make these potential advantages clear when counselling the more mature.

4 As incorrect insertion/malposition can cause every category of IUD problem, I will ensure that my own insertions are:
■ competent, careful, gentle and with sufficient pain relief
■ always preceded by my own bimanual examination and sounding
■ using the 'longest-lived' appropriate IUD (*see Qs 9.133, 9.136*).
In sum, I will endeavour to fit well the right device in the right woman, using the right technique; and I will maintain my skills by doing at least 12 insertions a year.

5 After the 6-week check I will maintain an 'open house' policy for users to discuss any symptoms with a healthcare professional by telephone or in person. Specifically, I will tell them that pain and bleeding are serious symptoms until proved otherwise, especially if sustained and intermenstrual.

6 More specifically, I will remember that any woman with menstrual irregularity and pelvic discomfort has an ectopic pregnancy until proved otherwise.

7 I will teach users that 'lost threads' means they are pregnant or at risk of pregnancy until proved otherwise.

8 In any continuing pregnancy I will ensure that the IUD is gently removed in the first trimester if feasible, and will teach users how to reduce the risks of abortion and preterm delivery. Moreover, I will follow the two equally important but opposite slogans in (9) and (10).

9 'Leave well alone' (often, after counselling, in asymptomatic long-term users).

10 'When in doubt, take it out' when the woman does have troublesome symptoms; and also for her own reasons upon her request, so the method is one over which she herself has full control. But then I must

not forget to take her relevant sexual and coital history and facilitate her plans for future contraception.

9.152 What problems of IUD use in the UK should be reported to the Medicines and Healthcare products Regulatory Agency (MHRA)?

The following should be reported:

- Extrauterine pregnancy
- All perforations/translocations
- Severe infections – most especially actinomycosis (*see* Q 9.72) or bacterial endocarditis (*see* Q 9.89)
- Apparent true allergy to any constituent of IUDs (*see* Q 9.87)
- Apparent interaction with a drug, or imaging technique (*see* Qs 9.127– 9.129)
- Exceptionally severe insertion reactions (*see* Q 9.118)
- Any unusual possibly related event.

PQ PATIENT QUESTIONS

QUESTIONS ASKED BY PROSPECTIVE OR CURRENT IUD-USERS

9.153 How does the IUD or the IUS work? Is it often causing an abortion?

The answer depends on your own definition of when pregnancy begins (*see* Qs 9.7, 10.3, 10.4). If your beliefs make you feel that contraception must never operate after fertilization, then this method is not for you.

9.154 Can the copper be absorbed from copper devices into the body?

A tiny amount is absorbed, but very little, so it is only just detectable in the blood. By far the majority of the small amount of copper that is lost over the years goes out in the vaginal fluid.

9.155 Why does the IUD or IUS have a tail? Can I pull it out myself?

Mainly to check that the device is present, but also to remove it when required. Deliberate self-removal is not recommended, but could be done. Removal by mistake has happened rarely, when chasing a 'lost' tampon perhaps.

9.156 Which is safer, the IUD or the ordinary pill? Could a woman die from using an IUD or IUS?

Overall, the risk of death or life-endangering disease is very low with both methods, but even lower with an IUD/IUS. Deaths have been caused but they are extremely rare. The problems are focused in the pelvic area and not all over the body, and they can all be minimized (*see* Q 9.151). The main problems have to do with future fertility (*see* Qs 9.21, 9.84, 9.86).

9.157 Does the IUD or IUS cause any kind of cancer?

There is no evidence for this, whether for copper or hormone-releasing varieties (*see* Q 9.20). Indeed, there is a hint of protection against cancer of the endometrium (lining of the womb), especially by using the LNG-IUS (*see* Q 9.18).

9.158 If I get pregnant, will the baby be harmed?

There is no evidence of this with copper IUDs, even if the pregnancy occurs with the IUD still in position. There is more uncertainty with the LNG-IUS (*see* Qs 9.100, 9.145). Either type of device should normally be removed in early pregnancy (*see* Qs 9.23, 9.145).

9.159 What has using the IUD or IUS got to do with the number of sexual partners I have?

A great deal, because the main problem with IUDs is pelvic infection, and nearly all IUD-linked infections are actually caught sexually. Also relevant is the number of sexual partners of your own partner, even if you are entirely faithful to him (see also the question in Q 9.120 *bullet 3*).

9.160 Do I need my partner's/husband's agreement to have an IUD or IUS?

No, the device can be inserted without his agreement. The threads can even be cut off if you so request, so he cannot know it is there unless you tell him. However, it is always ever so much better that any couple are both agreed, whatever method of family planning is chosen.

9.161 Should I ask to see which IUD or IUS I have before it is fitted?

Yes, most certainly, so you can't imagine something big and nasty. . . . Ideally, you should also write down its name and the date of fitting, in case you move to the care of a different doctor or clinic.

9.162 I think I'm allergic to copper; what should I do?

First, report the matter to your doctor. It might be possible to do special patch allergy tests. As most people who think they are allergic to copper turn out actually to be allergic to another metal, it might be all right to insert the device and see how you get on over the next few days. If you get marked discharge and pain within a very few days of insertion, you should return most promptly for advice (*see* Q 9.87).

9.163 I am told I have a cervical erosion (ectopy)/a tilted womb/a very tiny womb – can I have an IUD fitted?

If these are the only problems (i.e. there is no infection and the womb is not distorted congenitally or by fibroids) a device can normally be fitted (*see* Qs 9.85, 9.97, 9.142).

9.164   I have heard you can get very bad cramp-like pains when an IUD or IUS is fitted? What causes this and what can be done about it?

The pain people feel at insertion varies a great deal, from nothing to severe, and it is not easily predictable. Part of this is caused by the release of substances called prostaglandins, and you can ask your doctor for a specific painkiller that opposes their action. You should also discuss with him/her the possibility of having a local anaesthetic.

9.165   Does an IUD or IUS always have to be fitted during or just after a period?

No – not only can it be inserted later, provided contraception earlier in the insertion cycle has been brilliant, it is actually not good to insert during heavy bleeding (*see Qs 9.15–9.17*).

9.166   Does being an epileptic increase the chance of my having a fit during the insertion?

Yes it does, and your doctor should arrange to have available the treatment to prevent/stop an attack (*see also Qs 9.118, 9.119*). But take your usual medication up until you get to your appointment.

9.167   How soon can I have sex after having the IUD or IUS fitted?

The protection from pregnancy by a copper IUD, or from the LNG-IUS if fitted before day 8 of your cycle, is immediate, but although there is no proof that it is important, it is my recommendation that you wait for about 3 days, to reduce even more any infection risk (*see Q 9.121*). If it was the LNG-IUS that was fitted on/after day 8, you will be advised to use condoms to ensure effectiveness in the first month (*see Q 9.148*).

9.168   Can I use tampons internally after being fitted with an IUD or IUS?

My usual advice is to use only a sanitary towel at first, for the bleeding that follows immediately after IUD insertion, until 3 days have elapsed. Subsequently, sanitary protection can be entirely at your choice.

Prolonged use of the same tampon (more than 12 h) is always a bad idea, for fear of toxic shock syndrome (TSS).

9.169   Can an IUD or IUS fall out without my knowing?

Yes, this is certainly possible (*see Q 9.38*). The most likely time is during a heavy period, when it could be hidden within a large clot or on a tampon that is then flushed down the toilet. This is why it is best to check your threads after each period. Learning to feel for the strings is extra important with the GyneFix.

9.170   How often should I feel for the threads?

Once a month is sufficient – best right at the end of a period. If you have an LNG-IUS and are not seeing regular bleeds, then do this on the first day of each new month. This is so that you do not begin to rely on the method each new month, until you have checked that it is still in position.

9.171 How do I feel the threads of the IUD or IUS? What should I do if I now can't feel them any longer?

Either squat down or put one foot on a bathroom stool. Insert both your index and middle fingers into the vagina and feel more in a backwards than an upwards direction until you come across the cervix. This feels rather like a nose with only one nostril, and you should then be able to find emerging from the opening one or two little threads feeling like ends of nylon fishing line. If that is all you feel, well and good. If, however, you feel something hard, like the end of a matchstick, this could mean that the device is on its way out. In that case, or if you can no longer feel the threads at all, you must assume that you are no longer protected and start using another method (e.g. condoms). Contact your family doctor or clinic urgently in case emergency contraception is required – most likely by urgent reinsertion (*see* Q 10.22).

By the way, some women don't learn to do all this, instead their partner does it for them each month – which is fine!

9.172 Can my IUD or IUS get lost in my body (perforation)?

Extremely rarely. It is 999:1 against this happening in your case. It is a rare cause of the problem of 'lost threads' (*see* Q 9.42). Should it happen, the most that is normally required is a minor operation called a laparoscopy to retrieve it.

While your 'lost threads' problem is still being sorted out, and you are perhaps waiting for a hospital appointment, make sure that you use another method of family planning (because the womb itself might be empty) and also take immediate medical advice if you get any pain in the abdomen.

9.173 Can I go back to using an IUD or IUS after a perforation?

This depends on the cause; but an IUD can often be reinserted with success, since the tiny hole in the womb heals up so completely.

QUESTIONS ASKED BY CURRENT USERS

9.174 Do women have more vaginal discharge with an IUD?

Yes. Sometimes the discharge has a specific and treatable cause, so it should always be reported to your doctor. If testing shows nothing specific and treatable, like BV or thrush, then it is probably caused by an increase in the usual vaginal fluid (which includes mucus, the fluid of sexual arousal and even semen). That needs no treatment.

9.175 Someone has told me the IUD can break into pieces inside you, is this so?

Years ago there was one dud batch of Lippes loop devices, which were distributed worldwide and were liable to fracture. No modern device will break up, unless removal, which is normally very easy (*see Q 9.184*), were to be exceptionally difficult. In that case, a minor hysteroscopy operation might rarely be necessary to retrieve the missing portion.

9.176   My last period was very late and heavy; does this mean I might be miscarrying an early pregnancy?

Most probably not – heavy periods are not uncommon in regular use of an IUD, and the period could have been late just because your egg was released late in that cycle. However, you should visit the clinic for an examination and advice, partly in case your device was dislodged by the heavy flow. You might also ask about the LNG-IUS (Mirena).

9.177   Can my partner really feel the IUD or IUS during lovemaking as he says, and what can be done about it?

Some men notice the threads, depending on which way the cervix points and perhaps on the position of intercourse. Many couples just adapt their sex lives accordingly, but otherwise it is possible to have the threads cut right off (*see Q 9.126*).

9.178   Can I use a sunbed with an IUD in place, or have vibromassage?

Neither of these can affect your IUD in any way. *See also Qs 9.127–129* about 'deep heat' (short-wave diathermy) and whether vaginal treatments matter.

9.179   If my IUD contains metal, will it make an embarrassing 'bleep' when I pass through security devices at airports or large department stores?

Despite rumours, this does not appear to be a problem either with copper-bearing or steel devices (or with any of the clips used to sterilize people) – presumably because the amount of metal is too small.

Another rumour that can be discounted is the one that was started by the woman who accused the magician Yuri Geller of causing the failure of her copper IUD. She claimed that the pregnancy was conceived when she made love on the hearth-rug during a television demonstration by the above-mentioned showman of his metal-bending skills!

9.180   Can I cause my IUD or IUS to be expelled by vigorous aerobic exercises or intercourse in any unusual positions?

There is no evidence for this, and plenty of ordinary and sexual athletes use the method with success.

9.181   Are there any drugs that might interfere with the action of my IUD or IUS?

Tell your doctor about the IUD if you are to receive any treatment. Should this be a corticosteroid in high dose or other drug(s) that could interfere with immune responses, it might be better for you to transfer to another method of birth control. However, there is no current concern about either antibiotics or painkillers (*see Qs 9.86(18) and 9.88*), or other treatments (*see Qs 9.127–9.129*).

9.182 My girlfriend tells me I should have my device changed often, to prevent it getting infected or stuck inside me. My gynaecologist implies it would be better to have a new one before it officially runs out at 5 or 10 years, so as to keep it effective. Are these ideas true?

They are both 'urban myths', although still common, even what your gynaecologist is implying. Studies actually tend to show greater effectiveness the longer the same IUD or IUS is used, sometimes even beyond the end of the licensed time (*see Qs 9.130ff and 9.183*).

9.183 Do I really have to have my copper IUD changed at a set time, when it is suiting me well? And what about Mirena?

Nowadays this is becoming less and less necessary, and definitely not if your device was fitted above the age of 40 (*see Qs 9.130–9.137* for a full answer to this most important question, also *Q 9.150* about Mirena).

9.184 How is an IUD or the IUS removed? Is it ever difficult?

Normally there is no problem; there is much less discomfort than when having the device fitted in the first place. However, there are some situations in which it is more tricky and uncomfortable (*see Qs 9.34, 9.124*).

9.185 If my IUD or IUS is removed so that I can try for a baby, should I wait, using another method for a set time?

It is recommended, but not vital, that you wait for one period to 'clear the womb' first. Even women who conceive immediately the device comes out (so it was still in place during the last period before the pregnancy) seem to be as likely as anyone else to have a normal baby.

Emergency (postcoital) contraception

10

QUESTIONS ASKED BY PROSPECTIVE USERS OF POSTCOITAL CONTRACEPTION

PQ PATIENT QUESTIONS

BACKGROUND MECHANISMS

10.1 What is the definition of postcoital contraception, or emergency contraception (EC – the preferred term)?

In current usage this is any female method that is administered after intercourse but has its effects prior to the stage of implantation. The latter is believed to occur no earlier than 5 days after ovulation. Any method applied after intercourse that acts after implantation, even if this is before the next menses, should properly be called a postconceptional or contragestive agent.

The term 'morning-after pill' is not ideal because it could actually result in pregnancies by preventing women from presenting many hours later than the 'morning after' (*see* Q 10.7). Yet efficacy does appear to be greater the earlier hormone regimens are commenced (*see* Q 10.6).

10.2 Given all the new data and their implications, is there up-to-date guidance for clinicians about EC?

Yes, FSRH *Guidance, emergency contraception* was issued in April 2006 by the Clinical Effectiveness Unit of the Faculty of Sexual and Reproductive Healthcare [*Journal of Family Planning and Reproductive Healthcare* 2006;32:121–127]. In the rest of this chapter this is referred to as FSRH Guidance. As that document includes all the most important references, these will not be referenced individually here, aside from the two seminal WHO studies:

■ Multicentre, double-blind RCT of 1998 women randomized to one of two regimens:
  – LNG 0.75 mg stat, repeated 12 h later
  – two tablets of a contraceptive, each containing LNG 250 μg plus EE 50 μg, stat, repeated 12 h later.

This will be referred to as the 'WHO 1998 study' [*The Lancet* 1998;352:428–433].

■ Multicentre, double-blind RCT of 4136 women randomized to one of three regimens:
  – 10 mg mifepristone as a single dose
  – standard progestogen-only emergency contraception (LNG EC) – two doses of 0.75 mg LNG 12 h apart
  – a single dose of 1.5 mg LNG.

This will be called the 'WHO 2002 study' [*The Lancet* 2002;360:1803–1810].

10.3 Is it ethical and legal to use EC?

Yes. Legally, in the UK, a pregnancy is not recognized to exist until implantation is completed (Judicial Review of Emergency Contraception, Department of Health 2002; quoted in FSRH Guidance). Although the methods usually work by preventing fertilization, it is undeniable that the mechanism might often be through blocking implantation.

The question as to whether the prescriber and the woman concerned are happy to accept EC as ethical depends on accepting the view of most modern biologists and ethicists, that 'conception' is a process which certainly begins with the fusion of sperm and ovum but is not complete until implantation.

The situation is clarified by considering the status of the unimplanted blastocyst (*Fig. 10.1*). If it stays where it is in the cavity of the uterus, it is in a 100% 'no-go' situation – unless and until it can stop itself being washed away in the next menstrual flow by secreting enough hCG into the woman's circulation to maintain the corpus luteum. The all-destroying menses cannot be prevented without successful implantation.

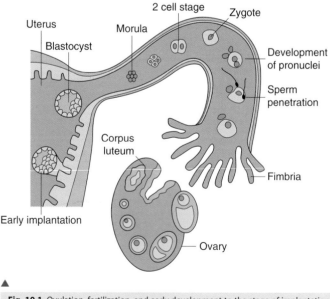

▲

Fig. 10.1 Ovulation, fertilization, and early development to the stage of implantation. *Q 10.3* considers the status of the unimplanted blastocyst, labelled above.

A second feature of the unimplanted situation is that the woman's physiology does not 'know' the blastocyst is present, yet. Only after implantation is there a two-way relationship, and for the first time 100% 'no-go' for the blastocyst becomes 'go'; now there is 'carriage'. As has been well said, at the earlier stage, when there is not yet 'carriage', how could application of any method of birth control be 'procuring a miscarriage'?

Finally, with at least 40% of blastocysts regularly failing to implant, there seems little logic in putting a high value on something with which Nature itself is so prodigal.

Prescribers must, of course, respect the views of their patients, and EC methods should not be used for any who are unhappy with the above interpretation. They should then, however, also understand the implications in relation to other methods (*see* Qs *9.7, 10.4*).

10.4 What are the implications of rejection of EC methods on ethical grounds?

In the main, this means that the woman concerned should also not use either IUDs or IUSs, or the old-type progestogen-only pill (*see* Q *7.75*). All these methods, although primarily working before fertilization, can operate – in a small minority of cycles – by blocking implantation.

10.5 What is the history of EC?

This is probably almost as old as the first recognition that semen is in some way responsible for pregnancy. Douching has been used since ancient times and remains in use today; 25% of women presenting for EC treatment in one UK study had first used a shower attachment, flannel or paper tissues, with or without a spermicide or household germicide. These methods are doomed to frequent failure; because sperm have been found in cervical mucus within 90 seconds of ejaculation.

The Persian physician Al-Razi suggested:

First immediately after ejaculation let the two come apart and let the woman arise roughly, sneeze and blow her nose several times and call out in a loud voice. She should jump violently backwards seven to nine times.

Jumping backwards supposedly dislodged the semen; jumping forwards would assure pregnancy.

A range of EC pessaries and douches have been described over the years, including wine and garlic with fennel, used in Egypt as early as 1500 BC; ground cabbage-blossoms in the fourth century; and culminating in Coca-Cola in some developing countries even today. Diet Coke may actually have had some spermicidal action – but then they removed the quinine!

The history of more effective methods begins in 1963 with trials of diethylstilbestrol (DES) at Yale University. Because of the risks to any pregnancy should the method fail, DES should now never be used. After the mid-1970s, the Yuzpe method (devised by a Canadian gynaecologist) became the first-choice method, using much less EE in combination with LNG.

Immediate insertion of a copper IUD is an alternative method first reported in 1972 and appropriate in some cases (*see Q 10.33*).

10.6   What are the currently accepted regimens of EC treatment?
See *Table 10.1*.

■ Immediate insertion of a copper-bearing IUD (*not* the LNG-IUS, *see Q 9.146*), not more than 5 days after the most probable calculated date of ovulation, even if there have been multiple acts of unprotected intercourse; or 5 days after any single (earliest) exposure.

■ The Yuzpe method: this is started within 72 h of the earliest act of unprotected intercourse, its efficacy being greatest in the first 24 h and

TABLE 10.1 Choice of methods for postcoital contraception – a brief summary

Copper IUD	Levonorgestrel (LNG) method (Levonelle 1500)	Combined hormone method
Intrauterine copper ions	Levonorgestrel 1.5 mg stat (single dose now preferred)	(Yuzpe: NB used only when LNG method not available) Microgynon 30 4 pills stat, 4 pills 12 h later
Normal timing		
Up to 5 days after earliest calculated day of ovulation or 5 days after earliest exposure in that cycle	Up to 72 h – but usable up to 120 h (see *Q 10.8* and *Appendix A*) after earliest act of intercourse	Up to 72 h
Efficacy		
Almost 100% (timing as above)	98.5%* (within 72 h)	97% (within 72 h)
Side-effects		
Pain, bleeding, risk of infection through insertion	Nausea 23% (15%)* and vomiting 6% (1.4%)*	Nausea 51% and vomiting 19%

References: 'WHO 1998 study' [*Lancet* 1998;352:428–433] and *'WHO 2002 study' [*Lancet* 2002;360:1803–1810].
Numbers rounded to one decimal place.

declining thereafter (although not to nil after 72 h). Two tablets of a contraceptive, each containing LNG 250 µg plus EE 50 µg, are given at once, followed by a further two tablets 12 h later. Although in the UK this has been supplanted completely by LNG EC and will be little discussed below, practitioners in some countries are forced – where there is no source of oral LNG (i.e. no appropriate POPs on the market) – to continue to recommend the Yuzpe method. This commonly entails using four tablets of Microgynon 30 or a local equivalent brand stat, repeated in 12 h.

◼ Use of LNG alone: this is referred to here and in the FSRH Guidance as LNG EC. If started within 72 h of the earliest exposure, it again has its greatest efficacy in the first 24 h, declining thereafter, but not to nil, at 72 h (*Q 10.12*). It requires 1500 µg LNG stat. In the WHO 1998 study (in divided doses) this proved to be more effective than the Yuzpe method, with fewer side-effects (especially vomiting, see *Table 10.2*, p. 483), and there are also fewer contraindications. In the UK this is now (2008) marketed to clinicians as Levonelle-1500 and to the public over-the-counter as Levonelle One Step.

In the US a version of LNG EC has the excellent brand name Plan B!

Outside Europe and the US, practitioners are usually forced to construct the dose from marketed POPs (e.g. by giving 50 tablets of the local equivalent of Norgeston stat). If this can be done it is still preferable (with much reassurance of the woman that 50 tablets is not an overdose!) to constructing the less effective and more nauseating Yuzpe regimen in bullet 2, above.

Other methods previously in use are now of historical interest only (*see also Qs 10.49 and 10.50* for variants being researched).

10.7 What is the mechanism of action of EC methods?

The IUD operates by blocking implantation (*see Q 9.7*) when, as it commonly is, inserted after ovulation. However, if applied earlier in the cycle, it will use its primary action (i.e. as in more usual long-term use): a toxic effect of copper on sperm that blocks fertilization. The mode of action of LNG EC is incompletely understood. If taken before the LH surge, it will usually inhibit or postpone ovulation, and it is probable that the uterine fluid/genital tract mucus can also be rendered hostile to the sperm.

After ovulation, other effects on LH levels and the length of the luteal phase might be important, but there is little evidence to support a direct anti-implantation effect (FSRH Guidance). Most authorities now believe that if LNG EC is not administered in time to block ovulation or fertilization, the method is much more likely to fail.

It is important to remember that fertile ovulation might simply be postponed in that cycle, hence the requirement to use a method such as the condom until the next period.

10.8 Will LNG EC work if given later than 72 h?

Yes, but less well, especially if that means treatment after midcycle. Although many prescribers have treated it as such, the 72-h time limit as licensed has never implied an absolute contraindication. From the data of the first WHO trial (1998), it appeared (although not well confirmed in the later 2002 trial) that LNG EC worked best if started in the first 24 h, and the failure rate increased with time thereafter.

In the second WHO (2002) trial, the two-dose LNG EC regimen had a 1.7% failure rate for treatment in the first 72 h, rising to 2.4% for treatment between 72 and 120 h. The results for the single dose were very similar at both time periods of the intervention, and if the two LNG regimens were pooled, treatment from 72 to 120 h had an overall failure rate of 8/314 cases or 2.5%. Given that so many would not have conceived anyway, calculations based on the best available data for conception risk by cycle day showed that this equates to prevention of 63% of actual conceptions expected, compared with preventing 84% of expected conceptions if treatment was within 72 h.

Most clients, if they have rejected the much more effective alternative of having a copper IUD inserted, will see those numbers as considerably better than doing nothing. Moreover, the WHO researchers concluded: 'Even if a declining trend in efficacy with time were verified, the regimens studied still prevent a high proportion of pregnancies even up to 5 days after coitus.'

10.9 Do you consider it is now adequately evidence-based (although unlicensed) to use LNG EC between 72 and 120 h after UPSI in selected cases?

Yes. However, only 12% of the WHO subjects were treated on days 4 and 5, confidence intervals were wide, including zero effect, so the FSRH Guidance says 'women should be informed of the limited evidence of efficacy . . . and of the alternative of a (copper) IUD'.

It should be recorded that the woman understands that:

■ She needs to be completely transparent about any possible earlier exposure, so that you can then proceed in good faith, in the belief that you will not be disturbing an already implanted pregnancy.
■ Insertion of a copper IUD would be more effective (indeed, I agree with the Faculty that that should always be said, even to women presenting within 72 h of exposure).

■ This late treatment ought certainly to be better than nothing, stopping at best around 6 out of 10 actual pregnancies to be expected with no treatment (contrast about 8 out of 10 if she had been treated earlier) and:

■ The treatment must, so long as this timing is unlicensed, be on a 'named-patient' basis (see *Appendix A*, p. 553).

10.10 Can LNG EC be given more than once in a cycle?

Yes and *see also Q 10.42*. The FSRH Guidance is in full agreement about this, though the manufacturer's SPC does not recommend it due to 'disturbances to the cycle'.

10.11 Might other progestogens or other drugs be effective?

Other progestogens such as desogestrel or gestodene, or even DMPA by injection, might well be effective, but neither their efficacy nor the best doses have so far been evaluated in proper trials.

The antiprogestogen mifepristone, in a single 10-mg dose, was shown definitively, in the third arm of the WHO 2002 study, to work as well as LNG EC; and other data suggest it is more effective up to 120 h (*but see Q 10.50*).

EFFECTIVENESS

10.12 What is the overall efficacy of the two main EC methods?

■ For the copper IUD method the failure rate is very low indeed. The FSRH Guidance quotes available data that postcoital copper IUDs will prevent at least 99% of expected pregnancies.

■ Data from the second (2002) WHO study of LNG EC has already been given in *Q 10.8*. The first, in 1998, was a randomized comparison, after single exposure, of the combined (Yuzpe) versus the LNG-only method. WHO calculated from that database that each 12-h delay raised the pregnancy risk by almost 50%. This has not been confirmed since, but earliest possible treatment is still definitely preferred. It was also clear that the Yuzpe method worked less well and it should now therefore only be used if LNG EC in some form is not available.

10.13 Should one be prepared to withhold EC treatment?

This can often be unwise. As the FSRH Guidance says, 'there is no time in the menstrual cycle when there is no risk of pregnancy following unprotected sexual intercourse (UPSI)'. As discussed at some length in *Q 2.13ff*, there is a fertile window of about 8 days, beginning about 7 days before the date of ovulation, but no woman can know when in a given cycle she will ovulate. The probability of conception in the first 3 days of the cycle appears to be negligible, but after taking an accurate menstrual and complete coital history the decision to treat depends on many factors, not least the amount of anxiety present.

The treatment is very safe, if not entirely risk-free, so if a woman is very anxious and wishes to use EC, in the words of the FSRH Guidance 2006, 'a pragmatic approach is often required'.

In future it might be possible to discover, simply and accurately in the clinic, what stage of the menstrual cycle the woman has reached. At present, although treatment is not always indicated, it is never easy to be sure that ovulation will not occur on a highly atypical day in that particular cycle. Your patient could be having an amazingly short, or long, menstrual cycle out of the blue.

So when in doubt, in the normal cycle, treat. When pills have been missed in the pill cycle, on the other hand, this treatment is much less often indicated (*see Q 10.22*).

10.14 What are the time limits for successful treatment?

■ *The IUD method with multiple exposure:* the time limit of 5 days relates either to 120 h after the first episode of UPSI at any time in the cycle (see below) OR after the most likely expected day of ovulation, i.e. expected date of next menses, subtract 14 days and add 5. This is calculated in good faith from the menstrual data given by the woman and *applies irrespective of the number of earlier acts of unprotected intercourse.*

Five days is well within the time limits from intercourse to the start of implantation, according to the consensus of medical opinion. It will not be construed in law as possibly procuring an abortion (*Judicial Review, Q 10.3*). My view is that the calculation should be based on the shortest likely cycle. This is strengthened by an earlier judgment that suggests some leeway: in the case of Regina *v.* Dhingra, 24 January 1991, Mr Justice Wright did not convict a GP accused of illegal abortion achieved by inserting an IUD 11 days after intercourse because it was day 18 and thus prior to implantation:

> I further hold, in accordance with the uncontroverted evidence that I have heard, that a pregnancy cannot come into existence until the fertilized ovum has become implanted in the womb, and that stage is not reached until, at the earliest, the 20th day of a normal 28-day cycle, and, in all probability, until the next period is missed.

■ *Single act of intercourse:* if this was after calculated ovulation, the copper IUD can be inserted (if indicated at all) up to 5 days after that unprotected act. But exposure once only at, say, day $x - 4$, before ovulation occurring on day x, allows treatment at $x + 5$ days (follows from bullet 1, above) i.e. 9 days (and it could be more) after the UPSI

10.15 Is it always preferable to treat at the earliest possible moment?

■ *The IUD method:* this is so effective that delay (so long as no later than 5 days after ovulation) is unlikely to lead to failure. This can be helpful in practice, if the facilities are not present for IUD insertion where and when the woman first presents (e.g. in a pharmacy or an evening surgery). Referral to an appropriate session a day or two later might be well within the time limit (*see Q 10.37*).

■ *The hormonal methods, specifically LNG EC:* given the 1998 WHO data (*see Q 10.6*), it is best practice to start treatment as soon as the woman presents.

10.16 What reasons can account for 'failure' of LNG EC?

1 Unasked-about or unadmitted other exposure earlier in the cycle. It is essential always to question each woman most closely about the possibility of inadequate contraception earlier than the index event.

2 Treatment initiated more than 72 h after first UPSI – or late in the cycle, when it has lost the chance to interfere with fertilization.

3 Vomiting within 2 h of tablet-taking (*see Q 10.24*). This is an obvious efficacy as well as comfort advantage of LNG EC compared with the old Yuzpe method, which was itself much more likely to cause vomiting. In practice it is a relatively rare cause of failure. Some authorities have argued that there is no need to replace the second two tablets if they are vomited back, because the occurrence of vomiting implies a particularly strong pharmacological effect. There are no data to support or refute this view. Women should be instructed to contact the clinician for consideration of some action, particularly in a high pregnancy-risk case. Such action could be the provision of further tablets along with an antiemetic (*see Q 10.25*) or more rarely in a coincidental severe stomach upset, the insertion of an IUD.

4 Non-compliance leading to inadequate dosage. For this reason, clinicians can sometimes prefer to see the LNG EC dose swallowed in their presence.

5 Unprotected intercourse subsequent to the treatment, which might have simply postponed ovulation (*see Q 10.16*). In the WHO 2002 study, after treatment within 5 days of a single UPSI, for the LNG EC and single-dose LNG groups combined, the conception rate was 6.6% among those who had unprotected sex between treatment and the expected menses but only 1.5% in those who claimed abstinence during that time.

In the real world, point (5) raises the important question of 'Quick start': should not a planned long-term method, such as the COC or injectable, be appropriately started immediately after the emergency method? *See Q 10.41.*

Points (1) and (5) are probably more common explanations than are true method failures.

10.17 What are the risks if the EC treatment fails? What about ectopic pregnancy?

This is a vitally important aspect of counselling. Whenever any of the methods operate at the uterine level, if the woman has pre-existing tubal damage (known or unknown), tubal implantation will clearly not be prevented. In other words, she will get her ectopic whether she has EC or not.

Additionally, there is the small possibility that the hormonal methods might interfere with tubal transport. This is disputed and, I would say, unlikely, given only one ectopic in 2712 women treated with either of the two LNG regimens in WHO 2002.

Actually, all the methods, including the IUD, much reduce the chance of fertilization, so the overall number of ectopics should be reduced, even if the percentage among the pregnancies goes up (*see Q 9.29*).

In practice, any woman presenting for EC might have tubal damage and, because she will be at risk with or without treatment, it is certainly safest to warn her to seek prompt advice if any pelvic pain occurs.

10.18 If the pregnancy is in the uterus, will it be harmed in any way (hormonal methods)?

A small teratogenic risk cannot be ruled out because insufficient pregnancies have gone to term after hormonal EC treatment failure, especially with LNG EC. In a series collected in the early 1990s by the then UK National Association of Family Planning Doctors/Faculty of SRH, there were 178 full-term pregnancies whose outcome was known following the previous (Yuzpe) EC therapy, which did of course contain the same progestogen LNG (along with EE). Reassuringly, the rate of and distribution of abnormalities was no different from what would be expected in a normal population, delivering without the Yuzpe EC therapy (Cardy, personal communication). Similarly, spontaneous reports to drug regulatory authorities after LNG EC do not suggest any consistent teratogenic effect.

Moreover, even if there were a potential adverse effect, exposure will be negligible if the hormonal methods are correctly used, and very little, if any, of the artificial hormone(s) could reach the blastocyst via the uterine secretions, because it is not yet implanted. Also:

■ The blastocyst is very resistant to partial damage by noxious agents. Research in animals suggests that it is either destroyed or else, because its cells are 'totipotent', it can recover and develop entirely normally.

■ It is very much accepted clinical practice for women to continue to full term when they have taken the combined or progestogen-only pill for several weeks during organogenesis: a more critical time (see first bullet, above), and there would also be more exposure. Yet meta-analyses and registers of fetal abnormality have failed even in those circumstances to show any significant increase in major fetal abnormalities.

In practice, the woman can be told:

The risk of a pregnancy being harmed is believed to be extremely small, less than that when the ordinary pill is inadvertently taken in early pregnancy – but no one can ever be guaranteed or promised a normal baby (1 in 50 have an important birth defect). Research so far, looking at babies born after failure of the emergency pill, has not proved any harmful effects. The risk is so low that after failed EC an abortion should never be recommended solely on fetal grounds.

The circumstances of the failed postcoital conception mean that, in UK practice, most women request a therapeutic abortion. If a woman wishes to continue to full term, very detailed records should be kept, documenting that she has fully understood the italicized statement above.

10.19 What about failure of the copper IUD method?

In the ultra-rare event of continuing pregnancy following EC insertion of an IUD, management should normally include removal of the device after a preliminary ultrasound scan, as discussed in *Q 9.23 (see also Qs 10.36, 10.39)*.

INDICATIONS AND ADVANTAGES OF POSTCOITAL CONTRACEPTION

10.20 What are the advantages of EC?

■ It provides a way of escape from an unwanted pregnancy at a time of high motivation after (for whatever reason) unprotected intercourse has taken place.

■ By definition, it is non-intercourse-related.

■ All three methods are effective; the copper IUD most.

■ The methods can be applied well after exposure to the risk, with a fair chance of success: up to 5 days after a single (earliest) UPSI if the hormone method is used and, in an extreme case, if an IUD is inserted, right up to 12 days (after exposure on, say, day 7 of a 28-day cycle).

■ The methods are very safe, although sharing the potential hazards of hormonal/intrauterine contraception, respectively. No deaths have been reported.

- Presentation for the EC treatment gives a welcome opportunity to discuss future contraception; in the case of the IUD, solving the woman's immediate problem can also provide for her long-term needs.
- The method is under a woman's control (i.e. its use cannot be prevented by her partner, if she can find a sympathetic provider).
- The method can be prescribed in advance in many cases, for example, a young woman about to travel abroad and anxious about rape or other circumstances of unprotected intercourse in foreign parts.

However, the present hormonal methods are not yet advised for regular ongoing use, for several reasons (*see Q 10.46*).

10.21 What are the indications for the treatment?

On presentation, depending on time of the cycle that exposure took place (*see Q 10.13*), whenever the clinician feels that the small risks of the method are outweighed by the risks of pregnancy and other relevant factors such as the woman's level of anxiety.

10.22 How do women present for treatment?

In the WHO 2002 study, 52% presented reporting that no contraception had been used, and 44% that there had been a condom failure. Outside of a research environment these would still be by far the most common groups, but there are numerous possible presentation categories to consider:

NO METHOD USED

1 'Moonlight and roses' summarizes the most common presentation in this category, where intercourse was consensual but unpremeditated. It is often with a new partner, especially first-time-ever intercourse or extramarital affairs (e.g. where the husband has had a vasectomy). Or there could have been an unexpected reconciliation with an ex-partner. Even today, and worldwide, far too few men consider that birth control is any of their business whatsoever.

2 Intercourse under the influence of alcohol or drugs.

3 Total misunderstanding of the 'safe period' approach, or disregard of the mucus signs (or red light of Persona) (*see Qs 2.28, 2.29*): these likewise equate to no method used.

4 Special situations:

    (a) Rape and sexual assault: here, counselling and management must be even more sensitive than usual, and continuing emotional support

is likely to be required. Involvement of the nearest Rape Crisis Centre and the local police force may be necessary. Avoid destroying forensic evidence if an accusation is to be made, and arrange tests and prophylaxis (and follow-up) for STIs.
(b) Incest.
(c) Women with learning disorders (taken advantage of).
(d) Recent use of teratogens: drugs, or live vaccine such as polio or yellow fever.

CONTRACEPTIVE FAILURE (OF THE METHOD OR OF ITS USE)

5 The most common category here is the split or slipped condom. In a study from the West Midlands no fewer than 48 out of 80 women reported a broken sheath. In more than one case a fragment of rubber was retrieved from the upper vagina, proving that not all such reports are fictions to appear respectable in the eyes of the provider.

In such cases, always discuss whether the (rubber) condom might have been exposed to any mineral or vegetable oil (*see Q 3.21*).

6 Complete or partial expulsion of an IUD or IUS, identified midcycle – or where midcycle removal of the device is deemed necessary (should be rare, *see Q 9.14*). Here, careful reinsertion of another IUD is preferable, especially if there has been repeated intercourse since the last menstrual period. But occasionally LNG EC might be preferred.
7 If there has been recent intercourse and deliberate removal of an IUD at midcycle is essential as part of therapy for infection (*see Q 9.14*).
8 Errors of cap use, e.g. the discovery after intercourse that it was in the anterior fornix; or its too-early removal.
9 *Gross prolongation of the pill-free week in a COC-user:* the woman should follow the advice of *Q 5.18 and Fig. 5.3,* namely that EC is usually advisable *if,* with sexual exposure since the last pack, the COC-user is a 'late restarter' by more than 2 days (meaning a 9-day pill-free interval); *or* more than two of pills 1–7 are missed.

What about midcycle or end-of-pill-cycle omissions?
■ Extra hormonal EC treatment is usually redundant for midcycle pill omissions, provided at least seven tablets were correctly taken; although I have suggested it be given empirically if five or more tablets were missed (*see Q 5.19*).
■ At the end of the pill cycle the standard advice to run on to the next pack will nearly always make the woman contraceptively even

safer than usual: having only had 'her own' pill-free interval (PFI).

■ However, the history of missed pills (e.g. through a severe vomiting attack) might sometimes not emerge until *after the next PFI has already been taken on top*: and this does indicate EC and also condom use for the next 7 days. *See also Q 5.25*, regarding the *very late pill-restarter*.

■ FSRH Guidance is also that LNG EC would be indicated if pills were 'effectively' missed *during use of liver enzyme-inducers and for 28 days afterwards (see Q 5.42)*: either side of, and thereby lengthening, the PFI, through inadequate additional contraception or UPSI.

10 In a POP-user:

(a) Sexual exposure: any time from the first missed tablet (late by 3 h, or 12 h if Cerazette) through until the mucus effect is expected to be restored after retaking the POP for 48 h, justifies hormone EC treatment, followed by condom use until pills have been taken correctly for a minimum of 2 days; but EC not normally needed during full lactation (*see Qs 7.22, 7.23*).

(b) If there has been a contraceptive accident or UPSI during, or in the 28 days following, use of liver enzyme-inducers (*see Q 5.42*).

11 In a DMPA user: here, the FSRH and UKMEC Guidance is to consider this only when it is more than 14 weeks since the previous injection. I prefer the more conservative protocol that first uses this at 13 weeks (*see Q 8.52*).

12 In a user of Implanon: inadequate additional contraception or UPSI during and for 28 days after use of liver enzyme-inducers.

13 Other contraceptive accidents involving, for example, spermicides or unsuccessful withdrawal.

DISADVANTAGES OF POSTCOITAL CONTRACEPTION

10.23 What are the disadvantages?

THE HORMONAL METHODS (ESSENTIALLY NOW JUST LNG EC)

■ Nausea, and rare (1.5%) vomiting (*see also Q 10.26*).

■ Failure rate, especially if the woman tries to use it frequently as her main long-term method.

■ Contraindications: very few (*see Q 10.27*). There is no age limit.

■ Further unprotected intercourse following therapy must be avoided, in case of postponement of ovulation (*see Q 10.7*).

■ The next menses are sometimes delayed beyond 7 days – in 5% of users of LNG EC according to WHO 2002 (*see Q 10.43*).

■ Interacting drugs must be allowed for (*see Q 10.29*).

COPPER IUD

- A 'surgical' procedure is involved, when what the woman is primarily requesting is a quick medical 'fix it'.
- Pain might be caused to the woman at insertion or subsequently.
- Risk of causing or exacerbating pelvic inflammatory disease (PID). Where the method must be used and the risk is judged high from a carefully taken sexual history, for whatever reason (including exposure through rape), then after the relevant tests – appreciating that the latter cannot identify *Chlamydia* for a minimum of 5 days after first exposure – antibiotic cover should be given (*see Qs 9.57, 9.58, 10.37*). And removal after the next menses might sometimes be best, after the woman is established on a more appropriate long-term method.
- There is a risk of causing all the other known complications of IUDs, because these are so often insertion-related (*see Qs 9.20, 9.21, 9.99*).

10.24 What is the incidence of nausea and vomiting after the currently used hormonal methods?

In the WHO studies, the mean incidence of these symptoms was as shown in *Table 10.2*. It is interesting that, for LNG EC, the WHO 2002 study results were different from those in 1998. But it is difficult to interpret this difference because there were very large variations around the means between the study centres in 2002: for example, nausea within 7 days of treatment was reported by only 2% in New Delhi but by 28% in Manchester!

The 2002 rate of vomiting (call it under 2%) seems a more accurate estimate than 5%, based on our clinical experience at the Margaret Pyke Centre.

10.25 What can be done to minimize the nausea/vomiting problem? Should one give antiemetics?

- In the first place, forewarned is forearmed.
- With respect to possible use of an antiemetic, domperidone maleate 10 mg is now recommended because it does not readily cross the blood–brain barrier or cause extrapyramidal side-effects.

TABLE 10.2 The incidence of nausea and vomiting after hormonal EC methods (WHO trials)

	Study year		
	1998	1998	2002
Nausea	Yuzpe 50.5%	LNG EC 23.1%	LNG EC 15%
Vomiting	Yuzpe 18.8%	LNG EC 5.6%	LNG EC 1.4%

But nausea and vomiting are so much rarer with LNG EC than with the old Yuzpe method (*see* Q *10.24*) that at the Margaret Pyke Centre and elsewhere, antiemetic treatment is given highly selectively, not routinely:

■ where there is a history of vomiting in the past following LNG EC
■ along with repeat dosing in the current cycle because vomiting occurred within 2 h
■ during a coincidental severe stomach upset (consider the IUD method).

10.26 What other symptoms are associated with EC treatment?

 'Fatigue' was reported by about 15% of all groups in the WHO studies. Fairly commonly reported is breast tenderness, plus a range of other symptoms including dizziness, headaches, eye symptoms, etc. The association with therapy is not necessarily causal.

A few women report a 'withdrawal bleed' following treatment even with LNG EC, and the woman should be instructed not to assume that this is her next period (unless she was treated very late in the cycle), but to take advice.

PATIENT SELECTION AND CHOICE OF METHOD

10.27 What are the absolute contraindications (WHO 4) to EC? And what factors might be classified WHO 3 (or 2)?

WHO and UKMEC say there are no absolute contraindications and I (almost) agree:

ALL METHODS – WHO 4
■ *Pregnancy:* WHO correctly states there is no known harm from EC to the fetus, but every effort should still be made to avoid exposure by taking a careful history, and, where indicated, doing the most sensitive pregnancy test available.
■ *Severe allergy to a constituent:* i.e. LNG or EE or an excipient in the tablets, or to copper (*see* Q *9.87*). A dubious history, or moderate allergy, is WHO 3. (The alternative method of the two is, of course, usable.)
■ *Patient's ethical objection to a method possibly operating after fertilization* (i.e. she disagrees with the UK legal view). This objection should not always be presumed to be absent because she has presented. Note also that if she presents at risk very early in the cycle, it could be explained that her ethical concern might not apply, because the method has then got to work by a pre-fertilization mechanism.

HORMONAL METHODS: LNG EC (COPPER IUD USABLE)

■ *Acute porphyria,* with past attack precipitated by sex hormones (WHO 4): predisposition alone is WHO 3 (*see Qs 6.43, 6.44*); other porphyrias are WHO 3 or 2.

■ *Current and sustained vomiting, out-of-control, from a severe stomach upset* (WHO 4 or 3).

■ *Current active and severe liver disease* with abnormal function tests (usually WHO 3).

■ *Current enzyme-inducer drug treatment* (WHO 3, might double dose but IUD better) – *see Q 10.29.*

There is no upper nor lower age limit (given sufficient risk of conception)

NON-HORMONAL METHOD: COPPER IUD

In addition to the three applicable absolute (WHO 4) contraindications listed above, the majority of all the IUD-related temporary and permanent absolute contraindications listed in *Qs 9.84–9.86* would also apply. However, it is acceptable practice in selected cases to insert a copper IUD with screening and full antibiotic cover (*see Q 10.23*) when PID has not been excluded; or in women at high risk (especially after rape).

If the IUD method is thought inappropriate for long-term use (e.g. in a nullipara who has had a previous ectopic pregnancy), it can always be removed after the next period when she is on a method such as DMPA.

10.28 What are not contraindications to the use of LNG EC?

■ Presentation more than 72 h after unprotected intercourse: this is an option, discussed above (*see Qs 10.8, 10.9*).

■ Previous ectopic pregnancy (*see Q 10.17*).

■ *Postpartum:* if an ovulation risk exists, which might be negligible if the LAM criteria apply (see next bullet and Q 2.36).

■ *Lactation:* the woman can also be reassured that LNG EC should not impair this. She might be concerned to avoid the vanishingly small but unquantified risk through the artificial hormones entering her breast milk. This can usually be done without prejudicing lactation by expressing the breast milk and bottle-feeding the infant for 24 h.

■ If hCG is persistent following trophoblastic disease: LNG EC is also usable (WHO 2, see Q 5.78).

■ *Current breast cancer:* this is WHO 2; an adverse effect is exceptionally unlikely with such short-term exposure.

10.29 What if a woman taking an enzyme-inducing drug (which could be by her own supply of St John's wort) should require hormonal EC?

See Qs 5.36–5.38 for a full discussion of this important question in relation to regular use of the COC. The solution here, in the FSRH Guidance of 2006, is simply to take two tablets (totalling 3 mg) of Levonelle 1500 – an unlicensed use (i.e. see *Appendix A*, p. 553).

The woman should also be advised of the alternative and more predictably effective choice of an IUD: indeed, the FSRH Guidance says this is the preferred option.

10.30 What if she is on a non-enzyme-inducing antibiotic?

There is not even a theoretical problem (*see Qs 5.36, 5.37*) with LNG EC, like all progestogen-only methods.

10.31 Can other drugs interact with LNG EC?

Concern has been raised in respect to warfarin and related coumarins (FSRH Guidance): the anticoagulant effect might be altered, more probably increased, so the woman should be warned and advised to have her INR test carefully checked, initially 3 days after the treatment.

10.32 What are the relative contraindications to EC IUD insertion?

■ All the relative contraindications listed in *Q 9.86* might apply if it is intended that the method will be used long term, but some (e.g. history of dysmenorrhoea or menorrhagia) are irrelevant to the very short-term option, just until the time of the next period with initiation of a different long-term method thereafter.

■ Past ectopic pregnancy: even in nulliparae this is only a weak relative contraindication (WHO 2) to very short-term use in selected cases (*see Q 10.17*).

10.33 Given that the majority of women presenting for EC prefer and expect oral treatment, when should the intrauterine method be offered instead?

As the question implies, LNG EC is indeed the normal first choice, but there are some special reasons for a copper IUD which are often not properly considered. These are:

■ Where she desires the most effective available option, which this is (*see Q 10.12*). The FSRH Guidance rightly makes a special point of this offer being made to *all* women attending for EC, even if they present within 72 h of UPSI, and especially when the assessed risk of conception is high (*e.g. 20–30% peri-ovulation* and additionally there is significant doubt that LNG EC works well post fertilization).

■ The woman's desire to use the IUD as her long-term method: this could be a very good indication in a parous woman with trouble-free periods, for instance, and also some who are nulliparous (*see Q 9.18ff*). However, it is always permissible (and sometimes to be recommended) that the device is used purely to solve the immediate problem, and is removed at the next menses. This also means STI screening and usually antibiotic cover, *see Q 10.37*.

■ Where there is an absolute (WHO 4) contraindication to the progestogen (i.e. severe allergy, acute porphyria with a previous attack, very severe liver disease); and sometimes in some less strong WHO 3 circumstances – e.g. the existence of enzyme induction (*see Q 10.29*).

■ Where there has been multiple exposure, and the clinician inserts the device in good faith no more than 5 days after the most probable calculated ovulation date (*see Q 10.14* and below).

■ Where presentation is more than 72 h since a single episode of unprotected intercourse: the upper time limit any time in the cycle being 5 days – but IUD insertion can be well beyond 5 days after UPSI so long as it is not beyond 5 days after calculated ovulation (length of shortest likely cycle, subtract 14 and add 5 days).

■ Rarely, as a result of vomiting. IUD insertion is only indicated if the woman is a high pregnancy-risk case and either
  – the vomiting occurs within 2 h of ingesting an LNG EC dose (but it is more usual to give an additional dose, perhaps along with an antiemetic (*see Q 10.25*)) or
  – there is an ongoing stomach upset that makes any oral method impractical.

See also Q 10.37 – for the practical details of EC use of a copper IUD.

COUNSELLING AND MANAGEMENT AT THE FIRST VISIT

10.34 How important is counselling for EC?

The treatment is simple and very safe: LNG EC has almost no absolute contraindications. Obviously, if there has been a simple condom rupture or dislodgement occurring in a stable relationship, the woman will just want her EC in a non-judgmental way with minimum delay and hassle. The amount of time and emotional support she needs will be far less than in cases of rape or incest, although the availability of such support should always be clear. In every case without exception:

■ Confidentiality must be real and must feel real, to every attender – most especially to young teenagers (*see Qs 11.5, 11.11*).

■ Every woman needs information and clear instructions sympathetically given. In practice, much of the information can be conveyed by a good leaflet and the discussion – including on the crucial subject of future contraception – most appropriately delegated to a family planning-trained nurse, and often now commercially by a pharmacist.

With Patient Group Directions, nurses (including school nurses) and pharmacists have been empowered to take the whole EC workload, which with good training they often do better than doctors – and this can also assist access for young women who feel they cannot afford the charge for normal over-the-counter provision by pharmacists.

The Faculty of SRH rightly stresses the importance of managed clinical care pathways to ensure 'joined-up' working between different service providers.

10.35 In summary, what aspects should be covered in taking the medical history?

1 Date of the last menstrual period, and whether it was in any way abnormal.
2 Details of the patient's normal menstrual cycles: shortest, longest and most usual lengths.
3 The calculated date of ovulation.
4 The day(s) in the cycle of all unprotected intercourse.
5 The number of hours since the first episode of unprotected intercourse.
6 The current method of contraception: LAM and 'natural' methods are particularly relevant (*see* Q *10.28, bullet 3*). In pill-takers who have missed pills, the timing relative to the PFI is critical (*see* Q *10.22(9)*).
7 Any contraindications (from the history), use of any enzyme-inducers (including St John's wort, *see* Q *10.29*), all risk factors for the COC (because it might be going to be used in future), and any past PID or ectopic pregnancy.
8 Take a sexual history in every case (*see* Q *1.14*) and 'offer STI screening to *all* [my emphasis] those attending for EC' (FSRH Guidance). Depending on the case, this might mean referral to a GUM department, or perhaps a *Chlamydia* test on site – and not only if she is choosing to have an IUD for EC.

It should be stressed that the whole 'contract' to give this kind of treatment depends on utmost mutual good faith and honesty, especially concerning the menstrual/coital history.

10.36 What are the ten main points to cover in counselling for EC?

1 Assess the menstrual and coital history and sexual history as in Q *10.35*, and hence whether any treatment is necessary. Offer the recommended STI screen.

2   Discuss, backed by a good leaflet, the methods available and their mode of action, medical risks and side-effects.

3   Advise her of the failure rate of each method, and the implications, i.e. the IUD being the most effective option, ectopic pregnancy risk (*see Qs 10.17 and 10.28*) and to return if she experiences any pain.

4   Explore her attitudes to possible failure of the regimen and continuance of the pregnancy: the small risk of fetal abnormality, which could happen although the method applied preimplantation is most unlikely to be causative (*see Q 10.18*).

5   Discuss the consequential importance of follow-up. Suggest that she brings an early morning urine sample if her next period is surprisingly light or absent.

6   *Above all*: let her make her own final decision – about whether to use EC treatment, and which method – when the above have been discussed.

7   If a hormonal method is selected, advise her to telephone the clinic or surgery for advice if she vomits within 2 h of either dose.

8   Discuss contraception for the rest of the current cycle (*see Q 10.7*): this is not a problem if the IUD is used.

9   Discuss long-term contraception. *See Q 10.40* for the advice to be given if the combined pill is selected.

10 Keep an accurate record, written at the time, dated and signed, especially (see *Appendix A*, p. 553) if the use will be unlicensed (e.g. use of LNG EC more than once per cycle).

10.37 What is different about insertion of a copper IUD as an emergency in this way rather than electively?

First, it is more like an elective insertion than some imagine, i.e. there is no rush, usually the 'emergency' pressure is off because there are several days until it would be 5 days after ovulation. So the actual procedure can and often should be done later in the day or the week, at a more convenient time and place – for the woman as well as the service.

The FSRH Guidance recommends:

1   'Ideally an emergency IUD should be fitted at first presentation': implying she has presented at a Level 2 service practitioner or clinic. Although even then she could have a sandwich and cup of coffee, and return for her premedication with a PGSI, possibly at the end of the surgery or clinic.

2   Give LNG EC as a 'holding manoeuvre' if there is to be a day or two's delay before the fitting.

The medical eligibility criteria are similar to routine IUD insertions *except* that nulliparity, young age, risk status for STIs and previous ectopic pregnancy are minor reasons for caution in such short-term use, balanced by risks of a likely pregnancy without the treatment. There can often be a plan to remove the IUD altogether when the woman is established on what might be a more appropriate long-term method.

If a carefully taken sexual history reveals the woman to be in a high-risk group – as it very often will among those attending for EC (FSRH Guidance says as much) – it is recommended, after screening at least for *Chlamydia*, to give either azithromycin 1 g stat or doxycycline 200 mg bd for 7 days and recommend abstinence pending results (FSRH Guidance).

However, if the woman is not in a high-risk group (monogamous, no recent partner change, condom accident) the use of prophylactic antibiotics *routinely* would not be recommended. This whole issue of infection risk at IUD insertion is discussed in some depth within and leading up to Q 9.58.

After the insertion, warn about any excessive pain or other manifestations of PID in the days ahead (*see* Q 9.59).

Which IUD?

If the woman is at all likely to become a long-term user, I would favour a banded copper IUD: i.e. the T-Safe™ Cu 380A or one of its clones for a parous woman. For a nulliparous woman:

■ First choice either the banded Mini TT 380 Slimline or the Flexi-T 380 where possible; or GyneFix if the uterus is very small or distorted.

■ Otherwise, a UT 380 Short or Flexi-T 300, which may be easier to fit through a narrow internal os, though a little less effective for long-term use.

10.38 Should these women always be examined vaginally?

No. It is obviously mandatory to allow safe assessment for and insertion of a copper IUD. But otherwise in my view the answer is normally 'no'; the anxiety so caused, for example, to a young teenager presenting after her first-ever sexual experience, rules it out. But there might be a clinical or screening indication:

■ To exclude a concealed (advanced) clinical pregnancy.

■ To screen opportunistically, as a minimum for *Chlamydia*, or more comprehensively at a GUM department. EC attenders under 25 or with more than one partner in the last year are high risk (FSRH Guidance). Pelvic tenderness or a purulent discharge suggestive of active infection might also be discovered.

Examination at follow-up is, similarly, only rarely required – on specific clinical grounds (*see* Q 10.44).

10.39 Should the woman be asked to sign any type of consent form?

This is deemed unnecessary, even for emergency IUD insertion, provided accurate contemporaneous records are kept, the clinician asserting that the woman gave verbal informed consent. It is most helpful to supplement the counselling, including about the chosen method for the future, with an appropriate leaflet – such as that produced by the fpa (*see Q 5.107*).

FOLLOW-UP

10.40 If the woman selects an oral contraceptive subsequent to EC treatment, when should she take the first tablet?

It is usual for both the COC and the POP to be commenced on the first day of the next menses. However, there is at times a light (and not relevant) withdrawal bleed just after the LNG EC hormones, and a light 'threatened abortion' loss might also occur very early in pregnancy. The FSRH Guidance states the woman should be advised about menstrual irregularity (*see Q 10.43*).

It has been practice at the Margaret Pyke Centre, therefore, that both the COC and POP should be started when the woman is convinced that the flow is within her own normal range, commonly on the second day rather than the first. This slight delay still allows the woman not to be required to use extra contraceptive precautions (*see Q 5.50, Table 5.4, Q 7.25 and Table 7.4*).

It is important, however, to ensure that, even if in doubt about her period, she does start the COC or POP before day 3 and then take advice – and that she knows that if started later, it would be best to use condoms additionally for 7 days.

10.41 Might she be instructed to start the combined pill or injectable immediately after EC treatment, i.e. a 'Quick start'?

This 'Quick start' approach might indeed be acceptable in selected cases. There is a minimal medico-legal concern: if the woman were to conceive, and the baby have an important fetal abnormality (as occurs in 2% of cases), a legal claim that the abnormality was caused by the extra packet of combined pills being given after implantation might be submitted. It would, of course, be highly unlikely that such an abnormality was truly caused by the COC (*see Q 6.47*) or injectable. However, it could be argued as being even more unlikely that teratogenesis would follow the LNG EC regimen alone, given, as it should only be, preimplantation (*see Q 10.18*).

There are definitely circumstances in which this would be good management – especially in a case where the risk of EC treatment failing is considered to be particularly low and the risk of conception through poor condom use before the next period is high – provided there has been a thorough and documented discussion of all the implications with the woman concerned.

See also Q 10.22(9) for a form of 'Quick start' that is already normal practice: if the PFI has been lengthened, an immediate (re-)start of the COC is routinely advised.

10.42 Can LNG EC be given more than once in a given cycle, if a woman has already received EC treatment and reports further exposure?

Yes. Because in clinical practice we cannot be sure when ovulation occurs, and it might have been postponed by earlier treatment, it might well be right to re-prescribe – repeatedly in the same cycle. At what interval? The Faculty Expert Group agreed, pending more data, that UPSI within just 12 h of a dose of LNG EC does not require a further dose. . . .

In support of the medical safety of repeated dosing, LNG 750 μg was marketed as Postinor in Hungary and elsewhere for many years, with a recommendation to use it postcoitally up to four times per month. The failure rate was reported as 0.8% for each treatment cycle and the only reported problem was irregular bleeding, about which women should be warned. Repeated use will not induce abortion if the woman were to be already pregnant.

Once again, this is an unlicensed use (see *Appendix A*, p. 553).

10.43 What is the usual time of onset of the next period after EC treatment?

In the WHO 2002 study, over half of the subjects had their next menses on the expected day plus or minus 2 days and all but 5% of the non-conceivers in the two LNG groups came on early or no later than 7 days late.

It is believed that late onset is more likely when treatment was early enough in the cycle to postpone ovulation. However, when it acts to block fertilization, the method tends to bring the next period on early. It is useful to be able to tell the woman that her next period is likely to be on time or early, so she will not need to be in suspense for too long.

No obvious impact on cycle length has been reported following postcoital IUD insertion.

10.44 How important is it to follow up EC women after treatment?

A defined follow-up visit is essential after IUD insertion, normally set for about 6 weeks but with a recommended telephone contact at about 1 week (*see Q 9.122*). Follow-up is not now the norm after hormonal EC, so long as the next period comes on normally. What matters is that the woman clearly understands that she can return without an appointment:

■ If she has any worrying symptoms, particularly pain or irregular bleeding.

■ If her menses are delayed by more than 7 days (*see Q 10.43*). A pregnancy test might then be necessary and, if there is any clinical doubt, especially concerning an ectopic, a pelvic examination and possible referral.

■ As needed to continue her ongoing contraceptive care – in all cases if she has been fitted with a copper IUD. Beware of the occasional pressure with the latter to 'leave well alone' in circumstances in which the IUD is a poor choice for long-term use (*see Qs 9.83–9.86 and 10.27*). The original and better plan to transfer to another method (such as DMPA or perhaps Implanon) might need to be encouraged.

10.45 What if the method does fail?

Good pregnancy-counselling should follow. After LNG EC there should be no real difference in the content of this counselling from that when any other method of birth control has failed (see the full discussion in *Q 10.18*).

Unless the woman is having a termination, if she is pregnant with an IUD in position, the device should normally be gently removed (*see Qs 9.23, 9.24*).

10.46 Should the LNG EC method sometimes be provided in advance of need?

Yes, indeed this is WHO 1 according to the WHO and UKMEC. As the FSRH Guidance reports and references, RCTs have shown that, for selected women, advance supply is safe. It does get used correctly by the majority of women, does not reduce the use of the more appropriate contraceptive methods and even (perhaps surprisingly) is not associated with an increase in unprotected sex. What has not yet been proved, however, is a reduction in abortion rates, seemingly because the women in the advance treatment group in the Lothian study [Glasier A et al 2004 *Contraception* 69:361–366] failed to recognize their need actually to use the provided EC method in the cycle in which they later conceived. This supports promoting more widespread use of the LARCs among young people in the UK!

If provided ahead of need, women need reminding that regular monthly use of EC is not highly effective. Even with very early use of the LNG EC method after UPSI, a lunar-monthly failure rate of, say, 0.4% would mean an annual failure rate of over 5%.

10.47 So what is your view on EC being now available additionally over-the-counter?

I consider that the advantages of over-the-counter supply of EC definitely outweigh its risks. For best practice, pharmacists should offer:

- ■ Excellent user-friendly labelling by leaflet and a checklist of important information for the client.
- ■ Adequate privacy for the pharmacy consultation.
- ■ Easy local arrangements for transfer for the insertion of a copper IUD, as is sometimes indicated, or for medical support if increased dosing is required, e.g. because of coincident enzyme-inducer drug treatment.
- ■ Easy arrangements for long-term contraceptive follow-up (via clinic, or family doctor) and to investigate STIs as required.
- ■ Details of a parallel location for free NHS supply, for those who might not be able to afford the retail product. *See also Q 10.34.*
- ■ Details of a 24-h telephone hot-line for clients' queries – NHS Direct now supplies this, and there is also the fpa's excellent service, accessed by telephone during working hours:
  - fpa UK: tel. 0845 310 1334, Monday to Friday 9 a.m. to 7 p.m.
  - fpa Scotland: tel. 0141 576 5088, Monday to Thursday 9 a.m. to 5 p.m., Friday 9 a.m. to 4.30 p.m.
  - fpa Northern Ireland: tel. 028 90 325 488 (Belfast) or 028 71 260 016 (Derry), Monday to Thursday 9 a.m. to 5 p.m., Friday 9 a.m. to 4.30 p.m.

10.48 What would be the features of an ideal future EC method?

These would be similar to those of any reversible birth control method (*see Q 1.15*), but the following aspects would require particular emphasis. The ideal EC treatment, not yet in prospect, would:

- ■ be so effective each cycle that on a cumulative basis the annual rate of failures was less than 1/100 woman-years (*see Q 10.46*)
- ■ be effective for the remainder of each cycle, maybe longer, as well as in relation to the particular act of intercourse
- ■ require only a single dose
- ■ have no contraindications (at all) – LNG EC gets very close
- ■ have a very low incidence of side-effects, whether dangerous or annoying (such as nausea)
- ■ cause no disturbance of the menstrual cycle
- ■ be free of teratogenic effects.

10.49 What are the prospects for the future of EC?

A really reliable postovulatory contraceptive agent with as many as possible of the features listed in *Q 10.48*, coupled with a simple and reliable method of determining whether the exposure had been before or after ovulation, would be a considerable advance. Indeed, in the distant future it might be possible for regular release of an EC agent (e.g. from an implant) to be actually triggered by a biological event such as the pre-midcycle estrogen surge.

Another potential approach, although one fraught with ethical and legal difficulties, is the regular use of a postconceptional or contragestive agent to be administrated only when the woman is just overdue her period. Given average fertility, this approach would mean exposure to the potential systemic risks of the agent only on a few (four to six) occasions each year; but it would be out of order for many because it would be seen as a regular early abortion.

10.50 Specifically, what agents are being studied?

The greatest current interest is in progesterone receptor-blocking agents, such as mifepristone. In the third arm of the WHO 2002 trial, a single 10-mg dose was shown to be as effective as either of the LNG regimens – and more recent work from Aberdeen shows it to be even more effective through to 5 days after exposure. However, delayed ovulation with menses delay beyond 7 days in almost twice as many women as with LNG EC poses a practical problem. Given also its 'aura' as an abortifacient, I fear that mifepristone is unlikely to be marketed for EC any time soon.

There would be particular interest in a product, perhaps an implant, effective if applied up to the time of nidation, which went on to give ongoing long-term contraception thereafter (on the model of copper IUD insertion).

PQ PATIENT QUESTIONS

QUESTIONS ASKED BY PROSPECTIVE USERS OF POSTCOITAL CONTRACEPTION

10.51 Is the 'emergency pill' the same as the 'morning-after pill'?

Yes, it is. The reason for the new name is that the treatment (although most effective when started in the first 24 h) can be given much later than the morning after – at least 72 h, and sometimes after many days if the IUD method is chosen. So the old name was extremely misleading. It should be abandoned!

10.52 And isn't the emergency pill just the same as the contraceptive pill?

One kind – still used abroad – can be constructed in most countries from marketed daily combined pills, in the way shown in *Table 10.1*. Levonelle One Step uses the same single hormone as one of the POPs. But both are given in a different way, i.e. in larger doses and following intercourse.

10.53 If my sex life is erratic, why can I not be given pills in advance for use on a regular basis?

A full answer to this common question is given in *Q 10.46*. There are some special reasons why it should not be used at all by some women, or why the alternative IUD method would be medically preferable (*see Qs 10.27, 10.33*). However, because the LNG EC pill method (Levonelle) is so remarkably safe, and there is such an epidemic of unplanned pregnancies in many countries, I feel the benefits outweigh the risks of it being much more available, including through school nurses and over-the-counter, supervised by pharmacists (*see Q 10.47*).

10.54 I shall be travelling alone in the Far East and South America for the next 6 months. Could I take a supply of EC treatment for emergency use?

It could certainly be appropriate for you to be prescribed a supply in advance (*see Q 10.46*) but you might, alternatively, consider arranging a regular method like the pill or even an IUD, along with a good supply of condoms of course!

10.55 Can I wait a few hours for my own or the surgery's convenience or should I be treated just as soon as possible?

There should not be any undue delay; treatment in the first 24 h is best for the pill method (LNG EC). Certainly there is no need to disturb anyone within a few minutes or an hour of intercourse!

If the best method for you is going to be the IUD (*see Qs 10.33, 10.60*), as *Q 10.37* points out, waiting at least for some hours is usually not a problem – it might even be recommended. If it will be on another day, you would often be given LNG EC first as well.

10.56 Should I mention any earlier times when we made love (since my last period), when I attend for EC advice?

Yes, this is essential. The decisions as to whether to treat and how to treat successfully all depend on you being entirely forthcoming about every relevant fact. This also includes telling the pharmacist/nurse/doctor the correct date of your last period and how normal it was. The whole 'contract' between you and the healthcare professional depends on what is called 'utmost good faith'.

10.57 Will I need to be examined before EC treatment?

Usually not (*see Q 10.38*) unless – after discussion – you choose the IUD method.

10.58 Why might the practitioner or pharmacist tell me the EC treatment is not necessary?

The main reason might be that, after considering the time of the month and every other aspect, they judge that there is an almost-nil risk of you conceiving; and that this does not justify the (small) risks of the EC treatment. This is mainly only true when COC pills have been missed, in the middle or at the end of a packet – as explained in *Q 10.22*.

10.59 What should I do if I vomit within 2 h of either of my doses, especially if I actually bring back pills?

Take urgent advice. If there is a high risk of conception in your case, it might be right then to insert an IUD. But more usually it will be enough just to give you an additional dose, perhaps with an antiemetic (*see Q 10.25*).

10.60 Why did the doctor/nurse recommend a copper IUD for me when I really wanted pills?

For one of the reasons in *Q 10.33*. Depending on you, this might be a good method to continue using long term, but remember that you can choose to have it removed after your next period if you then plan perhaps to transfer to another effective method such as the combined pill or an implant.

10.61 Why should I use another method of family planning between EC treatment and the start of my next period?

The reason is that sometimes the method might be working not by blocking the fertilized egg from establishing itself in your womb, but instead by blocking egg release. There is then a high risk of fertilizing that later egg if your partner does not use another method such as the condom.

10.62 Should I expect a period immediately after using EC pills?

A few women do get what is known as 'a withdrawal bleed' within a day or two of LNG EC treatment. This will not usually seem like a proper period and, unless you were due one so soon, it is important to continue using the condom or any other effective method you were recommended to use, until you do have a definite period – or you might need to arrange follow-up at the surgery or clinic.

Fortunately, your proper period normally arrives either on time or a little early. Be sure to come back for follow-up if your next period is delayed or unexpectedly light.

10.63 For what reasons should I see the doctor sooner than arranged, following EC treatment?

The main reason would be because of any pain in your abdomen, because of the small risk of pregnancy outside the womb in your fallopian tube (*see Q 10.17*).

10.64 Does EC treatment cause an abortion?

No, not according to the modern view of when pregnancy starts (*see Q 10.3* and *Fig. 10.1*).

10.65   Must I have an abortion if EC treatment fails?

Not necessarily. It is thought that this treatment will not significantly increase the risk of an abnormal baby above the surprisingly high 2% risk that all women run. So the decision (always very difficult) about what to do about the unplanned pregnancy is really just the same as it would be if any other method of family planning were to fail (*see* Q 10.18).

Contraception for the young, the not quite so young – and in future

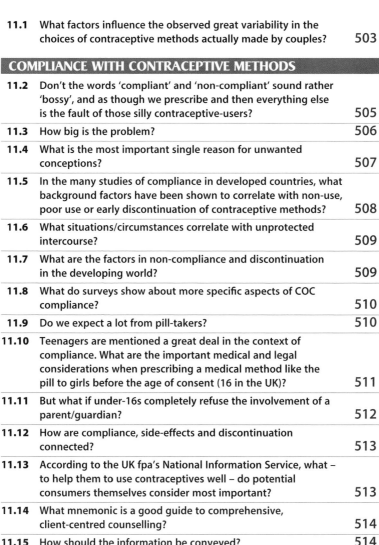

CONTRACEPTION FOR THE OLDER WOMAN – ABOVE AGE 40

This chapter includes much that is useful revision of the information elsewhere in the text. I am particularly indebted to Toni Belfield, Director of Information of the UK Family Planning Association (fpa). She has allowed me to use sections of her own text from an article in the *British Journal of Sexual Medicine,* but supplemented and much rearranged in this book's question-and-answer style. See also Belfield T 1999 in Kubba et al *Contraception and Office Gynecology* London: Saunders.

11.1 What factors influence the observed great variability in the choices of contraceptive methods actually made by couples?

Please refer to *Fig. 11.1* and *Table 11.1*, along with *Tables 1.1* (p. 12) and *1.2* (pp. 14–15).

The relative importance of the two main factors – maximum health safety as opposed to maximum effectiveness and independence from intercourse – and hence the appropriateness of different methods, varies greatly according to all the factors shown in Dr Christopher's 'factors wheel' (*Fig. 11.1*).

Choice, it seems, is seldom based on rational or objective information – the fact that a friend had a dreadful time with an IUD will weigh far more heavily than any amount of statistics that show this is not usually the case. It is also influenced by age and the particular stage of an individual couple's reproductive lifetime. Decisions are made at specific times:

- at the beginning of sexual experience
- after an accidental pregnancy or 'near miss'
- with life changes, e.g. a career change
- after a planned birth
- when there are problems with a particular method
- when the family is complete.

Initially, while the relationship is being established, a high degree of efficacy might be considered most important. However, if their sexual experience is infrequent or sporadic, male or female condoms may be ideal, provided they are used correctly, especially as they have the bonus of some protection against sexually transmitted diseases (STIs).

For child spacing, less efficient methods with reduced health risk might well be preferred. Once the family is established but the couple are not sure whether it is yet complete, the IUD can have particular merit. These points are summarized in *Table 11.1*, which is derived from Table 15 of my book *The Pill* and also looks forward to the near future.

This changing pattern of reproductive desire, in the couple's total life situation, places a big responsibility on the doctor or nurse to be themselves flexible and fully informed about the whole range of methods available. They must also be able and willing to spend time finding out

TABLE 11.1 The seven contraceptive ages of women

Age	Suggested method
0 Birth to puberty	No method required. Responsible sex and relationships education (SRE) is essential, *started by parents* and continuing through schooling
1 Puberty to marriage (or equivalent)	Either (a) a condom method, with emergency contraception back-up available; (b) the combined pill or combined options (skin patch or ring) or Cerazette; (c) a LARC, especially injectable or implant – for (b) and (c), always with a condom outside of mutual monogamy – or, if acceptable, (d) abstinence until the final life-partner if found. The choice depends on factors like religious views, perceived risk of sexually transmitted diseases, the frequency of partner changes and of intercourse
2 Marriage (or stable union equivalent) to first child	First choice probably a pill, but could be one of various patches/rings/injectables/implants followed perhaps by a fertility awareness method for some months before 'trying' for the first child
3 During breastfeeding	Either lactational amenorrhoea method (LAM) or any progestogen-only method with breastfeeding, or a simple barrier method. Intrauterine device or system, or male or female implant likely to be appropriate only if a long gap is expected between pregnancies
4 Family spacing after breastfeeding	Continue with any method started during 'age' 3, or shift to Cerazette/the combined pill/injectable/implant from an old-type progestogen-only pill, for greater effectiveness. Later, a banded copper IUD is progressively more appropriate, for a combination of the least long-term health hazards, efficacy and reversibility and cost; or of course the LNG-IUS if there are menstrual problems
5 After the (probable) last child	The first choice is an intrauterine device or system; other possibilities are any progestogen-only pill, or a combined hormonal method, if free of arterial or venous factors, or injectable/implant according to choice
6 Family complete, family growing up	First choice still as 5: banded copper IUD, or IUS if periods at all heavy or painful. Vasectomy would be generally preferable to female sterilization as more effective and easier to perform (*see Q 11.49*)
7 Perimenopausal (not sterilized)	*Contraceptive* hormone replacement therapy in some combination, e.g. the intrauterine system plus estrogen by any chosen route. Or, at this age, a weak contraceptive (e.g. spermicide or sponge), with or without standard non-contraceptive HRT, may be fully effective when combined with very reduced fertility. *See Q 11.33*

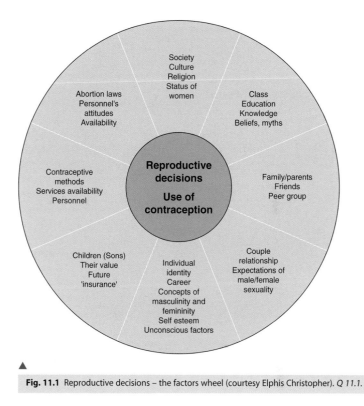

Fig. 11.1 Reproductive decisions – the factors wheel (courtesy Elphis Christopher). *Q 11.1.*

what sort of person they are actually dealing with, under the headings summarized in *Fig. 11.1*!

COMPLIANCE WITH CONTRACEPTIVE METHODS

11.2 Don't the words 'compliant' and 'non-compliant' sound rather 'bossy', and as though we prescribe and then everything else is the fault of those silly contraceptive-users?

Yes, but if we can ourselves agree not to mean anything of the sort, other words that are sometimes used – 'concordance' and 'adherence' – to me seem rather poor substitutes. What we are talking about is the user's responsibility to avoid user failure. More on the healthcare provider's responsibility follows later.

Regardless of whatever professional hat we wear, we are all also consumers when it comes to thinking about or using contraception, so our own experiences have the potential to make our counselling less objective than it should be. But how contraception is considered, discussed and, more importantly, delivered, will determine just how well it is accepted and used.

11.3   How big is the problem?

In a completely anonymous 1998 Sexual Health Matters survey, after a night on the town 1:5 young men admitted to sex that they now regretted, 1:7 had had totally unsafe sex and 1:10 were unable to remember if they had had sex!

Today, contraceptive choices and services are freely available, and research shows that people have the facts (in their heads) about contraception. Yet the behaviour that would be the logical outcome of that knowledge stubbornly refuses to follow!

Young people deserve encouragement to make sexually responsible choices, which start with either having or not having sex – and their views should be sought on all matters that affect their sexual health. Abstinence is one of the valid choices but, in surveys, applies to less than half of all girls who were 16 at their last birthday. Given the potential emotional and psychosocial trauma of very early coitarche, quite apart from the risk of STIs and cervical neoplasia, this group (and the boys too) should receive our encouragement – as providers – to continue to resist peer-group pressure and to wait for 'Mr or Ms Right'. They should not be labelled a minority group, because this has an implication of abnormality. Yet, if abstinence is fairly obviously the 'best', the best must not become the enemy of the good – which in the real world is to optimize the provision of sex and relationships education (SRE) and to provide totally confidential and appropriate reproductive and sexual health services.

Rates of unintended pregnancy and requests for abortion remain persistently high. Although the under-16s achieve more publicity, older teenagers and women aged 20–25 are together responsible for far more unplanned pregnancies. Cumulatively, about one woman in three in the UK now has at least one termination before the age of 30.

In a study of teenage mothers, 84% had had no intention of becoming pregnant but were using no contraception when they conceived.

Although in some studies where there was good compliance, the COC has had failure rates of well below 1/100 woman-years, in 'typical use', failure rates of 8% are commonly reported (see *Table 1.2*, p. 14), rising to up to 20% in inner-city areas. Worldwide, it has been calculated that if – by improved pill-taking – we could reduce the failure rate of this one method by 1%, at least 630 000 fewer women would have accidental pregnancies each year.

11.4 What is the most important single reason for unwanted conceptions?

Sex! It has been well said that the biggest sex organ is the head! The other reasons follow from that.

■ Sex is embarrassing: contraception is inextricably linked with emotional and sexual well-being and it is impossible to talk about contraception without addressing sexuality – the two are inseparable. Research shows that contraception continues to be a source of considerable embarrassment and anxiety for both men and women, and this has implications for its uptake and usage. It can have an inhibiting effect on people's willingness to seek information and advice from professionals.

■ Also, in Elphis Christopher's memorable phrase, 'sex is hot, and contraception is cold'. And any method that is chosen is always 'the least worst method'! Snowden wrote in 1990 that whereas it can be argued that the prevention of pregnancy is beneficial, the use of contraception is not a pleasant experience for most people, which is a marked contrast to the sexual behaviour that prompts its need! Actual choice results from a negative process of 'seeking the least bad' among the options. The methods not chosen were even more disliked than the method chosen.

■ Sex is now – the possible problems resulting from sex seem unimportant. As we have seen, 'head' knowledge can be superb but still does not affect behaviour in the heat of the moment. The brain and the genitalia are not often used at the same time (see the apocryphal story at p. 21)!

Risk-taking and AIDS are not unlike risk-taking and pregnancy. Neither AIDS infection nor fertilization are certain, the gambler often survives, and the penalty is remote: 9 months in the case of pregnancy, maybe years in the case of AIDS. (Malcolm Potts, 1988)

So, like safer sex, the built-in problem of family planning is the 'planning bit'. This highlights the potential advantages of the postcoital methods. But their potential is not being realized. A 1992 study by Nigel Bruce of unplanned pregnancies in North London showed that more than half of those who could have sought such emergency help because they (a) knew about it and (b) knew there had been a contraceptive risk, did not do so! Asked why, the reason given amounted to that they 'had got away with it before'. So, strong in matters of sex is the gambling instinct! Plus inertia . . .

■ The early years of reproductive life are not that fertile, through anovulation. In the first year after the menarche 85% of cycles are anovular, but this falls to an average of 30% after 5 years. So young people's experience of 'getting away with it' in early years is likely to catch them out a little later, as their fertility peaks in the late teens and early 20s.

■ Finally, 'the fact that contraception has to do with sex seems to set up an environment where health risks are exaggerated or misunderstood' (Malcolm Potts). Reinforced by the tabloid newspapers, this explains some of the risk-illiteracy of our clients about, say, the pill. Ordinary, unprotected sex and even the cigarette or spliff that follows: these all seem so natural and safe by comparison to the artificialness of contraception!

11.5 In the many studies of compliance in developed countries, what background factors have been shown to correlate with non-use, poor use or early discontinuation of contraceptive methods?

Here is a list, longish but doubtless not complete, relating mainly to the COC:

■ Young, immature: after the very first years, youth also means optimum fertility, hence a greater likelihood of not getting away with any of the more frequent compliance errors. According to Jones and Forrest in 1989, failure rates of the pill in the first 12 months of use are more than five times higher in the under-20s than in the 35–44 age group.

■ Unmarried.

■ Nulliparous.

■ Early coitarche.

■ Multiple sexual partners.

■ Previous contraceptive failure/abortion.

■ Perception of low personal risk of conception (especially because of previous 'scares' that resolved).

■ Erratic daily timetable.

■ Cultural or religious opposition to birth control.

■ Poor social conditions.

■ Parents not married.

■ Lack of parental support.

■ Low evaluation of personal health.

■ Low educational attainment and goals.

■ Feelings of lack of personal self-worth and self-determination.

■ Feelings of fatalism (babies happen, rather like death, 'when your number comes up').

■ Cigarette smoking (not only is unplanned conception more likely overall, but also, in several studies of young teenagers, smokers are likely to start sexual activity younger).

- Alcohol: 'drink in – wits out!': 53% of 16–24-year-olds in a study in the South-west of England felt they were more likely to forget about the risk of pregnancy after drinking alcohol. The same applies to other drugs of addiction.
- Media 'scare stories' and misinformation/myths.
- Fear of side-effects.
- Experience of side-effects: above all, bleeding side-effects. Also other side-effects, perceived or real, especially weight gain, headaches, nausea, depression, breast tenderness, acne.
- Wrong or incomplete information (e.g. about missed or vomited pills).
- Poor service delivery/counselling/advice, particularly when combined with lack of assurance of confidentiality for the client. This is the (preventable) provider contribution to compliance problems (*see Qs 11.16, 11.17*).

> There is some considerable overlap between these risk factors, but more importantly and very relevantly in practice, there is synergism. Ensure more time for counselling when combinations of the above apply!

11.6 What situations/circumstances correlate with unprotected intercourse?

Here are a few, which are well documented:

- First-ever intercourse (or first with a new partner).
- Around the start or the end of any relationship – another good argument for long-term relationships, because there will be fewer 'bust-ups' (when the pill packets are thrown away) and then rebound relationships which are unprotected. This also argues for the LARCs, long-term, 'forgettable' methods that, if there are no troublesome side-effects, are much more likely to be continued with across the gap between relationships.
- Times of major life stress, e.g. bereavement, unemployment.
- On holiday, or trips away from home: indeed any situation where the individual or couple feels anonymous, a bit mad and so liable to behave out of character.

11.7 What are the factors in non-compliance and discontinuation in the developing world?

Everything above, only more so – wrong information, for instance. In Rwanda I was told that it was widely disseminated and believed that the pill would cause permanent infertility. A recent survey in Egypt found that the most common error of providers, let alone users of the pill, was the belief (as often in the UK, *see Q 11.8*) that the next packet of pills should routinely be started on the fifth day of the withdrawal bleed! Fatalism and cultural and religious obstacles to good compliance are often very strong.

But the biggest single factor is the basic one of non-availability of the actual methods, or the drying up of supplies once a good method like DMPA has been initiated. Even when available, contraceptives are seen as an expense and inconvenient (as they are in many poor communities of the developed world, too).

11.8 What do surveys show about more specific aspects of COC compliance?

A 1986 general practice survey in a mainly low social class (inner-city) area showed that only 28% of women were taking the pill in accordance with the makers' instructions. Much of the confusion related (most crucially, *see Q 5.16*) to when to start the next packet after the pill-free interval (PFI):

- 12% believed they should wait until the fifth day of the withdrawal bleed
- 11% thought they should start the next packet only when the bleeding stopped, or after 1 week but only if the bleeding had stopped.

Starting late with the next packet was not perceived as anything to do with missing pills (*see Qs 5.16, 5.25*)! Two-thirds of the pill-takers in a similar GP study thought the most contraceptively risky pills to miss were in the middle of a pack. There is little to suggest any improvement since then in such settings.

By contrast, in 1988 in a semi-rural setting of higher social class, 89% were found to take their pills correctly. But could this in part be because those women had much more personal attention from the providers, explaining specifically things like the crucial importance of the PFI? We must admit that medical error – and especially not providing enough time for counselling and questions – can be significant components of user failure (*see Qs 11.15, 11.16*).

11.9 Do we expect a lot from pill-takers?

Yes!

Correct pill use means that a healthy woman has to take a pill daily for months or years at a time, whether her intention is to delay or prevent pregnancy, and whether she is consistently sexually active or not. She must know how long to wait between pill packets, how to make up missed pills, and when to use another method as a back-up. She then must have the back-up method available and actually use it. Finally, she must be confident about the pill's effectiveness and safety, despite frequent rumours and negative reports in the press. In short, the pill is a more complex method to deliver and use than we previously thought. (Linda Potter, Family Health International)

According to an NOP survey in the UK in 1991, 'on average women seem to forget a pill about eight times a year'. . . . And young teenagers seem to be regularly late with their pills, up to three times per month.

11.10 Teenagers are mentioned a great deal in the context of compliance. What are the important medical and legal considerations when prescribing a medical method like the pill to girls before the age of consent (16 in the UK)?

The General Medical Council (GMC) has issued (2007) invaluable guidance focusing on children and young people from birth through, in fact, to their 18th birthday, on the standards of competence, care and conduct expected – of all doctors registered with the GMC. See www.gmc-uk.org/guidance/ethical_guidance/children_guidance/index.asp.

MEDICAL

In my view we should try to avoid the term 'sex education', as it invites the response 'So you are teaching them to have sex!' What we should say, and promote, is sex and relationships education (SRE), and, importantly, for both genders. When seeking advice on sex, relationships, contraception, pregnancy and parenthood, young people are entitled to accessible, confidential, non-judgmental and unbiased support and guidance – recognizing the diversity of their cultural and faith traditions. We should listen to their views and respect their opinions and choices. It is crazy to pay lip-service to *choice* without accepting that one valid choice is 'saving sex', i.e. waiting (not yet having) sex: as well as, if that is rejected, having safer and well-contracepted sex. As in the Netherlands, SRE should promote the societal norm that sex may be a feature of a good relationship if and when adequate contraception exists (combined – wherever there is not assured mutual monogamy – with condoms for safer sex).

Because a significant proportion of early postpubertal menstrual cycles are not fertile, young women – who now tend to have their coitarche earlier than in the past – may discover that they can 'get away with it' for several cycles. An unhelpful learning experience which means that all too often the young do not seek advice until they have already conceived. . . . Ready access to emergency contraception is an obvious priority.

Aside from the conception risk, there is the risk of STIs, cervical neoplasia and much potential emotional trauma. But it must be made clear that the risks are those of precocious sexual activity and multiple partners, not of the pill or any other contraceptive.

A modern low-estrogen combined pill is commonly offered, although its 'default state' (i.e. of conception if errors are made) is far from ideal. In common with all hormonal contraceptives, once periods are established the pill poses no special medical problems in adolescents, as compared with women in their 20s (including with respect to breast cancer or cervical cancer, *see Qs 5.80, 5.82, 6.57*).

The chaos of many teenagers' lives means that the LARCs are often best: *they should be seen as first-choice methods along with, and often preferable to, the COC.* Injectables and implants (especially perhaps Implanon, *see Q 8.57ff*) are somewhat preferable to IUDs or the LNG-IUS because of the pelvic infection anxieties and anticipated insertion difficulties of the intrauterine methods. Yet these are exaggerated and the latter methods are definite options. Regarding the concern about bone density and DMPA, *see Q 8.24.*

Because this age group are now the most at risk for all sexually transmitted agents, including *Chlamydia* and HIV, it is essential to promote use of the condom in addition, often, to the selected main contraceptive ('Double Dutch' – so-called because the Dutch give the lead here, as they do in so much to do with teenage reproductive health). Unfortunately, reliance on the condom alone for pregnancy prevention by teenagers usually gives poor results. If it is nevertheless selected, take every opportunity to remind users about the emergency pill.

LEGAL AND SOCIO-ETHICAL

Sexual intercourse before the age of consent still represents a category of technical law-breaking, not by the girl but by the male partner(s). Yet prosecutions are very rare if they are about the same age.

Any GP faced with an under-16-year-old needs first, as appropriate, opportunely and non-patronizingly, to raise the advantages – both psychological and physical – of 'saving sex' as defined above. If this rings no bells, seek next the agreement by the young person that they will tell, or be happy for you to tell, at least one parent. This is vastly preferable.

11.11 But what if under-16s completely refuse the involvement of a parent/guardian?

In 1985 the House of Lords overturned an Appeal Court judgment in the celebrated case brought by Victoria Gillick. In the ruling, Lord Fraser of Tullybelton produced the 'Fraser Guidelines', which are still the basis in the UK for assessing what is sometimes termed a young person's 'Gillick competence'. They are also in the revised DHSS *Memorandum of Guidance* (DHSS HC(FP)86). In the summary below, note that the **highlighted** initial letters part spell out the words:

UnProtected SSexual InterCourse

It is good practice to proceed to prescribe a medical contraceptive without parental knowledge and consent if:

1 The girl, although under 16 years of age, will **U**nderstand the doctor's advice.

2 She cannot be persuaded to inform the **P**arents or allow the doctor to inform them.

3 She is very likely to begin or to continue having **S**exual intercourse with or without contraceptive treatment.

4 Her physical or mental health or both are likely to **S**uffer unless she receives contraceptive advice or treatment.

5 Her best **I**nterests (therefore) require the doctor to proceed without parental consent.

6 At all times the young woman's entitlement to 100% assurance of **C**onfidentiality is the same as for any adult. This must not only be real, as goes without saying, but it must also be explicit to her, e.g. even if she recognizes that the receptionist is a friend of her mother's!

11.12 How are compliance, side-effects and discontinuation connected?

In a complex way. To quote Linda Potter again, referring primarily to pill-users in poor communities (i.e. in inner cities of rich countries as much as in the developing world):

Poor compliance can lead directly to pregnancy. However, incorrect use can also contribute to discontinuation. Studies indicate that as many as 60% of new OC users discontinue use before the end of the first year, most within the first 6 months, and most of these because of menstrual irregularities and other side-effects.

The side-effects may be either the cause or effect of incorrectly taken pills, and may lead to either discontinuation or failure, making the relationship a complex one. For example, nausea in the first few months may lead to intermittent use, which in turn may provoke breakthrough bleeding, which in turn may lead to discontinuation.

11.13 According to the UK fpa's National Information Service, what – to help them to use contraceptives well – do potential consumers themselves consider most important?

Above all, information. Some professionals feel consumers cannot deal with 'too much information' but the number of enquiries to the fpa (about 100 000 per year) suggest that consumers want more information, not less.

Sadly, in the fpa's experience, too many professionals do not provide full information about the range of options, fully explain the side-effects or discuss risks and benefits of contraceptive methods.

Many professionals make assumptions, often underestimating a person's degree of motivation, ability or needs and so 'censor' or limit information, and many use a variety of ways to pressure a woman to use certain methods. In a word, paying lip-service to 'client choice'; they are much more into 'provider choice'. So women often express to the fpa feelings of anger, frustration and powerlessness because they feel they are not listened to, not spoken to on equal terms and given neither time nor 'permission' to voice fears or anxieties.

Family planning advisers need to be aware of how far they might go in determining choice rather than influencing it, i.e. there is a need to consider the differences between informed consent and informed choice.

There are fears, worries and doubts about potential, perceived and currently known side-effects. What consumers consider important when choosing a method are:

- effectiveness – will it work? (emphasis on failure rather than success)
- suitability – how are they going to feel?
- risks and benefits
- how to use a particular method
- how the method works.

11.14 What mnemonic is a good guide to comprehensive, client-centred counselling?

In US Family Planning circles, the recommended word is 'GATHER'. This stands for:

G: **greet** each young person warmly.

A: **ask** the young person about herself (himself) and why they have come.

T: **tell** the young person about each available family planning method. Then demonstrate the method(s) that most interest her.

H: **help** her to choose the method she feels will best suit her and her partner.

E: **explain** how to use the chosen method, using a user-friendly leaflet to be taken away and for reference.

R: **return** for follow-up. Agree on a time to meet again routinely *or* at short notice upon request.

The very word 'greet', coming first in this approach, conveys a client-centred approach beautifully. It is worth remembering the response from members of a Focus Group (run by Brook, who provide user-friendly services for young people) to the question 'Who would you want to see for advice about sex and contraception?': 'Someone with a SMILE would be your best bet' was the reply. What an implied indictment that implies, about the providers those particular young people had previously encountered. . . .

11.15 How should the information be conveyed?

Verbally and by the written word, supplemented these days by videos, computer games and websites. The onus is on providers to give information that is accurate. It should update, reassure and demythologize – all without embarrassment. Knowledge is power.

Providing written information, and currently the best brief source in the UK is the fpa leaflets, offers privacy, anonymity and time to absorb information at leisure. People can remember only 20% of what they hear and only 50% of what they hear and see.

The length of the text is not a barrier to communication for consumers, provided the material is well organized, well laid out and well signposted. Indeed, the more comprehensive fpa leaflets that are now available should be given with the words 'Keep this in a safe place for reference'.

Contraceptive manufacturers and family planning organizations are at last actively working together to standardize and simplify the information given. Providers can already choose, selectively, to offer some of the better manufacturers' literature, which has been much improved in recent years. Possibly even more important is creative packaging, whereby user-friendly design assists compliance, and some companies' packets now convey valuable information like what to do in the event of missed or vomited pills. The increasing use of video and audio recordings is also to be welcomed because they can save time and be discussion-openers, ensuring the ground is covered fully, especially the bits the provider might find 'boring' and so forget to mention at the crucial first visit.

11.16 As an overstretched but well-intentioned family practitioner, how might I improve my family planning service?

Generally, more people attend GPs for contraception than community-based family planning clinics. But availability of the choice of service is paramount – including the clinic service, which is, moreover, an essential resource for the practical training of doctors and nurses in this field. Availability of complementary (not rival) and accessible services is important; at present, with repeated 're-disorganizations' of the NHS, potential users of contraception have to run a bit of an obstacle race to find the service that meets their specific needs.

Doctors and nurses tend to put birth control methods into five major categories: barrier, hormonal, intrauterine, sterilization and termination of pregnancy. But to our clients there are primarily just two categories: those methods you can get on with yourself and those where you have to involve (get 'permission' from) other people, possibly rather bossy people, and so lose privacy and control. Given this context, therefore, in our own services we must set aside any illness-oriented style and adopt an information-providing and counselling mode for these healthy couples.

There are a number of very practical questions you might consider:

FAMILY PLANNING, THE SCOPE

In our practice, do we provide:

■ A full range of contraceptive methods, on site or easily arranged, including all the LARCs, as first-choice options, and postcoital contraception and, yes, condoms (some GPs do contrive somehow to provide them free to clients on site . . .)?

■ Pregnancy testing and support and counselling for unplanned pregnancy?

■ Counselling and referral for male and female sterilization?

■ Advice and help with regard to 'safer sex'?

■ Help or referral for sexual and relationship problems?

■ Advice, treatment or referral for STIs?

■ Advice, help or referral for infertility?

■ Comprehensive well-woman/well-man services?

SERVICE PROVISION

Do we:

■ Work as a joined-up team (I include here receptionist, health visitor, school nurse, practice nurse, partners)?

■ Provide flexible clinical services, with rapid access/walk-in facility for urgent first visits (postcoitally) and adequate support to those with follow-up problems (e.g. side-effects of IUDs or pills)?

■ Provide sufficient time for all family planning consultations, especially the first or the postcoital visit? Have we fully thought through the pros and cons of a dedicated session?

■ Provide an assurance – especially to the young – of confidentiality in visits, communications and record keeping? In short, from reception onwards, can we consider ourselves to be fully teenage-friendly? (The RCGP and RCN provide an excellent green laminated card for practices, issued in 2002, including a brief questionnaire to assess this).

■ Provide (where possible) a choice of male or female doctor?

TRAINING

Do we ensure that all staff (including reception/clerical staff, but most especially nursing staff) are appropriately trained?

INFORMATION

Do we:

■ Always provide standardized, complete, up-to-date and objective information? That is, the information we ourselves would expect to receive?

■ Use suitable language that both enables and informs? Thus, do not talk about coils, rhythm method or morning-after contraception, but do talk about IUDs, natural family planning and emergency (postcoital) contraception.

■ Make it clear during counselling for pills and barrier methods that there is a profound difference between the failure rates for 'perfect' use and typical use?

■ Always discuss risks and benefits?

■ Recognize that people are not always comfortable and might feel too shy to ask questions? (It can help to 'ventriloquize' some questions, and to ask certain others to check that the most important facts have been retained.)

■ Always provide good written information that backs up and reinforces any verbal advice?

■ Publicize our services so people know about them? Possibly, for about-to-be teenagers, arranging a 'milestone meeting' with the Practice Nurse for all on the practice list – timed for just after they have their 12th birthdays: about healthy lifestyles, sex and contraception? Ideally backed by a dedicated practice leaflet for teenagers?

Ensuring compliance is, after all, not about professionals 'telling' consumers what to do – it is about enabling consumers to make informed choices through a partnership with health professionals. (Toni Belfield)

IATROGENIC CAUSES OF UNPLANNED PREGNANCIES

11.17 How wrong can we, the providers, sometimes be? Can a doctor or nurse be an accessory in causing 'iatrogenic' unplanned pregnancies?

Very much so. We have just been reviewing, in a contraceptive context, plenty of evidence for the saying: 'You can take the horse to the water but you cannot make it drink'. But is it not also clear already that we as providers can fail in the first place to 'take the horse to the water'?

Many 'sins of omission and of commission' by providers are obvious in *Qs 11.13–11.16*. The list that follows, of over 30 more specific errors, primarily medical or prescribing errors, is by no means complete. Indeed, I would be interested to receive other examples to use in the next edition! What is probably more important than all of them is summarized in that Focus Group response 'Someone with a SMILE would be your best bet' (*see Q 11.14*).

The provider can 'cause an iatrogenic and unwanted pregnancy' in any one of the following ways:

1 First and foremost, by not allowing enough quality time for the contraceptive consultation, possibly as two visits in the first week (*see Q*

5.106) – backed by good literature. This leads to one of the most common – most basic – errors, which is when the practitioner simply says 'You must stop the pill' without any adequate discussion of the future method.

2 When changing methods, by not ensuring an appropriate overlap. For instance, when changing from progestogen-only pill (POP) or IUD to condom, failing to advise use of the condom for 7 days before the POP is discontinued or device removed. Or if a woman is transferring to a (for her) untried method like the diaphragm or Femidom (*see* Q 4.55), removing an IUD before she has found the new method to be satisfactory. And, prior to female sterilization, failing to advise abstinence or extra care with barrier methods for the cycle leading up to the surgery risks a clip-induced ectopic or an intrauterine conception (*see also* Qs 9.13, 9.14).

3 Especially postpartum, if any amenorrhoeic sexually active woman wants to start using a hormonal or intrauterine contraceptive, by insisting on waiting (a) for a 6-week postnatal visit (*see* Q 11.22) or (b) for the next period (which then never comes because she conceives during the wait!) – when there other are ways of minimizing the risk of fetal exposure (*see* Qs 8.52, 11.22).

Many studies have shown that confusion about irregular bleeding, and its nuisance-value as a side-effect, are among the most frequent causes of pill-taking errors, discontinuations and unwanted conceptions.

CHAPTERS 1–4

4 After a bad attack of PID, overstressing that the woman might be infertile – so she is inefficient with subsequent contraception.

5 Overstressing the ineffectiveness of coitus interruptus (*see* Q 3.6) so that it is not used when it would be a very great deal better than nothing in an 'emergency' situation.

6 Failure to warn about the 300+ million sperm in each man's ejaculate, and the unpredictability of sperm survival in the female genital tract. Hence failure to explain the consequences: that a tiny 'leak' of semen can cause pregnancy, and that the postmenstrual 'safe period' is of a completely different order of potential efficacy from the properly identified postovulatory phase (*see* Qs 2.4–2.17).

7 With Persona, recommending the method to the 'wrong' kind of couple ('limiters', when they should be 'spacers'); failure to offer the option of relying only on the second infertile phase (as described in *Qs 2.31 and*

2.32) and failure to explain the preliminary need for two natural cycles of barrier method use after any hormones (including for emergency contraception).

8 Failure to advise about effective condom use, and especially about common chemicals/prescriptions that damage rubber (*see Q 3.21*).

9 Regarding diaphragms and caps, wrong case selection: these are only suitable for 'spacers' of pregnancy within monogamy. Also by giving such a profusion of other instructions about spermicide, etc. (most of which have never been validated) that the woman fails to get the most important message: namely that she should make a secondary check that her cervix is covered following every insertion of her diaphragm or cap, however comfortable it feels.

CHAPTER 10 (CONSIDERED HERE BECAUSE EMERGENCY CONTRACEPTION IS SO OFTEN INDICATED THROUGH FAILED USE OF ABOVE METHODS)

10 Failure to inform male and female users of barrier contraceptive about the existence of emergency contraception, and failure to offer it when appropriate (e.g. if an IUD has to be removed midcycle, *see Q 9.14*).

11 Use of the misleading term 'morning-after pill' (*see Q 10.1*).

12 Failure to inform women that the postcoital 'emergency pill' can be used up to 72 h after exposure.

13 Not being prepared to insert an IUD postcoitally up to 5 days after ovulation, as calculated in good faith (*see Q 10.14*). With exposure on day 7, this could mean, quite legally and ethically, insertion up to 12 days after unprotected intercourse! And with a solitary exposure, 5 days after intercourse is acceptable at any time in the cycle.

CHAPTERS 5–8

14 Giving erroneous starting instructions for the combined pill (*see Q 5.50* for the correct ones, including the 'Quick start' option in selected cases (*Table 5.4*, p. 145, and *Q 10.41*)).

15 Failure to explain the significance of the pill-free (or patch-free or ring-free) week in the initial consultation, in advance and alongside the relevant fpa leaflet about a combined hormonal method (*see Qs 5.16–5.28*) as well as supplying the manufacturer's PIL. Understanding at the outset the simple idea that the COC and its relatives are bound to work least well at the end of the regular time when they haven't been taken at all (i.e. the contraceptive-free time), helps to stop the common notion that 'being a bit late starting' is not 'missing a pill'! Detailed examples:

(a) Not stating clearly that starting the new packet on time is critically important and that the first pill is the most 'dangerous' if missed.

(b) Not explaining that, if pills are missed at the end of a packet, the next following PFI should be shortened or eliminated.

(c) Giving implicitly wrong instructions for subsequent packs, e.g. 'The doctor said [he/she probably didn't, but was the point clarified?] that I should wait until the fifth day of my next period – or until it is finished – before I restart each packet.'

(d) Instructing the woman to start a new brand of pill on day 1 of the WTB after the last one without advising her what to do if, by chance, she gets no WTB in that cycle. She might well then wait beyond 7 days unless otherwise instructed.

16 Failure to check at follow-up whether pill-takers still have a copy of the fpa leaflet as well as the PIL and if they have lost it, replacing as necessary at follow-up.

17 Simply represcribing the COC (perhaps with a 'pep-talk' about compliance) after true pill method failures, or even when only one or two tablets have been missed. Instead, one of the LARC methods should usually be offered (*see Qs 5.28, 5.32*).

18 Inadequate explanations at pill discontinuation. Examples:

(a) Failure to inform a woman that the pill-free week is only a safe time for unprotected intercourse if she does in fact restart a new packet. If she is discontinuing the method, it is very common for a woman to assume that the condom is unnecessary for the first week. In reality she might well ovulate early in the second week (*see Qs 5.16, 5.25*).

(b) Failure to explain that calendar calculations, of even the potentially safer second phase of the safe period, are completely invalidated during the first cycle following pill discontinuation, which can be very variably prolonged.

(c) Failure to dispel the myth: 'I heard that women often take a long time to get pregnant after stopping the pill, so I thought I would be safe.'

19 Failure to forewarn and explain that the occurrence of BTB should not be considered as a period (and the pill therefore stopped abruptly) – and that it might subside over time. Choosing a brand that produces good cycle control is obviously helpful too.

20 Failure to demolish the myth that you should not restart with a new pack until a 'period' has occurred. Not explaining, in fact, that absent WTB is very rarely because a pregnancy has occurred. (Some women become pregnant through failure to restart the pill after the first episode of absent WTB and hence become unnecessarily pregnant solely because they thought they already were.) A useful check of good pill-taking is to ask the user which day of the week she regularly starts each new pack: beware if she says 'It all depends!'

21 Ovulation induction in a woman who presents with oligo-/amenorrhoea but definitely does not (yet) want to be pregnant (*see Q 5.65*). '*No-one ever asked me if I wanted a baby yet!*'

22 Unnecessarily avoiding the COC in cases of past secondary amenorrhoea from which there has been a complete recovery (*see Qs 5.64, 5.68*).

23 Unnecessarily instructing the woman to discontinue/avoid the COC because of the medical myths in *Qs 6.57, 6.78 and 6.79*, including for minor surgery like laparoscopy (*see Q 6.15*).

24 In the case of a healthy woman who really wants to continue pill-taking, agreeing too readily to her 'taking a break' when the idea comes only from a friend (*see Qs 6.73, 6.74*).

25 Unnecessarily instructing a woman to stop the POP (or any EE-free method) before any surgery, however major (*see Qs 7.41, 7.72*).

26 Telling the woman – correctly – to stop the COC before major surgery (*see Q 6.14*) or because of migraine with focal aura or other valid reasons, but failing to discuss and organize an alternative such as DMPA.

27 Failing to explain to a woman transferring to the POP that she should cease to take 7-day breaks.

28 Failing to discuss with a lactating user of an old-type POP that her chance of breakthrough conception will greatly increase whenever she begins weaning her baby. So if efficacy is very important to a woman, she should be offered Cerazette or advised to start the COC in good time, as explained very specifically at *Q 7.56*.

29 Starting any enzyme-inducer treatment with absolutely no special contraceptive advice in users of a hormonal method from *Chapters 5, 6, 7 and 8*. Or the mirror image, failure to advise appropriately when prescribing a hormone method to an existing user of an interacting drug, whether short term (e.g. rifampicin just for 2 days plus 28 days thereafter) or long term (*see Qs 5.36, 7.28, 8.11*).

30 Telling a woman who is over 2 weeks late with her DMPA injection 'Go away until you have your next period' among other errors of management of the late injection (*see Q 8.52*).

31 Bad handwriting (a real problem in practice). One of the most dangerous examples of this is when Femodene is intended but Femulen is read by the person issuing the pills. I am aware of at least one pregnancy caused this way because the woman continued to take routine pill-free breaks of a week's duration! Preventive recommendation, as practised at the Margaret Pyke Centre: always write Femodene-30 or Femulen POP. Also easily misread: Marvelon-30/Mercilon-20 and Evra/Evorel.

CHAPTER 9

32 Failure to observe the 'do not rely on the IUD for 7 days pre-removal' rule recommended in Q 9.14. Avoidable intrauterine or 'iatrogenic' extrauterine pregnancies in IUD-users following clip sterilization can also result. Barrier method-users should abstain during the same 7 preoperative days.

33 Failure to insert an IUD on presentation around midcycle, if necessary up to day 5 following the most probable day of ovulation. As explained in Q 9.15, a much more generous interpretation of the term 'postmenstrual' could lead to a worthwhile reduction in the number of conceptions caused by clinicians who wait for the woman's elusive next period. Let alone always insisting on inserting IUDs during menses as, despite the very strong counter-arguments (*see* Q 9.15), according to the fpa's helpline, many doctors still do!

34 Failure to warn women that, if they fail to feel the threads of an IUD, until proved otherwise their uterine cavity is IUD-free (*see* Q 9.33).

CONTRACEPTION/STERILIZATION AFTER PREGNANCY

11.18 When should counselling start?

It should not be an afterthought: it should be initiated antenatally. Counselling should be non-directive, with the doctor or midwife acting as an adviser and facilitator and never making the decisions. It is true that most women are more motivated towards family planning just after childbirth than at any other time, and in many parts of the world postnatal follow-up is weak or non-existent. However, although it might be correct to 'strike while the iron is hot', caution is necessary, especially regarding sterilization, and all kinds of pressure are to be avoided. For all women this is a time of emotional turmoil as well as one of rapidly changing hormonal status.

11.19 What is known about sexual activity in the puerperium?

See the brilliant section on this in the book by Esther Sapire (see Further Reading). According to Masters and Johnson, writing in 1966, after delivery almost 50% of women have low levels of sexual interest for at least 3 months. In another study, the same percentage had resumed sexual activity as soon as 6 weeks, but possibly with little enthusiasm on the woman's part. However that may be, the onset of sexual dysfunction reported much later can often be traced back to this time. Sleepless nights, exhaustion and limited time together can affect both partners. The man might resent exclusion from the intense bond between mother and baby, compounded by the woman's fatigue and diminished libido. In the woman, there might be multiple anxieties about the baby and about adjustment to motherhood. All these can be worse if there is a true postpartum depression.

Physical problems include breast and nipple tenderness, or dyspareunia from the site of perineal suturing, monilial vaginitis and diminished vaginal lubrication.

11.20 When does fertility return after pregnancy? What is the earliest postpartum day on which ovulation can occur, without and with breastfeeding?

Despite much research it remains impossible to predict this accurately for any individual woman. This is due not only to normal biological variation, racial or genetic factors, but also to the effects of:

- the nutritional status of the woman
- the stage of gestation at which the pregnancy ended
- whether indeed she is breastfeeding – and in that case the timing, frequency and duration of nipple stimulation, the amount of supplementary feeding and the time elapsed since delivery.

Although fertilization is the only proof that an ovulation is fertile, research suggests that, in the absence of breastfeeding, fertile ovulation could possibly and very rarely occur on day 28, and contraception of some kind should therefore be started by then (*see Q 5.50*).

It is even more difficult when attempting to answer the same question for lactating women, because the variability in intensity of baby-induced nipple stimulation is superimposed on woman-to-woman variation. But avoiding all freak ovulation events is perhaps asking too much: a better question is 'For how long can lactation be expected to provide the same kind of contraceptive protection as other acceptable birth control methods, such as the IUD?' (one answer is contained in LAM, *see Q 2.36*).

The essential caveat is that LAM still has a 2% failure rate even when well applied: no promise of complete efficacy should be implied – as should be the case with all methods.

11.21 Isn't there a two-way interaction between lactation and contraception?

Yes. Lactation can affect contraceptives, primarily by greatly increasing the efficacy of the old-type POP and all non-hormonal methods like barriers and spermicides. Conversely, the COC, for example, can affect lactation adversely by altering the quantity and constituents of breast milk.

Breastfeeding should also be advocated and promoted by clinicians because it is so good for babies – and might give some protection against breast cancer.

11.22 In an amenorrhoeic woman – for example, postpartum, say at 6 weeks, if not breastfeeding and contraception has been questionable – how can a provider be reasonably sure the woman has neither conceived nor is on the point of conceiving?

Some doctors are so paranoid that they insist on the arrival of a period before allowing the woman to start a hormonal method or IUD. But in the possibly long wait for this, they thereby risk an 'iatrogenic' conception (*see Q 11.17(3)*).

For starters, in this evaluation, WHO has produced a useful clinical checklist, see Box.

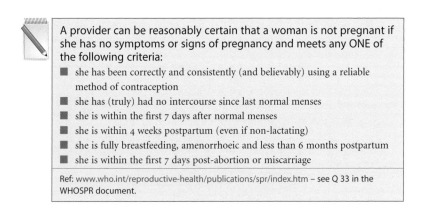

A provider can be reasonably certain that a woman is not pregnant if she has no symptoms or signs of pregnancy and meets any ONE of the following criteria:

- she has been correctly and consistently (and believably) using a reliable method of contraception
- she has (truly) had no intercourse since last normal menses
- she is within the first 7 days after normal menses
- she is within 4 weeks postpartum (even if non-lactating)
- she is fully breastfeeding, amenorrhoeic and less than 6 months postpartum
- she is within the first 7 days post-abortion or miscarriage

Ref: www.who.int/reproductive-health/publications/spr/index.htm – see Q 33 in the WHOSPR document.

Postnatal checks Based on the 4ᵗʰ bullet here: why do we perpetuate the tradition of postnatal checks at 6 weeks? They could be arranged instead routinely at or just before 4 weeks, when the risk of a fertile ovulation having occurred is negligible (*see Q 11.20*), even if the woman has not managed to breastfeed?

Availability of one of the ultrasensitive slide or dipstick pregnancy tests now marketed for use in the surgery is invaluable here (e.g. Clearview). On an early morning urine this will diagnose pregnancy at or before the 14th day after ovulation; but not of course one very recently conceived, due to fertilization within that time. If that is a relevant possibility, one useful protocol is the following, based on the very similar situation of a grossly late DMPA injection (*see Q 8.52*):

■ If possible, reach an agreement with the woman that she will either abstain or use condoms with greater care than ever before, UNTIL there has been a total of 14 days since the last sexual exposure. If a *sensitive* (20 IU/L) pregnancy test on an early morning urine is *then* negative, the chances of a conception are negligible and:

- the proposed medical method can be started plus (except for the copper IUD) the usual advice for 7 further days of added barrier contraception; and
- a follow-up pregnancy test in a further 2 weeks would be wise.

■ NB: If, however, the woman and her partner are *not* prepared to abstain or use condoms safely for the necessary days to reach 14 since her last sex, a useful compromise is to provide the POP (e.g. Cerazette) for that time and then proceed as above. (The teratogenic risks to a fetus exposed to the POP have been established as very low.)

In all circumstances, counsel the woman regarding possible failure and the need for later pregnancy testing if there is doubt.

11.23 Can natural family planning be used successfully after childbirth (after LAM, *see Q 2.36*)?

The fundamental problem, throughout reproductive life, is how to recognize fertile ovulation far enough in advance to allow for the capriciousness of survival of the very best among the millions of sperm deposited at intercourse. The problem is compounded after pregnancy by the very variable effects of lactation, as discussed above.

With or without breastfeeding, postpartum the estrogenic changes of increased quantity, clarity, fluidity, slipperiness, elasticity and good Spinnbarkeit occur well in advance of the first fertile ovulation. Hence, if cervical mucus is used, there are numerous false alarms.

Users of natural family planning who begin mucus observations from the cessation of lochia and who do abstain or switch to another method from the very first appearance of estrogenic mucus onwards will most probably avoid pregnancy. But they will also be avoiding intercourse for an unnecessarily long time. Changes in the cervix – dilatation, softening and elevation away from the introitus – might help (*see Q 2.36*).

To date, newer techniques using various biochemical changes are still disappointing for accurate ovulation prediction without those false alarms and far enough ahead.

11.24 Do you recommend an IUD/IUS for family spacing?

Yes, and also when the family might prove to be complete but the couple aren't sure yet. See *Chapter 9* for more details. Particularly relevant points at this postpartum time are:

■ *Infection:* this can be caused by lack of screening or poor technique during insertion (*see Q 9.55*) or exacerbated if uterine tenderness due to postpartum endometritis is overlooked. The individual's risk of sexually transmitted conditions still poses the main threat for the future, however.

■ *Perforation:* this has been a particular concern in relation to postpartum IUD insertion. However, no significant additional risk for T-shaped IUDs was shown by Chi [*Contraception* 1993;48:81–108]: rate 1 in 1632 during lactation. Perforation postpartum seems to be primarily a problem of linear (e.g. Lippes loop) devices and can be almost eliminated by withdrawal insertion techniques – and by extra care by an experienced inserting doctor. Ideally, postpartum clinics should not be used routinely for training purposes because lack of expertise markedly increases this risk.

11.25 What is your advice on the timing of postpartum IUD/IUS insertions?

See Qs 9.101 and 9.102. Good results are reported whenever this is between 4 and 8 weeks after delivery. I favour 4 weeks to avoid all the contraception 'hassle' discussed in *Q 11.22*, although the postcoital contraceptive action of the IUD method does offer useful leeway.

After lower segment caesarean section (LSCS) the scar will have healed by 4 weeks and is situated at the level of the internal os. So there is no need to delay insertion beyond say 6 weeks. After elective LSCS the cervical canal might require gentle dilatation, often with local anaesthesia, as for nulliparae. These insertions are not for beginners. An option reported with good results from China is to insert via the lower segment incision immediately the placenta has been delivered.

IMMEDIATE POST-ABORTION INSERTION

This can be appropriate (*see Qs 9.103, 9.142*).

11.26 Are COCs suitable immediately postpartum?

Despite their efficacy, convenience and many other advantages, COCs should not be used during lactation (WHO 4). Most studies report some adverse impact on breastfeeding performance and milk volume composition. And, in any case, the COC cannot improve upon the near 100% efficacy of the POP plus full lactation.

11.27 When should the COC be started in women who do not breastfeed?

If a COC is started too late, some women will become pregnant before their first period. If it is started too early, there is the risk that the estrogen content will increase the already increased risk of thromboembolism in the puerperium. So, ideally, COC-taking should not begin until the changes induced by pregnancy have returned to normality. This starts with delivery of the placenta, but fibrinogen concentrations actually increase at first until a decline starts around day 5. Dahlman and others found that both blood coagulation and fibrinolysis were significantly increased during the first 2 weeks, but by 3 weeks both were, in general, normal. This literature supports UK practice, which is that estrogen-containing pills (or patches/ rings) are normally started no sooner than day 21 of the puerperium (*see Q 5.50*).

Selective delay beyond 4 weeks using an alternative contraceptive might be safest where known risks apply, particularly in combination. These factors are obesity, preceding severe pregnancy-related hypertension, the HELLP syndrome, operative delivery, especially caesarean section, restricted activity, age above 35 and grande multiparity. A good rule is to wait until full mobility, plus normality of any previously abnormal biochemical or other tests.

11.28 What if the woman had pregnancy-related hypertension?

It used to be thought that women with hypertension in a preceding pregnancy would be unusually prone to oral contraceptive-induced hypertension. This was disproved by Pritchard and Pritchard in 1977. However, it is definitely a relative contraindication (*see Q 5.138, bullet 1*), requiring extra care in use of the COC method (WHO 3).

Why? Because the RCGP study showed that this past history is linked, for unknown reasons, with an increased risk of arterial thrombosis – and very seriously so if they also smoke (risk ratio of over 40!). If no alternative to the COC is acceptable and pre-eclampsia was severe at the preceding delivery, starting the COC should be delayed for at least 8 weeks.

11.29 Where should the POP fit into any scheme for postpartum contraception?

It remains the first-choice hormonal method during lactation. This is discussed in detail at *Qs 7.53–7.57*. Unlike the combined pill, POPs, including Cerazette, have not been found to impair the quantity or the quality of breast milk.

■ *Timing of postpartum use:* as there is no anxiety about enhancing the risk of thrombosis, it is medically safe to start the POP almost immediately. However, UKMEC recommends that, as with the COC, women (whether or not breastfeeding) should begin to take the POP on about day 21 following delivery.

■ *Amenorrhoeic women* (later than above): with but especially without breastfeeding, once risk of cyesis has definitely been excluded, if necessary by the protocol described above (*see Q 11.22*), they may start the POP at any time, with 7 days additional contraceptive precautions.

■ *Efficacy:* it is important to bear in mind that because there is the additional contraceptive effect of breastfeeding, less than perfectly compliant takers of old-type POPs will 'get away with it': until, perhaps, weaning and hence fertile ovulation commences (*see Q 7.56*). Two successive women in one of my own clinics gave the history that their next baby came 'too soon' that way, because the suggestion that they might prefer to switch to the COC at weaning had not been made to them! This point needs making in advance: if efficacy is very important to a woman, she should be prescribed Cerazette or the COC so she can start in good time (details at *Q 7.56*).

11.30 What about injectable contraception postpartum? Does the same apply as with the POP?

Most studies of DMPA show either no change or an improvement in both quantity of milk and duration of lactation. Both DMPA and NET-EN and their metabolites cross from maternal plasma into breast milk, and to a greater extent than with the POP, so it is not a first or frequent choice in the UK. Yet it has been calculated that a child would have to breastfeed for 3 years to receive as much DMPA as the mother receives in 1 day. And, to date, no morbidity and no adverse effects on growth have been found.

■ *Timing of the first dose:* because, in some countries, contact with medical personnel is limited to delivery, the first dose of DMPA is sometimes given within 48 h of delivery. Injectables do not increase the risk of puerperal thrombosis, yet UKMEC classifies administration before 6 weeks as WHO 2 because:
  – the immature baby might have problems metabolizing the DMPA
  – this is much earlier than necessary for contraception
  – there is a hint from the literature that early administration increases the likelihood of heavy and prolonged bleeding.

Hence, in the UK, the first dose is now preferably (but not always) delayed to 5–6 weeks postpartum.

In a woman who is *not* breastfeeding I would be quite happy to give DMPA at any mutually convenient time before day 21 – so it could be sure to prevent the earliest likely ovulation – but with forewarning about the possibly increased risk of bleeding.

■ *Efficacy:* here there is no concern that the method will become less effective as breastfeeding frequency diminishes. Instead, the woman must be warned to plan well ahead if she wants another baby, because of the well-recognized delay in return of fertility – although this has often been exaggerated (*see Q 8.38*).

11.31 What is the policy about hormonal methods if there was trophoblastic disease in the last pregnancy?

This is fully discussed in Q 5.78. In brief, all of these are WHO 3 except the COC, ring and patch (which are WHO 4) and emergency contraception (which is WHO 2).

11.32 What considerations apply to male or female sterilization in the early puerperium?

It often appears convenient for all concerned if the woman is sterilized at this time. But Professor Robert Winston showed many years ago that the decision is more commonly regretted at this time of emotional instability for many couples. So there is a welcome trend to offering laparoscopic sterilization as an interval procedure about 12 weeks postpartum. The inadvisability of routine postpartum procedures is well shown by the observation that a distinct minority, around 15%, change their minds during that 12 weeks, preferring to keep their contraceptive options open longer.

There then still remains the risk of early death of the latest child (e.g. by the sudden infant death syndrome). Many vasectomy services therefore prefer to defer the procedure until the youngest child is at least 6 months of age. It is not clear why such admirable caution is less commonly observed by obstetricians with regard to female sterilization, especially as there is a strong suspicion that the procedure fails more often when clips are applied to the thick 'juicy' tubes of the puerperium. Indeed, the excellent RCOG guideline at www.rcog.org.uk recommends a modified Pomeroy procedure at this time.

CONTRACEPTION FOR THE OLDER WOMAN – ABOVE AGE 40

Background factors

11.33 What is the intrinsic fertility of older women, above age 40?

The available evidence suggests, as shown and discussed in *Table 1.2* (p. 14), that the intrinsic fertility of such women is reduced to about half what it was at the age of 25, with a further decline accelerating above 45. An unknown part of this is due to reduced frequency of intercourse. Whatever the explanation, the conclusion is that a method with an accidental pregnancy rate unacceptable in a younger woman might well be satisfactory for use in the 40s. For example, in the Oxford/FPA study, above age 45 the POP had a failure rate (0.3 per 100 woman-years) that is indistinguishable from that to be expected in a younger woman using the combined pill. Another example is the recommendation above 50 to use simple methods like spermicides or the contraceptive sponge (*see Q 4.64*).

Some older women, however, might have actual or preventable gynaecological morbidity to weigh up against the risks of the combined pill (*see Q 11.37*) and so might be better off because of its beneficial effects, although not really needing such a high-efficacy method.

11.34 How can one normally diagnose physiological infertility after the menopause?

Despite much research, there is no simple answer to the question 'When can I stop all contraception?' Long spells of amenorrhoea in women under 45 can indicate the arrival of a premature menopause, but they might also be due to other spontaneously reversible causes. Even above that age, prolonged amenorrhoea does not rule out the chance of a later ovulation, although the risk is less if there are definite vasomotor symptoms.

We now know that FSH measurements alone are most misleading – they only mean reduced feedback of ovarian hormones on the pituitary *at that time*, the ovaries might well still have potentially fertile ova to release. Occasionally, women with many months of amenorrhoea, symptoms of the menopause and even elevated FSH levels subsequently ovulate and even conceive!

- It is accepted that women above the age of 50 years who have had amenorrhoea for over 12 months, unmodified by hormones, can abandon alternative contraception. During the 1-year wait any simple method (e.g. contraceptive foam) is adequate.
- At a younger age there is a greater risk of spontaneous late ovulations, so 2 years of amenorrhoea with extra precautions is recommended.

Below 40 this is 'secondary amenorrhoea' and needs to be investigated fully by standard tests.

The classic rule is as above: 2 years of amenorrhoea are required for the diagnosis of final ovarian failure right up to age 50. This age limit seems to have been chosen rather arbitrarily, without hard data. Some authorities have been prepared to lower the full 2-years no-bleeding requirement for added contraception to under 45 in recent years, if vasomotor symptoms are prominent: this is minimally less secure, but perhaps acceptably so.

But there still remains the problem, discussed later (*see Qs 11.41, 11.42*), that so many women have their menopause masked by the use of hormones (combined or progestogen-only or HRT).

11.35 What are the medical risks associated with pregnancy above age 40?

Although it might be easier to prevent, unintended pregnancy is in many ways a greater catastrophe at this age. Both maternal and perinatal mortality are much higher. There is also a steady increase in the risk of chromosome abnormalities with maternal age. Hence, whereas we should certainly avoid using too 'strong' a method, the woman needs to be reassured that any chosen method will prove to be effective in her own case.

11.36 What is the 'best' method for women above 40?

There is no such thing as a single best method. Individualization is the key, as usual – see on:

Hormonal methods

11.37 What are the desirable features of contraception at the climacteric?

Table 11.2 summarizes these. It is clear that only the combined pill/patch/ring – or some other combination of progestogen with estrogen, including HRT – is capable of providing all the first six features in that table. But at some risk (mentioned at (8)), masking of the menopause (7) being relatively simple to deal with, *see Q 11.42*).

It is now clear that there is often some symptomatic loss of ovarian function starting 5–10 years before the actual menopause. Women in these years would derive additional non-contraceptive benefits if (upon their request) they were allowed by their physicians to use some form of combined therapy. Many of the desirable features listed in *Table 11.2* would then be provided, at least in theory. The first manifestations of climacteric symptoms can be suppressed. Many women suffer preventable hot flushes, and in some osteoporosis might begin, before they see their last period. Symptoms of the so-called 'normal' menstrual cycle (premenstrual syndrome, heavy and painful periods) are often controlled.

Perhaps most important is the reduced risk of those gynaecological disorders that are related to the menstrual cycle, listed at (5) in the table. It might be that use of an appropriate COC – or of course the LNG-IUS, without or, as indicated, with added estrogen – will eliminate the need for and risk of other medical or surgical treatments. *Yet the circulatory risks, which are increasing all the time, and the increasing risk of breast cancer with age must also be put into the equation.*

TABLE 11.2 Desirable or 'ideal' features of any contraceptive for use during the climacteric (before and as required after the menopause)

1 Effective in this age group
2 Improves sex life by:
   (a) perceived effectiveness and reassuring period pattern, or amenorrhoea
   (b) not being an intercourse-related method
   (c) possible estrogenic slowing of skin ageing, improved body image and libido, and treatment of vaginal dryness
3 Controls climacteric symptoms (especially vasomotor and psychological symptoms, and the urethral syndrome)
4 Controls symptoms of 'normal' cycle (especially the premenstrual syndrome, and irregular, heavy or painful periods)
5 Reduces incidence or manifestations of gynaecological pathology. This potential benefit applies to pelvic infection, extrauterine pregnancy, fibroids, dysfunctional haemorrhage, endometriosis, functional ovarian cysts, and, above all, carcinoma of the ovary and uterus
   (Consequent reduction in the risks of treatment for these conditions, especially hysterectomy)
6 Estrogenic protection against osteoporosis
7 Absence of masking of the menopause
8 Absence of systemic adverse effects:
   (a) known serious circulatory conditions such as hypertension, arterial or venous disease
   (b) other serious conditions, particularly breast cancer

Note: **Only the combined pill/ring/patch or some other combination of estrogen and progestogen is capable of providing all the above desirable features (*excepting numbers (7) and (8)*). The remaining options chiefly act as contraceptives – usually without a positive benefit on the conditions shown.** *See Q 11.37.*

11.38 *Table 11.2* **suggests that the known benefits of the COC are greater in the older age group and so in highly selected women may still outweigh the risks, although they are also increasing with age. But which pill should be used?**

■ First, it needs to be clear that this permissiveness regarding the COC applies only to women who are entirely healthy and *completely* free of arterial and venous risk factors. 'Completely' includes being migraine-free and taking regular exercise.

■ Second, enthusiasm for the COC must be tempered with caution as regards breast cancer risk, which does go up with age (*see Qs 5.92, 5.93*), by probably about an added 30 cases per 10 000 women for use to age 45 (see *Table 5.6*, p. 166), although this is balanced by protection against ovarian, endometrial and colorectal cancer.

■ Third, the COC is not the only estrogen/progestogen combined contraceptive option anyway – *see Q 11.44*.

Ideally, the minimum acceptable dose of any progestogen and the estrogen should always be used, to produce the fewest possible metabolic effects on both lipids and clotting factors. At present, the choice normally lies between Mercilon, Femodette/Katya 30/75 (new generic marketed in UK since last edition) and Loestrin 20, as the only 20-µg combined products available in the UK.

11.39 Is it ever appropriate to give a cyclical HRT regimen before the menopause, might this suffice for contraception?

No. None of the recommended regimens at this time which give estrogen alone at some point in their cycle is reliable. Only the LNG-IUS plus HRT combination is currently licensed for use before final ovarian failure without the method causing (usually) unacceptable bleeding.

A useful unlicensed possibility is the 'Good Practice Point' in the Faculty of SRH Guidance document *Contraception for women aged over 40 years* [*Journal of Family Planning and Reproductive Health Care* 2005;31:51–63] quoted earlier at *Q 7.64*:

Women can be advised that a POP can be used with HRT to provide effective contraception.

Note that this implies, as well as following the advice at *Appendix A*, p. 553, using a standard suitable HRT product and then *adding* either an old-type POP or Cerazette – i.e. supplementary to, not instead of, the progestogen regimen of the licensed HRT product.

Otherwise, standard HRT products are best reserved (and then usefully) for those with estrogen deficiency symptoms who are not at risk of pregnancy through abstaining, relying on sterilization or vasectomy, or happy to use as well some non-hormonal contraceptive such as condoms, a contraceptive sponge or spermicide.

11.40 Why do we not use natural estrogens for contraception in all women, with or without risk factors, before the menopause?

Mainly because of the need for contraception and cycle control, which EE does so well. Because natural estrogens are less completely or predictably absorbed and have lower potency, they have until now not proved so effective in either capacity. This might change through further research.

11.41 If the combined pill, cyclical HRT and other hormonal products are used in a woman's late 40s, will they not mask the menopause?

Yes. The 'standard' teaching has been as at *Q 11.34*, to switch to a non-hormonal method and only discontinue all contraception after the occurrence of complete amenorrhoea for 12 months (or 2 years if under age 50). But this precludes use of cyclical HRT or the COC (whose withdrawal bleeds will indefinitely mask the menopause) and HRT alone is not safely contraceptive, at the very time when vasomotor symptoms might most be benefited. And other hormonal methods such as the LNG-IUS and Cerazette may mask the menopause through amenorrhoea.

11.42 How can infertility at the menopause be diagnosed in women still using the COC or other masking hormones, including HRT?

In fact, it is not always necessary to know the precise time of this (*see Qs 7.63, 11.43*). Since, as we have already seen above, FSH levels are unreliable for diagnosis of sustained loss of ovarian function, one of the options in the Boxes below should be followed, the first of which implies simply stopping the (masking effect of) current hormone treatment:

> **Plan A** *Contraception may cease: after waiting for the 'officially approved' 1 year of amenorrhoea above age 50, having stopped all hormones*
> This is the obvious plan for current users or switchers at this age to:
> - copper IUDs
> - condoms
> - sponges or spermicides (which, unlike in younger women, do appear to be adequate in the presence of such drastically reduced – progressing to absent – fertility).

But what to do if the woman is using one of the hormonal methods or HRT, which mask the menopause?

■ DMPA or COC (or Evra patch or NuvaRing): age 50–51, the average age of ovarian failure, is the time to stop these. By this time they are needlessly strong, contraceptively, so their known risks – which increase with age – are no longer justified.

■ The POP, or an implant, or the LNG-IUS, or a sponge/spermicide with ongoing HRT: as contraceptives these add almost negligible medical risks that increase with age. Therefore, one of these (usually the POP, a good choice for users of one of the methods at bullet 1 to switch to, or the barrier contraceptive with HRT) may simply be continued until the latest age of potential fertility has been reached: then the woman just stops all contraception (no tests!).

When is that age?

A good estimate is age 55. The Faculty of SRH, in their Guidance (reference at Q 11.39), quote Treloar's population-based evidence that 95.9% have ceased menstruation for ever by then. Such bleeds as may happen later, in the other 4.1%, would be extremely unlikely to occur in cycles that were fertile. (It is true that the *Guinness Book of Records* has reported one or two older mothers (into their early 60s!), but authentication is uncertain.)

However, the policy in Plan B below should be tailored to the individual, and any (rare) woman who experiences *regular* menses above age 55 should continue a simple method of contraception.

Plan B *Contraception may cease: at age 55 after having switched to, or having continued with, a progestogen-only method – most commonly a POP (old type) – with due warning that initially, without the passage of more time (i.e. Plan A), there can be no cast-iron certainty*

■ If she develops pronounced vasomotor symptoms she could stop earlier than this, to follow Plan C below, perhaps with added HRT.

■ If a remote risk of fertility is still a source of anxiety, there is always an option, even after stopping the POP at age 55, to transfer to using a sponge or spermicide for one final year – and certainly if regular menses ensue.

What if to age 55 seems too long to wait?

> **Plan C** *Contraception may cease: above age 50 if three other criteria also apply*
> Such older users of hormonal contraception may cease using any method *IF* they have indeed passed their 50th birthday, *AND*, after a trial of 2 months' discontinuation (using barriers or spermicides) they have:
> 1 Vasomotor symptoms
> 2 Two high FSH levels (>30 U/L) when off all treatment, separated by 1 month. In combination with the other criteria here, FSH levels are useful, despite their unreliability on their own . . .
> 3 Continuing amenorrhoea indefinitely beyond this trial period (she should report back urgently if not so!)
> With due warnings about lack of certainty, these women may cease all contraception before the approved '1 year's amenorrhoea post 50' has occurred. Or, as before, just use a sponge or spermicide for one final year.

There are useful *clues* for COC-users and POP-users that discontinuation to follow the protocol in the above Box is worth a try, namely:

- if COC-users start getting 'hot flushes' at the end of their PFI – especially if a high FSH result is obtained then
- if users of an old-type POP develop vasomotor symptoms with amenorrhoea while still taking it (NB: Q *7.62* has more on this).

11.43 Is it always important to establish precisely when the menopause takes/took place?

No, not in my opinion. If contraception is not an issue or the woman is on any form of HRT with natural estrogen, or using the LNG-IUS with estrogen, or she is happy to stay on the POP or Implanon until beyond age 55, the diagnosis of the precise time of the menopause can be considered to be of academic interest only.

The COC and DMPA are, however, different. There is a cross-over between diminishing contraceptive need by such strong methods and increasing risk with age (osteoporosis in the case of DMPA), which occurs, surely, about the average time of the menopause (50–51).

11.44 How about the LNG-IUS for the older woman (*see Qs 9.143–9.149*)?

This is a fantastic option. Not only can it protect against most of the gynaecological problems to be expected, especially menorrhagia (which is so common in this age group, whether or not related to fibroids or endometriosis), but also it provides local progestogen protection against endometrial hyperplasia and cancer.

Furthermore, NICE has stated that any woman who had her LNG-IUS inserted above the age of 45 and who has complete amenorrhoea may continue to use the same LNG-IUS 'until contraception is no longer needed' – i.e. essentially after age 55 (see Q 9.150).

Using the LNG-IUS also permits estrogen hormone replacement to be given later if and when it is indicated (though then with replacement every 4 years, *see* Q 9.150), systemically, while almost completely avoiding the side-effects of systemic progestogens. It is contraceptive, ultra-low progestogen, PMS-free and 'no-period HRT', usable before proof of ovarian failure!

Non-hormonal methods above age 40

11.45 Is the copper IUD underutilized at this age?

Yes, definitely (*see* Q 9.19). It is suitable not only because the banded IUDs are as effective as sterilization, especially when combined with reducing fertility, but also because infection and expulsion rates decline with age and are lowest in the 40s. In the absence of intermenstrual or very heavy bleeding, it can be highly acceptable. Moreover, there is no need routinely to change any copper IUD fitted after the 40th birthday, until after the menopause (*see* Q 9.136).

11.46 What about the condom and vaginal contraceptives?

These options are as appropriate at this age as at any other, and have their own obvious advantages. But in my experience condoms are not sufficiently 'user-friendly' to be accepted for the first time by couples who have not used them regularly earlier in their reproductive life. Many women introduced to the diaphragm, however, are surprised by its ease and convenience.

Condom tip: older men in couples where the condom is the truly best choice after counselling, may sometimes have medical grounds, in my opinion, for using a phosphodiesterase type-5 inhibitor (such as Viagra or Cialis). The improved and sustained erection can enormously increase acceptability and regular use of the condom method, sometimes even in younger men also with a degree of situational erectile dysfunction.

The use of spermicides alone is not recommended in the '*younger* older' years. But spermicides and sponges are sufficient contraception and very acceptable: for that necessary time of 1 or 2 years of amenorrhoea following what appears to be the menopause (*see Qs 11.34, 11.42*) – which can only ever be finally diagnosed in retrospect.

11.47 Can the methods based on fertility awareness be recommended leading up to the climacteric?

No. At present, for those whose views make this the only acceptable approach, the mucus and cervical assessment methods (*see Qs 2.25ff, 2.36*), or Persona, all require a lot of unnecessary abstinence by older women. This is because during the climacteric there is follicular activity with estrogenic mucus and estrone-3-glucuronide in the urine – but without necessarily being followed by a fertile ovulation.

For the future, in an older woman who ovulates only (say) once every 4 months, a most useful new technology would be a means to predict each actual ovulation, far enough ahead to allow for sperm survival. Just three short spells of abstinence per year and she could avoid all the risks of the artificial methods of birth control.

11.48 Isn't postcoital contraception (as in *Chapter 10*) best avoided in this age group?

Not so, it might be entirely justifiable. There should be no hesitation, well above age 40, in using the hormonal method whenever there is a pregnancy risk, even if small.

11.49 Surely either male or female sterilization is the ideal answer, for many older couples above age 35?

It certainly can be, for many; more than 210 million couples worldwide rely on female sterilization (WHO 2003). According to recent surveys, around 40% of couples above age 40 in the UK rely on sterilization of one or other partner. The methods are effective and highly convenient, free of all proven long-term risks after the initial operation.

This book, as you know, majors on the reversible contraceptive methods. But a superb fully up-to-date and comprehensive Guideline No 4 with review of both male and female sterilization is obtainable from the RCOG Bookshop as a paper publication – and also on their website: http://www.rcog.org.uk/index.asp?PageID=699.

Female sterilization, specifically, is likely to be used much less in developed countries in the future. This is because of what I term a 'push' and a 'pull'. The 'push' is that we now know it doesn't work very well (CREST study, *see Q 11.50*) and is prone to late failures; the 'pull' is from all the new reversible methods that are at least as effective (*see Q 11.51*).

Most authorities consider any association of bleeding problems with female sterilization by tubal occlusion using clips or rings to be coincidental, not causal. The principal explanation is that after sterilization the woman discontinues the COC, or other hormonal contraceptive, which had been controlling the pain and bleeding of her 'normal' or abnormal menstrual cycle for years without her knowing it. This is how I can ask medical students my catch question: how is it that vasectomy might be able to cause both menorrhagia and dysmenorrhoea?!

Female sterilization appears to give a so-far unexplained protection against ovarian cancer.

There are many traps for the unwary clinician, however. An infrequent but real example is the sterilization-clip-induced ectopic in the cycle of the procedure, caused because the woman was not warned of the danger of less than perfectly protected intercourse in the 7 days before surgery which happens to take place before a blastocyst has travelled far enough down the tube.

More serious, because affecting far more people, is the problem of relationship/marriage breakdown, now that it is so frequent. Requests for reversal are more frequent after vasectomy, because the man often remarries a younger woman. Careful counselling is therefore mandatory, including an assessment of both the general and the sexual relationship of the couple, and a consideration of relevant aspects of gynaecology even if vasectomy is the operation proposed. And then there is the late failure risk, now quantified as much higher than used to be thought (*see* Q 11.50).

11.50 What is the risk of late failure? Can total reassurance be given after, say, 1–2 years?

Unfortunately, no. Such late failures do occur, even after vasectomy with two subsequent negative sperm counts. Our estimate from the Elliot-Smith clinic in Oxford (at which I have operated since 1970) was around 1:2000. This still makes vasectomy much more effective than female sterilization: the American CREST study (in which over 10 000 women were followed-up for up to 10 years) showed a surprisingly high overall failure rate of 1.8% [*American Journal of Obstetrics and Gynecology* 1996;174:1161–1170], or 1.4% by 7 years (which is indistinguishable from the failure rate of the banded copper-T and the LNG-IUS in long-term studies). For every sterilization method assessed by CREST, up to 50% more failures were ascertained after 10 years as had been identified by the end of the first year, meaning that many were true re-canalizations.

CREST did not have available to study the more effective Filshie clip, which is standard in the UK. However, on the CREST 'model', the 2-year failure rate of Filshie clips, which in 2003 was estimated as around 2:1000, would need increasing to about 3:1000 after 10 years. Currently, therefore, we should inform young women at counselling that the lifetime failure rate of Filshie clip sterilization is estimated at about 1:300 (contrast vasectomy: 1:2000) and that 1:3 of all those sterilization failures is ectopic.

The outpatient hysteroscopic method called Essure is also highly effective, but has other disadvantages:

- Experts admit it is not always feasible on the day.
- The tubal damage caused is *completely* irreversible.

Obviously, all failure risks decline dramatically with diminishing fertility approaching the menopause.

11.51 Are the alternatives to sterilization offered often enough?

I think not. Many couples would actually prefer to avoid surgery and there are plenty of ways of doing so, as outlined above. Before referral for sterilization, especially of relatively young couples, in my experience three important choices are far too often not even mentioned. These are Implanon (*see Q 8.63*), the modern banded copper IUDs and the LNG-IUS (*see Chapter 9*). The gold standard among copper IUDs is the T-Safe Cu 380A (*see Q 9.10*). But GyneFix and the LNG-IUS have their own merits.

Certainly, another method would be preferable to sterilization when the woman is past the age of about 48, because sterilization will not provide 'value for money'. (The chance of pregnancy is so low and her 'auto-sterilization' by the menopause is imminent.) Indeed, depending on the regularity or otherwise of her menstrual cycle and vasomotor symptoms, a simple method like a contraceptive sponge might already be equivalent, for efficacy.

Interfacing issues for the older woman

11.52 What about hysterectomy?

A hysterectomy is sometimes appropriate, and indeed might be essential gynaecological treatment. Hence the vital importance before vasectomy of diagnosing in the female partner large fibroids, all adnexal masses and stress incontinence.

However, even by the most modern minimal techniques, the morbidity and mortality of hysterectomy greatly exceed those of the other sterilizing options above; and the LNG-IUS deals of course with most of the bleeding and the pain indications that formerly justified such surgery.

11.53 Is transcervical resection or ablation of the endometrium for menorrhagia contraceptive?

Unfortunately, not so. Blastocysts can even implant in the ovary or on the peritoneum, so the absence of (most of) the endometrium is not enough.

Younger women conceive with surprising ease. Moreover, important risks are emerging:

■ The pregnancy has a high chance of being a tubal ectopic.
■ The fetus might have a major malformation.
■ There might be serious intrauterine growth retardation.
■ There might be varying degrees of placenta accreta.

11.54 So what contraception is recommended for a woman following endometrial resection or any of the modern ablation therapies?

It is normally preferable that laparoscopic sterilization is performed under the same anaesthetic. Otherwise, one of the above effective methods could and should be initiated, not excluding an IUD. However, according to the experts in this field, copper IUDs are relatively contraindicated (WHO 3), and if used are best fitted immediately, with great care and antibiotic cover. And it must be understood that the device can sometimes be almost impossible to remove, stuck among adhesions in a shrunken uterine cavity. The LNG-IUS is a much better option (WHO 2) as maintenance follow-up after any form of ablation (Alfred Cutner, personal communication, 2002).

The LNG-IUS (*see Q 9.143*), of course, might remove the need for this surgery in the first place – especially as it often helps pain, which is not usually improved by the ablative techniques. Furthermore, it may be used as a preventive, to reduce the risk of recurrence of symptoms, by being inserted at the time of ablation, or after resection of submucous fibroids – or at follow-up hysteroscopy if the original symptoms do not resolve.

11.55 So what is your conclusion – what practical guidelines are there regarding contraception for the older woman?

■ As usual, the choice will depend on the outcome of non-directive counselling, considering all the options discussed briefly here and more thoroughly earlier in this book. It begins to look as though no contraceptive method is necessarily contraindicated on the basis of age alone.

■ One of the very best modern options to emerge clearly, though, is the LNG-IUS – alone, or with estrogen if needed as HRT to treat relevant symptoms.

11.56 What else is important in discussing contraception around the climacteric?

It is important to remember that contraception is often a 'ticket' to see the doctor. In reality there might be many basic anxieties concerned with sexuality, the woman's relationship to her partner, the 'empty nest' syndrome, new health problems, ageing, and low self-esteem with the 'finality' of the approaching menopause. Moreover, even if, as so often, the woman tries to assume sole responsibility, her partner's caring involvement should be sought – and nurtured if found!

THE FUTURE (SEE ALSO Q 8.73)

11.57 Will we ever have a pill for men?

At long last a marketed systemic male contraceptive appears on the horizon, perhaps – though one hesitates to say it after so many false dawns – even within the next 10 years. The most promising approaches are:

1 a long-acting testosterone ester by injection or implant, coupled with an injectable or more probably implanted progestogen
2 the pharmacological semen-blocking method, or 'dry orgasm' pill.

Approach (1)

The first approach is one of *suppressing spermatogenesis* by pituitary inhibition (similar to the effect of the COC in women) but maintaining masculinity and libido through the androgen component. It has proved difficult to get the right dosing balance in all men, so as to provide efficacy through azoospermia, or sufficiently marked oligospermia, plus normal masculinity; and yet avoid unwanted hyperandrogenic manifestations such as acne, aggression, prostatic hypertrophy or increasing the already-present male susceptibility to arterial disease.

Approach (2) – the 'dry orgasm' pill

This is a novel non-hormonal approach based on the same highly unusual side-effect of two drugs with quite different main actions – and first reported many decades ago. As far back as 1961, American psychiatrists were reporting the side-effect, succinctly put in the title of a 1968 case report about this particular phenothiazine: 'Thioridazine-induced inhibition of masturbatory ejaculation in an adolescent'.

Later – acting on reports going back even further to the mid-1950s – workers in Israel published [Homonnai ZT et al 1984 *Contraception* 29:479–491] a pilot study in 13 men of the identical strange effect of an alpha-adrenergic blocker, under the title 'Phenoxybenzamine – an effective male contraceptive pill'. This title was not perhaps an overstatement, since at no time did any of the volunteers produce any semen at all at ejaculation, while on treatment with 10–30 mg of the drug, yet with apparently complete restoration of semen volume and quality on discontinuation. There was no evidence of retrograde ejaculation nor of effects on testosterone, FSH, LH or prolactin. Of greatest interest is that none of the men reported any adverse effects on libido, erection, sexual performance or on their sensations of orgasm and ejaculation – despite no fluid emission.

Where has this interesting possibility got to, in the 24 years since that pilot study? The original drugs had too many reported side-effects; indeed, thioridazine is no longer in the *British National Formulary* and phenoxybenzamine has a very restricted use as a hypotensive in the treatment of phaeochromocytoma. But the pharmacologists Amobi and Smith at King's College Hospital have continued working systematically on our excised vasectomy specimens from the Margaret Pyke (London) and Elliot-Smith (Oxford) clinics, and have identified the mechanism of action (on the vas and also, necessarily to result in dry ejaculations, 'downstream' from the prostate). The original drugs, some new ones they have identified, and also tailored ones that have been synthesized with the same 'chemical signature', all if given at the right (low) dosage contrive to paralyse the longitudinal muscles of the Wolffian duct system while still permitting the circular muscles to contract. This leads to loss of the usual coordinated ejaculatory 'Mexican wave'; instead there is a sphincter action, reversibly preventing emission of both sperm and seminal fluid.

At the time of writing we are seeking funding to take the most promising candidate drugs forward through all the required preliminary phases of clinical testing for efficacy and safety. This will certainly cost millions of dollars and take at least 10 more years – 60 years since those first reports. Watch this space!

11.58 Would a male pill make a vas deferens?

Apologies for the corn in the question: but it is a serious concern of many women, that they would never trust a man who *said* he was using any form of 'male pill' – or even if he really was, would he ever remember, since he has no personal 'investment' in contraception, to take it sufficiently conscientiously?

Both the approaches outlined in Q 11.57 have advantages here:

■ The first is likely to be an implant, and as this is likely to be in the upper arm like Implanon, a user's sexual partner can confirm for herself its presence and likely ongoing action, by simple palpation! Moreover:

■ The 'dry orgasm' method has the potential to be a 'pre-coital' pill – i.e. possibly working at full efficacy say in about 2–4 h after it is swallowed. This also could help to reassure the anxious wife or partner, since she could supervise him taking the tablet at supper-time ready for action at bed-time! (But there should still be the option for greater spontaneity of taking it daily.)

Survey data of men from many different cultures report a uniform majority around 60% who claim they would be prepared to use a male pill-type method if it was available, medically safe and did not alter sexual function or masculinity. In short, I am confident that male systemic methods would be a useful addition to the range of contraceptive choices, primarily in stable relationships.

It would be good if I could take the 'pill' or use an implant for a year or two, then my wife maybe also for a further year or two: being able to share (like we do most other things) the risks and side-effects of contraception!

11.59 What should be the direction of future contraceptive research?

Fig. 11.2 displays elegantly, although simply, the primary sites of action both of the existing methods and of those currently under study.

Inspection of this figure confirms an obvious fact: that the major scientific interest in birth control research has been directed at relatively high-technology, interventionist methods that have the potential or the reality of systemic side-effects.

Regrettably, most contraceptive researchers in recent years have concentrated mainly on attempts to 'tinker' with the existing COCs or progestogen-only methods, by using new routes like implants or skin patches or vaginal rings. Much less research effort has been directed to devising innovative systemic agents: I have personally been disappointed that there have not been spin-offs from all the endeavour into artificial reproduction techniques. These could be mirror-image methods, which use the same advances in basic science to help to prevent conception as much as to promote it. I consider this an example of how humankind is 'hard-wired' to breed and how family planning will always play second fiddle to pro-natalism – shown as much in funding priorities by grant-givers as in the choice of PhD research projects by enthusiastic young scientists. . . .

Yet both the above approaches (*see Q 11.57*) are about adapting or replicating *systemic methods*, which in either gender by whatever route – whether cutaneous or subcutaneous, rectal or vaginal, nasal or retinal! – can never (obviously, since they must get into the bloodstream) be totally free of all risk, nor easily shown to be safe *enough*. This is the heart of the problem to which Carl Djerassi drew attention in his classic book *The Politics of Contraception*. How do we prove that the unwanted effects of a systemic agent are acceptable or (hopefully) do not exist? It is because this process is so difficult, so expensive and with such long lead-times (*see Q 11.57* for what may very well be the best example of that!) that Djerassi was so pessimistic about the future of contraceptive research.

Perhaps we should be starting somewhere else. Far more research should concentrate on producing a method, empowering women and men, which is as effective and 'user-friendly' as the LNG-IUS but as medically

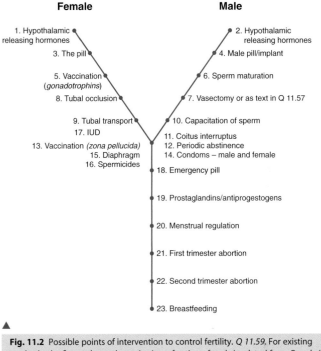

Female   **Male**

1. Hypothalamic releasing hormones
2. Hypothalamic releasing hormones
3. The pill
4. Male pill/implant
5. Vaccination (*gonadotrophins*)
6. Sperm maturation
8. Tubal occlusion
7. Vasectomy or as text in Q 11.57
9. Tubal transport
10. Capacitation of sperm
17. IUD
11. Coitus interruptus
12. Periodic abstinence
13. Vaccination (*zona pellucida*)
14. Condoms – male and female
15. Diaphragm
16. Spermicides
18. Emergency pill

19. Prostaglandins/antiprogestogens

20. Menstrual regulation

21. First trimester abortion

22. Second trimester abortion

23. Breastfeeding

Fig. 11.2 Possible points of intervention to control fertility. *Q 11.59.* For existing methods, the figure shows the main sites of action of each (updated from *People* (IPPF) 1981;8(4):6–7).

safe and STI-protective as the condom. We badly need something like a contraceptive microbicide, fully effective in both roles!

Meantime, to return to a theme with which we began the book (see *Table 1.1*, p. 12), currently the main choice for women is between (a) the efficacy and convenience of systemic methods like the COC but with the associated risk of both annoying and serious side-effects, and (b) the relative lack of efficacy and inconvenience of methods like the diaphragm, coupled with their virtual absence of risk.

And for truly 'safer sex' for the foreseeable future, given the 'world shortage' of monogamy, most people in most settings will have to continue to use two methods: i.e. an effective systemic or intrauterine contraceptive combined with a male or female condom.

FURTHER READING

Main sources of references* and quotations

Carter Y, Moss C, Weyman A 1998 RCGP handbook of sexual health in primary care. RCGP: London

Filshie M, Guillebaud J 1989 Contraception: science and practice. Butterworths: London

*Guillebaud J 2003 Contraception. In: McPherson A, Waller D (eds) Women's Health (formerly Women's problems in general practice), 5th edn. Oxford University Press: Oxford

Guillebaud J 2007 Contraception today. A pocketbook for general practitioners. Informa Healthcare (Martin Dunitz): London

The INFO Project of Johns Hopkins Bloomberg School of Public Health, Center for Communication Programs and WHO, 2007 Family planning: A global handbook for providers. CCP and WHO: Baltimore and Geneva. [Also available complete and searchable on line at www.fphandbook.org]

*Kubba A, Sanfilippo J, Hampton N (eds) 1999 Contraception and office gynecology: choices in reproductive healthcare. WB Saunders: London

*Penney G, Brechin S, Glasier A 2006 Family planning masterclass: evidence-based answers to 1000 questions. RCOG Press: London

*Potts M, Diggory P 1983 Textbook of contraceptive practice. Cambridge University Press: Cambridge

Sapire E 1990 Contraception and sexuality in health and disease. McGraw-Hill: Isando

*WHO 2004 Medical eligibility criteria for contraceptive use. WHO/RHR/00.02. WHO: Geneva

*WHO 2005 Selected practice recommendations for contraceptive use. WHO: Geneva

Or, more simply for latest versions of above WHOMEC and WHOSPR, visit the WHO website; or for UKMEC and numerous other invaluable Guidance documents, the website of the Faculty of SRH; also the websites of NICE for the Guideline on LARCs; and of the RCOG for Guideline on Male and Female Sterilization.

Important background reading – plus titles for a general readership

Cooper A, Guillebaud J 1999 Sexuality and disability. Radcliffe Medical Press: London

Djerassi C 1981 The politics of contraception: birth control in the year 2001, 2nd edn. Freeman: Oxford

Ehrlich P, Ehrlich A 1991 The population explosion. Arrow Books: London

Guillebaud J 2005 The pill, 6th edn. Oxford University Press: Oxford

Montford H, Skrine R 1993 Psychosexual medicine series 6. Contraceptive care: meeting individual needs. Chapman & Hall: London

*Population reports (various years to 2008) [Excellent comprehensive reviews of the literature on developments in population, contraceptives and sterilization. Obtainable from the Population Information Program, Johns Hopkins School of Public Health, 111 Market Place, Suite 310, Baltimore, MD 21202, USA. Website: www.jhuccp.org]

Skrine R, Montford H 2001 Psychosexual medicine – an introduction. Edward Arnold: London

BELIEVABLE WEBSITES FOR RESOURCES/REFERENCES IN SEXUAL AND REPRODUCTIVE HEALTH

www.gmc-uk.org/guidance/ethical_guidance/children_guidance/index.asp
This guidance, on the standards of competence, care and conduct expected of all GMC-registered doctors, focuses on children and young people from birth until their 18th birthday

www.margaretpyke.org
Local services and superb training courses on offer

www.ippf.org.uk
Online version of the *Directory of Hormonal Contraception*, with names of (equivalent) pill brands used throughout the world; also books and guidance papers with a developing world emphasis

www.who.int/reproductive-health
WHO Medical Eligibility Criteria (WHOMEC) and Practice Recommendations (WHOSPR) for contraceptive use plus other guidance documents

www.rcog.org.uk
Evidence-based RCOG Guidelines on male and female sterilization; and many gynaecological topics that interface with contraception, such as infertility, induced abortion and menorrhagia. Also: answers to FAQs; a wide range of patient information leaflets; and RCOG on-line bookshop for almost any publication in the field

www.fsrh.org
UK Medical Eligibility Criteria (UKMEC) and Selected Practice Recommendations (UKSPR) which are UK-adapted from WHO; also Faculty of SRH guidance and FACT reviews on numerous contraceptive topics such as Emergency Contraception and access to the invaluable *Journal of Family Planning and Reproductive Health Care*

www.nice.org.uk/guidance/CG30
Specific URL for access to valuable Guideline from NICE on the long-acting reversible contraceptives, 2005

www.jhuccp.org
Website of Johns Hopkins School of Public Health Information Program: produces the excellent Population Reports (see Further Reading)

www.fertilityuk.org
The fertility awareness and NFP service, including teachers available locally – a brilliant website, factual and non-sectarian

www.bashh.org
National guidelines for the management of all STIs and contact details for GUM clinics throughout the UK

www.fpa.org.uk
Patient information plus those essential leaflets! There is also an invaluable helpline: 0845 310 1334

www.everychildmatters.gov.uk/teenagepregnancy
The Teenage Pregnancy Unit's site to brief service providers, journalists etc: for all publications, FAQs, helplines. The parallel website for young people themselves is www.ruthinking.co.uk below

Excellent direct-access websites for young people:

www.brook.org.uk
Similar to the fpa website but for under-25s; plus a really secure confidential online enquiry service. Helpline: 0800 0185023

www.likeitis.org.uk
Reproductive health for lay persons by Marie Stopes. Brilliantly teenage-friendly and matter-of-factual

www.ruthinking.co.uk
'Sex – are you thinking about it, *enough*?' Factual website that fully informs plus helps teens to access services in own local area. Sexwise line: 0800 282930. There is also 0800 567123 for similar safe-sex advice for the older age group (primarily 20–30s).

www.teenagehealthfreak.com
FAQs as asked by teenagers, on all health subjects, not just reproductive health – from anorexia to zits!

Regarding hormone-replacement therapy (HRT):

www.the-bms.org
Research-based advice about the menopause and HRT

Regarding sexual and relationship problems:

www.ipm.org.uk
Website of the Institute of Psychosexual Medicine

www.basrt.org.uk
Website of the British Association for Sexual and Relationship Therapy; provides a list of therapists

www.relate.org.uk
Enter postcode to get nearest Relate centre for relationship counselling and psychosexual therapy. Many publications also available.

John Guillebaud's website on the Environment Timecapsule project – and related sites:

www.ecotimecapsule.com
www.populationandsustainability.org
www.optimumpopulation.org
www.popconnect.org – source of the dramatic DVD 'Population Dots'
www.peopleandplanet.net

APPENDIX A
Use of licensed products in an unlicensed way

Often, licensing procedures have not yet caught up with what is widely considered the best evidence-based practice. Such use is legitimate medically and legally – and may indeed be necessary for optimal contraceptive care, provided certain criteria are observed. These are now well established (see Faculty of SRH Guidance July 2005. *Journal of Family Planning and Reproductive Health Care* 2005;31:225–242). In brief:

The prescribing physician must accept full liability and:

- Be adopting an evidence-based practice endorsed by a responsible body of professional opinion
- *Assess the individual's priorities and preferences,* giving a clear account of known and possible risks and the benefits
- *Explain to her that it is an unlicensed prescription*
- *Obtain informed (verbal) consent and record this*
- Ensure good practice, including follow-up, to comply fully with professional indemnity requirements: along with meticulous record-keeping
- Note that this will often mean the doctor providing dedicated written materials, because the manufacturer's PIL insert may not apply in one or more respects.

This protocol (the bullets with *italics* above) is generally termed 'named-patient' prescribing.

Notes:

1 Attention to detail is important – as, in the (unlikely) event of a claim, the manufacturer can be excused from any liability. But keeping a separate dedicated list of patients' details is no longer considered necessary.
2 *Nurse prescribers* cannot *prescribe* medicines outside the terms of the licence, but they may *supply and administer them as above*, within fully agreed and authorized Patient Group Directions (and as agreed with their insurer, such as the Royal College of Nursing).

Some common examples of named-patient prescribing:

- Advising more than the usual dosage, such as when enzyme-inducer drugs are being used with:
    - the COC (*Qs 5.39, 5.40*) or any POP (*Q 7.28*)
    - hormonal emergency contraception (*Q 10.29*)

■ Sustained use of COC over many cycles (i.e. more than just to cover a holiday):
  – long-term tricycling (Q 5.32) or, now:
  – 365/365 use (Q 5.34)
■ Use of banded copper IUDs for longer than licensed duration:
  – under the age of 40 (e.g. T-Safe Cu 380A for more than 10 years (Q 9.135)
  – continuing use to post-menopause of *any* copper device that was fitted after age 40 (9.136)
■ Continuing use of the same LNG-IUS for contraception:
  – in an older woman (i.e. where fitted above age 35) for up to 7 years rather than the licensed 5 years, if desired, at a patient's fully informed request (Q 9.150)
  – indefinitely if she had it fitted above 45 and she is amenorrhoeic (NICE advice) and not using it as part of HRT (Q 9.150)
■ Use of hormonal EC:
  – beyond 72 h after the earliest exposure or
  – more than once in a cycle (Q 10.8)
■ *Use of 'Quick start'.* This means, with appropriate safeguards (including, as relevant, using the protocols in the Boxes in Q 11.22), commencement of pills or other medical methods of contraception:
  – late in the menstrual cycle or
  – immediately after hormonal EC

There are other examples that may be found elsewhere in this book, as well as in the Faculty of SRH guidance referenced above. Yet during the currency of this edition, future updates to the relevant licence and the summary of product characteristics may remove the need to follow the above 'named-patient' protocol in some instances – indeed, hopefully, all of them in due course.

APPENDIX B
UKMEC summary sheets: common reversible methods

UK Category 1 includes conditions for which there is no restriction for use and Category 4 includes conditions which represent an unacceptable health risk if the method is used. UK Category 2 indicates that a method can generally be used, but more careful follow-up may be required. The provision of a method with a conditions given a UK Category 3 requires **expert clinical judgment and/or referral to a specialist contraceptive provider**, since use of the method is not usually recommended unless other methods are not available or not acceptable.

UK Category	Hormonal contraception, intrauterine devices and barrier methods
1	A condition for which there is **no restriction for the use** of the contraceptive method
2	A condition where the **advantages of using the method generally outweigh the theoretical or proven risks**
3	A condition where the theoretical or **proven risks usually outweigh the advantages** of using the method
4	A condition which represents an **unacceptable health risk** if the contraceptive method is used

Initiation (I)	Starting a method of contraception by a woman with a specific medical condition.
Continuation (C)	Continuing with the method already being used by a woman who develops a new medical condition.

NB: The categories in the following table – on the above 1–4 scale, which is the same as that initially devised by WHO (*Q 5.121*) – are not always identical to those I have proposed earlier in this book. The differences are generally explained in my text and also are very rarely greater than a single category above or below what UKMEC proposes.

CONDITION	CHC	POP	**COMMON REVERSIBLE METHODS**			
			DMPA/NET-EN	IMP	Cu-IUD	LNG-IUD
PERSONAL CHARACTERISTICS AND REPRODUCTIVE HISTORY						
Age	Menarche to <40 = 1 >40 = 2	Menarche to <18 = 1 18–45 = 1 >45 = 1	Menarche to <18 = 2 18–45 = 1 >45 = 2	Menarche to <18 = 1 18–45 = 1 >45 = 1	Menarche to <20 = 2 >20 = 1	Menarche to <20 = 2 >20 = 1
Parity						
(a) Nulliparous	1	1	1	1	1	1
(b) Parous	1	1	1	1	1	1
Breastfeeding						
(a) <6 weeks postpartum	4	1	2	1		
(b) 6 weeks to <6 months (fully or almost fully breastfeeding)	3	1	1	1		
(c) ≥6 weeks to <6 months postpartum (partial breastfeeding medium to low)	2	1	1	1		
(d) ≥6 months postpartum	1	1	1	1		
Postpartum (non-breastfeeding women)						
(a) <21 days	3	1	1	1		
(b) ≥21 days	1	1	1	1		

	C	I
Postpartum (breastfeeding or including post-caesarean section)		
(a) 48 hours to <4 weeks	3	3
(b) ≥4 weeks	1	1
(c) Puerperal sepsis	4	4
Post-abortion		
(a) First trimester	1	1
(b) Second trimester	1	2
(c) Immediate post-septic abortion	1	4
Past ectopic pregnancy	1	1
History of pelvic surgery (including caesarean section) (see also postpartum section)	1	1

UKMEC

DEFINITION OF CATEGORY

CATEGORY 1 A condition for which there is no restriction for the use of the contraceptive method

CATEGORY 2 A condition where the advantages of using the method generally outweigh the theoretical or proven risks

CATEGORY 3 A condition where the theoretical or proven risks usually outweigh the advantages of using the method

CATEGORY 4 A condition which represents an unacceptable health risk if the contraceptive method is used

Abbreviations: I, Initiation; C, Continuation; CHC, Combined hormonal contraceptive; POP, Progestogen-only pill; DMPA, Depot medroxyprogesterone acetate; NET-EN, Norethisterone enantate; IMP, Implanon; Cu-IUD, Copper intrauterine device; LNG-IUD, Levonorgestrel intrauterine device

CONDITION	CHC	POP	DMPA/NET-EN	IMP	Cu-IUD	LNG-IUD
Smoking						
(a) Age <35 years	2	1	1	1	1	1
(b) Age ≥35 years						
(i) <15 cigarettes / day	3	1	1	1	1	1
(ii) ≥15 cigarettes / day	4	1	1	1	1	1
(iii) Stopped smoking <1 year ago	3	1	1	1	1	1
(iv) Stopped smoking ≥1 year ago	2	1	1	1	1	1
Obesity						
(a) Body mass index ≥30–34 kg/m²	2	1	1	1	1	1
(b) Body mass index 35–39 kg/m²	3	1	1	1	1	1
(c) Body mass index ≥40 kg/m²	4	1	1	1	1	1
CARDIOVASCULAR DISEASE						
Multiple risk factors for arterial cardiovascular disease (such as older age, smoking, diabetes and hypertension)	3/4	2	3	2	1	2

COMMON REVERSIBLE METHODS

Hypertension					
(a) Adequately controlled hypertension	3	1	2	1	1
(b) Consistently elevated blood pressure levels (properly taken measurements)					
(i) systolic >140 to 159 mmHg or diastolic >90 to 94 mmHg	3	1	1	1	1
(ii) systolic ≥160 or diastolic ≥95 mmHg	4	1	2	1	1
(c) Vascular disease	4	2	3	2	2
History of high blood pressure during pregnancy (where current blood pressure is normal)	2	1	1	1	1

UKMEC

DEFINITION OF CATEGORY

CATEGORY 1 A condition for which there is no restriction for the use of the contraceptive method

CATEGORY 2 A condition where the advantages of using the method generally outweigh the theoretical or proven risks

CATEGORY 3 A condition where the theoretical or proven risks usually outweigh the advantages of using the method

CATEGORY 4 A condition which represents an unacceptable health risk if the contraceptive method is used

Abbreviations: I, Initiation; C, Continuation; CHC, Combined hormonal contraceptive; POP, Progestogen-only pill; DMPA, Depot medroxyprogesterone acetate; NET-EN, Norethisterone enantate; IMP, Implanon; Cu-IUD, Copper intrauterine device; LNG-IUD, Levonorgestrel intrauterine device

CONDITION	CHC	POP	DMPA/NET-EN	IMP	Cu-IUD	LNG-IUD
Venous thrombo-embolism (VTE) (includes deep vein thrombosis (DVT) and pulmonary embolism (PE))						
(a) History of VTE	4	2	2	2	1	2
(b) Current VTE (on anticoagulants)	4	2	3	3	3	3
(c) Family history of VTE						
(i) First degree relative aged <45 years	3	1	1	1	1	1
(ii) First degree relative aged ≥45 years	2	1	1	1	1	1
(d) Major surgery						
(i) With prolonged immobilization	4	2	2	2	1	2
(ii) Without prolonged immobilization	2	1	1	1	1	1
(e) Minor surgery without immobilization	1	1	1	1	1	1
(f) Immobility (unrelated to surgery) e.g. – wheelchair use, debilitating illness	3	1	1	1	1	1
Known thrombogenic mutations (e.g. factor V Leiden; prothrombin mutation; protein S, protein C and antithrombin deficiencies)	4	2	2	2	1	2

COMMON REVERSIBLE METHODS

Condition	CHC	POP (I / C)	DMPA	IMP (I / C)	Cu-IUD	LNG-IUD (I / C)
Superficial venous thrombosis						
(a) Varicose veins	1	1	1	1	1	1
(b) Superficial thrombophlebitis	2	1	1	1	1	1
Current and history of ischaemic heart disease	4	2 / 3	3	2 / 3	1	2 / 3
Stroke (history of cerebrovascular accident)	4	2 / 3	3	2 / 3	1	2
Known hyperlipidaemias (screening is NOT necessary for safe use of contraceptive methods)	2/3	2	2	2	1	2
Valvular and congenital heart disease						
(a) Uncomplicated	2	1	1	1	1	1
(b) Complicated (e.g. with pulmonary hypertension, atrial fibrillation, or a history of subacute bacterial endocarditis)	4	1	1	1	2	2

UKMEC

DEFINITION OF CATEGORY

CATEGORY 1   A condition for which there is no restriction for the use of the contraceptive method

CATEGORY 2   A condition where the advantages of using the method generally outweigh the theoretical or proven risks

CATEGORY 3   A condition where the theoretical or proven risks usually outweigh the advantages of using the method

CATEGORY 4   A condition which represents an unacceptable health risk if the contraceptive method is used

Abbreviations: I, Initiation; C, Continuation; CHC, Combined hormonal contraceptive; POP, Progestogen-only pill; DMPA, Depot medroxyprogesterone acetate; NET-EN, Norethisterone enantate; IMP, Implanon; Cu-IUD, Copper intrauterine device; LNG-IUD, Levonorgestrel intrauterine device

	CHC		POP		DMPA/NET-EN		IMP		Cu-IUD	LNG-IUD	
CONDITION	I	C	I	C	I	C	I	C		I	C
NEUROLOGIC CONDITIONS											
Headaches											
(a) Non-migrainous (mild or severe)	1	2	1	1	1	1	1	1	1	1	1
(b) Migraine											
(i) Without aura, age <35 years	2	3	1	2	2	2	2	2	1	2	2
(ii) Without aura, age ≥35 years	3	4	1	2	2	2	2	2	1	2	2
(iii) With aura, at any age	4	4	2	3	2	3	2	3	1	2	3
(c) Past history of migraine with aura at any age	3		2		2		2		1	2	
Epilepsy	1		1		1		1		1	1	
Depressive disorders	1		1		1		1		1	1	
REPRODUCTIVE TRACT INFECTIONS AND DISORDERS											
Vaginal bleeding patterns											
(a) Irregular pattern without heavy bleeding	1		2		2		2		1	1	1
(b) Heavy or prolonged bleeding (includes regular and irregular patterns)	1		2		2		2		2	1	2

Condition	CHC	POP	DMPA/NET-EN	IMP	Cu-IUD (I / C)	LNG-IUD (I / C)
Unexplained vaginal bleeding (suspicious for serious condition) Before evaluation	2	2	3	3	4 / 2	4 / 2
Endometriosis	1	1	1	1	2	1
Benign ovarian tumours (including cysts)	1	1	1	1	1	1
Severe dysmenorrhoea	1	1	1	1	2	1
Gestational trophoblastic neoplasia (GTN) (includes hydatidiform mole, invasive mole, placental site trophoblastic tumour) (a) hCG normal	1	1	1	1	3	3
(b) hCG abnormal	1	1	1	1	4	4
Cervical ectropion	1	1	1	1	1	1
Cervical intraepithelial neoplasia (CIN)	2	1	2	2	1	2
Cervical cancer (awaiting treatment)	2	1	2	2	4 / 2	4 / 2

UKMEC

DEFINITION OF CATEGORY

CATEGORY 1 A condition for which there is no restriction for the use of the contraceptive method

CATEGORY 2 A condition where the advantages of using the method generally outweigh the theoretical or proven risks

CATEGORY 3 A condition where the theoretical or proven risks usually outweigh the advantages of using the method

CATEGORY 4 A condition which represents an unacceptable health risk if the contraceptive method is used

Abbreviations: I, Initiation; C, Continuation; CHC, Combined hormonal contraceptive; POP, Progestogen-only pill; DMPA, Depot medroxyprogesterone acetate; NET-EN, Norethisterone enantate; IMP, Implanon; Cu-IUD, Copper intrauterine device; LNG-IUD, Levonorgestrel intrauterine device

CONDITION	COMMON REVERSIBLE METHODS					
	CHC	POP	DMPA/NET-EN	IMP	Cu-IUD	LNG-IUD
Breast disease						
(a) Undiagnosed mass	I 3 / C 2	2	2	2	1	2
(b) Benign breast disease	1	1	1	1	1	1
(c) Family history of cancer	1	1	1	1	1	1
(d) Carriers of known gene mutations associated with breast cancer (e.g. *BRCA1*)	3	2	2	2	1	2
(e) Breast cancer						
(i) Current	4	4	4	4	1	4
(ii) Past and no evidence of current disease for 5 years	3	3	3	3	1	3
Endometrial cancer	1	1	1	1	I 4 / C 2	I 4 / C 2
Ovarian cancer	1	1	1	1	I 3 / C 2	I 3 / C 2
Uterine fibroids						
(a) Without distortion of the uterine cavity	1	1	1	1	1	1
(b) With distortion of the uterine cavity	1	1	1	1	4	4

Anatomical abnormalities		
(a) Distorted uterine cavity (any congenital or acquired uterine abnormality distorting the uterine cavity in a manner that is incompatible with IUD insertion)	4	4
(b) Other abnormalities (including cervical stenosis or cervical lacerations) not distorting the uterine cavity or interfering with IUD insertion	2	2

UKMEC	DEFINITION OF CATEGORY
CATEGORY 1	A condition for which there is no restriction for the use of the contraceptive method
CATEGORY 2	A condition where the advantages of using the method generally outweigh the theoretical or proven risks
CATEGORY 3	A condition where the theoretical or proven risks usually outweigh the advantages of using the method
CATEGORY 4	A condition which represents an unacceptable health risk if the contraceptive method is used

Abbreviations: I, Initiation; C, Continuation; CHC, Combined hormonal contraceptive; POP, Progestogen-only pill; DMPA, Depot medroxyprogesterone acetate; NET-EN, Norethisterone enantate; IMP, Implanon; Cu-IUD, Copper intrauterine device; LNG-IUD, Levonorgestrel intrauterine device

	COMMON REVERSIBLE METHODS					
CONDITION	CHC	POP	DMPA/NET-EN	IMP	Cu-IUD	LNG-IUD
Pelvic inflammatory disease						
(a) Past PID (assuming no current risk factors of STIs)						
(i) With subsequent pregnancy	1	1	1	1	I 1 / C 1	I 1 / C 1
(ii) Without subsequent pregnancy	1	1	1	1	I 2 / C 2	I 2 / C 2
(b) PID – current	1	1	1	1	I 4 / C 2	I 4 / C 2
STIs						
(a) Current purulent cervicitis or chlamydial infection or gonorrhoea	1	1	1	1	I 4 / C 2	I 4 / C 2
(b) Other STIs (excluding HIV and hepatitis)	1	1	1	1	I 2 / C 2	I 2 / C 2
(c) Vaginitis (including *Trichomonas vaginalis* and bacterial vaginosis)	1	1	1	1	I 2 / C 2	I 2 / C 2
(d) Increased risk of STIs	1	1	1	1	I 2/3 / C 2	I 2/3 / C 2

HIV / AIDS

					I	C
High risk of HIV	1	1	1	2	2	2
HIV infected						
(a) Not using anti-retroviral therapy	1	1	2	2	2	2
(b) Using anti-retroviral therapy	2	2	1	2	2	2
AIDS and using HAART	2	2	2	2	2	2

OTHER INFECTIONS

					I	C
Schistosomiasis						
(a) Uncomplicated	1	1	1	1	1	1
(b) Fibrosis of the liver	1	1	1	1	1	1
Tuberculosis						
(a) Non-pelvic	1	1	1	1	1	1
(b) Known pelvic	1	1	1	4	4 3	4 3
Malaria	1	1	1	1	1	1

UKMEC

DEFINITION OF CATEGORY

CATEGORY 1 A condition for which there is no restriction for the use of the contraceptive method

CATEGORY 2 A condition where the advantages of using the method generally outweigh the theoretical or proven risks

CATEGORY 3 A condition where the theoretical or proven risks usually outweigh the advantages of using the method

CATEGORY 4 A condition which represents an unacceptable health risk if the contraceptive method is used

Abbreviations: I, Initiation; C, Continuation; CHC, Combined hormonal contraceptive; POP, Progestogen-only pill; DMPA, Depot medroxyprogesterone acetate; NET-EN, Norethisterone enantate; IMP, Implanon; Cu-IUD, Copper intrauterine device; LNG-IUD, Levonorgestrel intrauterine device

CONDITION	COMMON REVERSIBLE METHODS					
	CHC	POP	DMPA/NET-EN	IMP	Cu-IUD	LNG-IUD
ENDOCRINE CONDITIONS						
Diabetes						
(a) History of gestational disease	1	1	1	1	1	1
(b) Non-vascular disease						
(i) non-insulin dependent	2	2	2	2	1	2
(ii) insulin dependent	2	2	2	2	1	2
(c) Nephropathy/ retinopathy/ neuropathy	3/4	2	3	2	1	2
(d) Other vascular disease or diabetes of >20 years' duration	3/4	2	3	2	1	2
Thyroid disorders						
(a) Simple goitre	1	1	1	1	1	1
(b) Hyperthyroid	1	1	1	1	1	1
(c) Hypothyroid	1	1	1	1	1	1
GASTROINTESTINAL CONDITIONS						
Gall bladder disease						
(a) Symptomatic						
(i) treated by cholecystectomy	2	2	2	2	1	2
(ii) medically treated	3	2	2	2	1	2
(iii) current	3	2	2	2	1	2
(b) Asymptomatic	2	2	2	2	1	2

History of cholestasis					
(a) Pregnancy-related	2	1	1	1	1
(b) Past COC-related	3	2	2	1	2
Viral hepatitis					
(a) Active	4	3	3	1	3
(b) Carrier	1	1	1	1	1
Cirrhosis					
(a) Mild (compensated)	3	2	2	1	2
(b) Severe (decompensated)	4	3	3	1	3
Liver tumours					
(a) Benign (adenoma)	4	3	3	1	3
(b) Malignant (hepatoma)	4	3	3	1	3

UKMEC

DEFINITION OF CATEGORY

CATEGORY 1 A condition for which there is no restriction for the use of the contraceptive method

CATEGORY 2 A condition where the advantages of using the method generally outweigh the theoretical or proven risks

CATEGORY 3 A condition where the theoretical or proven risks usually outweigh the advantages of using the method

CATEGORY 4 A condition which represents an unacceptable health risk if the contraceptive method is used

Abbreviations: I, Initiation; C, Continuation; CHC, Combined hormonal contraceptive; POP, Progestogen-only pill; DMPA, Depot medroxyprogesterone acetate; NET-EN, Norethisterone enantate; IMP, Implanon; Cu-IUD, Copper intrauterine device; LNG-IUD, Levonorgestrel intrauterine device

CONDITION	COMMON REVERSIBLE METHODS					
	CHC	POP	DMPA/NET-EN	IMP	Cu-IUD	LNG-IUD
Inflammatory bowel disease (includes Crohn's disease, ulcerative colitis)	2	2		1	1	1
ANAEMIAS						
Thalassaemia	1	1	1	1	2	1
Sickle cell disease	2	1	1	1	2	1
Iron deficiency anaemia	1	1	1	1	2	1
Raynaud's disease						
(a) Primary	1	1	1	1	1	1
(b) Secondary						
(i) without lupus anticoagulant	2	1	1	1	1	1
(ii) with lupus anticoagulant	4	2	2	2	1	2

DRUG INTERACTIONS

Drugs which affect liver enzymes					
For example rifampicin, rifabutin, St John's wort, griseofulvin, certain anticonvulsants (phenytoin, carmazepine, barbiturates, primidone, topiramate, oxcarbazepine)	3	3	1	3	1
Non-liver enzyme inducing antibiotics	2	1	1	1	1
Highly active antiretroviral therapy (HAART)	2	2	**I** 2/3 **C** 2		**I** 2/3 **C** 2

UKMEC

DEFINITION OF CATEGORY

CATEGORY 1 A condition for which there is no restriction for the use of the contraceptive method

CATEGORY 2 A condition where the advantages of using the method generally outweigh the theoretical or proven risks

CATEGORY 3 A condition where the theoretical or proven risks usually outweigh the advantages of using the method

CATEGORY 4 A condition which represents an unacceptable health risk if the contraceptive method is used

Abbreviations: I, Initiation; C, Continuation; CHC, Combined hormonal contraceptive; POP, Progestogen-only pill; DMPA, Depot medroxyprogesterone acetate; NET-EN, Norethisterone enantate; IMP, Implanon; Cu-IUD, Copper intrauterine device; LNG-IUD, Levonorgestrel intrauterine device

Index

Note: Page numbers in **bold** refer to figures and tables.

E

P

T

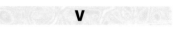

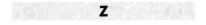